Sports Injury and Rehabilitation

Sports Injury and Rehabilitation

Edited by **Pablo De Souza**

SYRAWOOD
PUBLISHING HOUSE

New York

Published by Syrawood Publishing House,
750 Third Avenue, 9th Floor,
New York, NY 10017, USA
www.syrawoodpublishinghouse.com

Sports Injury and Rehabilitation
Edited by Pablo De Souza

International Standard Book Number: 978-1-68286-113-4 (Hardback)

Printed in the United States of America.

Contents

Preface

The purpose of the book is to provide a glimpse into the dynamics and to present opinions and studies of some of the scientists engaged in the development of new ideas in the field from very different standpoints. This book will prove useful to students and researchers owing to its high content quality.

Sports nutrition has emerged as an independent discipline in the recent years. It is focused on dietary advancements to help improve the performance of athletes along with minimizing the risk for diseases. This book focuses on the dietary requirements of athletes and how to fulfil it for best results. It comprises researches which shed light on the significant aspects of human body such as the physiological principles, metabolism etc. This book discusses the effects of various organic and inorganic substances on the strength, endurance and immunity of the athletes. It aims to enlighten the readers with the most innovative nutritional strategies and also provide insights into different body compositions to understand the functioning and metabolism of an athlete and thus device the most suitable dietary plan. This book will serve as a resource guide for nutritionists, dieticians, students and anyone else associated with the field of sports nutrition.

At the end, I would like to appreciate all the efforts made by the authors in completing their chapters professionally. I express my deepest gratitude to all of them for contributing to this book by sharing their valuable works. A special thanks to my family and friends for their constant support in this journey.

Editor

The role of physical activity and diet on bone mineral indices in young men: a cross-sectional study

Selma C Liberato[1*], Josefina Bressan[2] and Andrew P Hills[3]

Abstract

Background: Osteoporotic fractures are a significant cause of morbidity and mortality, particularly in developed countries. Increasing peak bone mass in young people may be the most important primary prevention strategy to reduce the risk of osteoporosis. This study aimed to examine the relationship between dietary factors and physical activity on bone mineralization in young men.

Methods: Thirty-five healthy men aged 18–25 y had anthropometric measures, body composition, resting metabolic rate, blood pressure, blood lipids, food intake, physical activity and cardiorespiratory fitness assessed.

Results: Participants who consumed more than 1000 mg/d of calcium were taller and had higher levels of whole body mineral content than participants who consumed less than 1000 mg/d of calcium. Similarly, participants who expended more than 20% of total daily energy engaged in moderate- to vigorous-intensity physical activity had higher cardiorespiratory fitness and higher levels of body mass adjusted bone mineral content than participants who did not meet this level of energy expenditure. There were no differences in blood pressure or blood lipids between participants in calcium or in physical activity energy expenditure categories.

Conclusions: A high intake of dietary calcium and high daily energy expenditure engaged in moderate- to vigorous-intensity physical activity were positively associated with bone mineralization in young men, particularly in the lumbar region.

Keywords: Dietary intake, Physical activity, DXA, BMC, BMD, Body composition

Background

Osteoporotic fractures, particularly in the most susceptible areas of the spine and hip [1], are a significant cause of morbidity and mortality in developed countries [2]. Osteoporosis is defined as a reduction in bone mineral density (BMD) 2.5 standard deviation (SD) below the mean for healthy young people at the age of attainment of peak bone mass, in general using a reference population matched for age, sex and race (and expressed as a T-score) [3].

Osteoporotic fractures may have their genesis during the growing years [2] as bone mass and strength are gained during this period [4] with peak bone mass being a major determinant of osteoporosis in later life [5,6]. Therefore, increasing peak bone mass in young people during the time of skeletal maturation may be the 'best bet' primary prevention strategy to reduce the likelihood of this disease [6].

While bone and body size have been identified as the main determinants of bone mineral content (BMC) [7], physical activity (PA), nutritional factors, sex hormones and drugs have also been found to play a role in bone mineralization [6-8].

Positive relationships between dairy product intake and total BMC and BMD have been reported in women aged 18–50 y [6,9]. However, it is uncertain which nutrient or combination of nutrients is responsible for changes in bone mass when dairy products are consumed because

* Correspondence: Selma.liberato@gmail.com
[1]Menzies School of Health Research, Charles Darwin University, Darwin, NT, Australia
Full list of author information is available at the end of the article

protein, calcium, phosphorus and vitamin D are known to be associated with bone health [6].

There is limited evidence of an effect of dietary calcium intake on BMC in children [10], young women aged 19–35 y [11] and perimenopausal women aged 45 to 58 y with amenorrhoea for 2–24 months [12]. In adolescents aged 12 to 16 y [8], dietary calcium had no effect on BMC [8].

Physical activity (PA) on the other hand, has been shown to contribute to bone mass in many studies [10,11,13-16]. For example, BMC was found to be higher in the dominant arm of female tennis players [14] and in pre- and early-pubertal children with the highest levels of habitual PA [10] or involvement in a 2-year school-based exercise program [5]. A study with 2384 young men attending the mandatory tests for selection to compulsory military service in Sweden found that history of regular physical was the strongest predictor and could explain 10.1% of the variation in BMD [17].

Type of PA has also been shown to contribute to bone mineralization. Whereas vigorous-intensity PA, including resistance training programs and high-impact exercise has been shown to influence bone mass in some studies [7,15,18-20], others have shown that a minimum intake of calcium seems to be essential for PA to have an impact on bone mass [4,21]. In contrast, strength training 3 d/wk for 12 months had no benefit on bone mineralization in postmenopausal women [21] and there was no association between bone mineralization and level and frequency of sports participation in adolescents aged 12 to 16 y [8].

Calcium and weight-bearing PA have been suggested to have their greatest effect early in life [4,16,22] and with consistently high calcium intake [4,21,23]. The recommended dietary intake (RDA) of calcium for men aged 19–30 y is 1000 mg/d [24] with most young men able to meet the RDA by consuming at least three servings of milk, cheese or yogurt daily. In Australia, the median intake of calcium in men 19–24 y was only 961.5 mg/d [25].

There is limited evidence of an effect of dietary calcium intake on bone mineralization in young men. Studies examining the effects of calcium intake and level of physical activity in free living conditions on bone mineralization are also limited, particularly in young men. In addition, intake of dairy products, which are the main source of calcium [26], may be associated with a dietary fat intake [6] and adversely affect blood lipids [24] or blood pressure. Only one study with girls examining effect of calcium and bone mineralization has investigated the effects of calcium intake on blood lipids.

This study aimed to examine the relationship between dietary factors, physical activity and bone mineralization in young men. Blood lipids were also assessed in the current study.

Methods

Thirty-five healthy men aged 18–25 y, recruited from the local community in the city of Brisbane, Australia volunteered for the study. Participants were recruited by flyers posted in shopping centers and education centers as well advertisement in local newspapers. Inclusion criteria to participate in the study were age between 18 and 25 years and absence of any chronic disease. Queensland University of Technology Human Research Ethics Committee approved the participant recruitment and data collection procedures. The methods of this cross-sectional study have been previously described in detail [27] and are here described in brief. Anthropometric measures including body weight and height, body composition, and waist and hip circumferences were undertaken. Body mass index (BMI) was calculated as weight (kg) divided by height (m^2). Body composition, including BMC, BMD and lean body mass, was measured by dual-energy X-ray absorptiometry (DXA) (DPX-Plus; Lunar Corp, Madison, WI).

Resting metabolic rate (RMR) was assessed by continuous open-circuit indirect calorimetry using a Deltatrac II metabolic cart (Datex-Ohmeda Corp., Helsinki, Finland http://www.hospitalnetwork.com/doc/Deltatrac-II-Metabolic-Monitor-0001) in half of the participants. Due to technical problems, the MOXUS O_2 system (AEI Technologies, Pennsylvania, USA) was used to assess RMR of the remaining participants. In our laboratories we have consistently found measured RMR values are less than 100 kcal lower using the Deltatrac compared to MOXUS system. A similar proportion of lean and overweight participants were assessed using each of the methods and therefore likelihood of measurement bias was reduced.

Sitting blood pressure (BP) was assessed after a 10-min rest using a standard sphygmomanometer. Following an overnight fast of at least 8 h, a blood sample was collected for later total cholesterol (TC), high density lipoprotein cholesterol (HDL-C), low density lipoprotein cholesterol (LDL-C) and triglycerides (TG) determination using reagents from Roche Diagnostics (Indianapolis, IN). The measurement of TC and LDL-C were based on the determination of Δ^4-cholestenone after enzymatic cleavage of the cholesterol ester by cholesterol esterase, conversion of cholesterol by cholesterol oxidase, and subsequent measurement by Trinder reaction of the hydrogen peroxide formed [28]. A combination of a sugar compound with detergent was used to selectively determine LDL-C in serum [28]. The HDL-C was determined directly in serum using polyethylene glycol-modified enzymes and dextran sulfate [28].

Both food intake and PA were assessed over four days. Food intake was assessed using household estimates in a food record, and entered into the Foodworks (v.3.02) nutrient analysis software (Xris software Pty Ltd. Brisbane,

Australia, http://www.xyris.com.au). Protein and fat were expressed as source of energy intake (EI). As PA has been shown to have no effect with calcium intake <1000 mg/d [21], an average daily intake of 1000 mg of calcium was used as the cut-off to divide participants into low- and high-intake of calcium groups.

Physical activity was assessed based on activity records using nine categories of PA intensity (1–9) to account for each 15-min period throughout the day. The four-day PA record scores 1, 2, 3, 4, 5, 6, 7, 8 and 9 correspond to 1, 1.5, 2.3, 2.8, 3.3, 4.8, 5.6, 6 and 7.8 metabolic equivalents (METs), respectively [29]. Using measured RMR, the total daily energy expenditure (TDEE) was calculated for each participant after accounting for each of the 96 15-min periods of a day and multiplying the score by its specific MET value. Physical activity level was calculated by dividing TDEE by RMR. For each participant, 15-min periods were classified into three PA levels, according to the Center for Disease Control and Prevention and the American College of Sports Medicine Position Statement [30]: a) light (TDEE < 3 METs), moderate (3–6 METs) and vigorous (TDEE ≥ 6 METs). The B-PAR scores 1 to 4, 5 to 7 and 8 to 9 correspond to light, moderate and vigorous PA, respectively [29,31]. A median 20% percent of TDEE engaged in moderate- to vigorous-intensity PA served as the cut-off for high vs. lower level PA groups.

Cardiorespiratory fitness was measured by a continuous speed, incremental grade running test on a treadmill. Participants were fitted with a Polar Coded Transmitter™ and receiver (Polar Electro, Kempele, Finland), a Hans-Rudolf headset (with two-way breathing valve and pneumotach) and a nose-clip. After a 4-min warm-up at 3.5 mph, 0% grade, speed was increased to a previously determined comfortable speed, which was the same until the end of the test. Thereafter, the treadmill slope was increased by 2% every min, until the participant reached exhaustion. Rating of perceived exertion using the Borg scale was obtained during each stage and participants were encouraged to achieve a rating of 18 or higher as an indicator of maximal effort. Maximal oxygen uptake (VO_{2max}) was assessed using a MOXUS Modular O_2 System (AEI Technologies, Pennsylvania, USA). VO_{2max} was achieved when the difference between the last 2 completed stages determined by the average of the last 30-sec period before the load increased was <1.6 ml/kg.min or when both heart rate ±10 bpm of 220 − age and respiratory exchange ratio >1.15, were achieved. VO_{2max} was defined as the highest observed value averaged across 15 seconds in a completed stage. When the participant did not reach VO_{2max}, VO_2 peak oxygen uptake, the highest observed value of VO_2, was considered in analysis.

All measurements were undertaken by the same investigator in two sessions of two hours each. In the first session, after receiving a detailed explanation of the study requirements and measurements to be collected, the participants provided written consent to participate in the study, had anthropometric data and blood pressure collected and had 1-hour session with a dietitian about how to record the dietary intake data. The participants were asked to attend the biochemical laboratory at their convenience to have blood sample collected after a fasting period for the lipids measurements. In the second session, the participants discussed in detail the dietary intake data recorded to clarify any doubts and had the body composition, resting metabolic rate and the cardiorespiratory fitness measured. A technician helped with the body composition and cardiorespiratory fitness assessment.

A two factor, between-subjects analysis of variance was performed. The factorial analysis of variance (ANOVA) is an inferential statistical test that allows testing if each of several independent variables has an effect on the dependent variable. It also allows determination of the independence of main effects (i.e., if two more independent variables interact with each other).

Participants in the current study were divided according to their calcium intake (low and high calcium intake refers to less or more than 1000 g/d, respectively) and percentage of TDEE engaged in moderate-to-vigorous PA (low and high PA refers to expending less or more than 20% of TDEE engaged in moderate-to-vigorous PA, respectively) in a 2 × 2 between-subjects, factorial design. If there was no interaction between independent variables (p > 0.05 for all dependent variables) the variables were independently analysed by T test.

Results

Factorial analysis considering calcium as one factor and PA as the other factor was not significant (p > 0.05) for all variables tested. Therefore, the mean for calcium intake as well as for PA were compared by T test.

Anthropometric, PA, fitness, dietary and DXA measurements according to calcium intake and energy expended of the participants are shown in Table 1. Participants who consumed more than 1000 mg/d of calcium were taller and energy-adjusted calcium intake, calcium/phosphorus ratio, and lean mass adjustment calcium intake were higher than participants who consumed less than 1000 mg/d of calcium. Participants who expended more than 20% of the TDEE engaged in moderate- to vigorous-intensity PA had higher VO_2 max than participants who expended less (Table 1).

Table 2 contains mean values of whole body and regional BMC and BMD according to participants' calcium intake and energy expenditure engaged in moderate- to vigorous-intensity PA. Participants who consumed more than 1000 mg/d of calcium had higher levels of whole

Table 1 Anthropometric, physical activity (PA), fitness (VO$_2$ max), dietary and DXA measurements of the participants (mean ± SD) according to calcium dietary intake and PA level

	Low calcium	High calcium	P values[1]	Low PA	High PA	P values[1]
Anthropometric						
Height (m)	1.73 ± 0.07	1.78 ± 0.06	0.03	1.74 ± 0.06	1.77 ± 0.08	0.18
Body mass (kg)	74.89 ± 14.50	79.83 ± 12.03	0.28	79.39 ± 13.39	76.12 ± 13.45	0.48
Lean mass (kg)	56.42 ± 8.41	61.47 ± 7.72	0.07	57.37 ± 8.30	60.11 ± 8.39	0.34
BMI (kg/m^2)	24.79 ± 3.99	25.03 ± 3.03	0.84	26.15 ± 3.77	24.09 ± 3.09	0.09
Waist circumference	82.21 ± 9.06	83.06 ± 7.72	0.77	85.32 ± 9.18	80.86 ± 7.31	0.12
Physical activity						
EE doing moderate to vigorous PA (kcal)	744.62 ± 410.72	988.04 ± 412.21	0.09	477.91 ± 179.90	1131.08 ± 324.14	0.09
VO$_2$ max (ml of O$_2$)	50.84 ± 8.30	53.26 ± 6.41	0.37	47.38 ± 7.94	54.93 ± 5.48	0.01
Dietary						
Calcium (mg)	757.91	1458.57		1008.20 ± 555.12	1191.62 ± 399.24	0.26
Calcium/energy (mg/kcal)	0.32 ± 0.09	0.50 ± 0.12	< 0.001	0.40 ± 0.19	0.42 ± 0.10	0.64
Calcium/phosphorus	0.49 ± 0.12	0.68 ± 0.10	< 0.001	0.57 ± 0.17	0.61 ± 0.13	0.52
Calcium/lean mass (mg/kg)	0.0135 ± 0.0035	0.0241 ± 0.0070	< 0.001	0.0177 ± 0.0099	0.02 ± 0.01	0.48
Protein (%)	16.92 ± 4.74	16.68 ± 2.52	0.85	17.26 ± 5.04	16.49 ± 2.58	0.61
Fat (%)	32.36 ± 5.79	32.17 ± 4.85	0.92	32.86 ± 6.46	31.86 ± 4.38	0.59

Abbreviations: BMI, Body mass index; EE, energy expenditure.
[1] T test.

Table 2 Mean values ± SD of body composition parameters in young men having low and high intake of calcium and expending low and high percentage of daily energy engaged in moderate- to vigorous intensity physical activity (PA)

	Low calcium intake	High calcium intake	P values[1]	Low PA	High PA	P values[1]
BMC (g)						
Whole body	3191.26 ± 555.27	3611.15 ± 486.94	0.02	3263.56 ± 473.83	3502.97 ± 596.04	0.21
Whole body/height	1833.41 ± 267.85	2021.94 ± 239.81	0.04	1872.64 ± 242.08	1968.86 ± 282.55	0.30
Whole body/body mass	42.97 ± 4.61	45.44 ± 3.23	0.07	41.41 ± 3.73	46.13 ± 3.18	<0.001
Whole body/BMI	129.67 ± 12.82	144.57 ± 19.10	0.01	125.39 ± 12.25	145.30 ± 16.26	<0.001
Arms	434.18 ± 85.41	470.52 ± 93.25	0.24	436.66 ± 80.28	463.67 ± 96.48	0.39
Legs	1269.27 ± 251.31	1335.26 ± 232.11	0.43	1266.74 ± 224.37	1327.52 ± 252.87	0.47
Trunk	1056.90 ± 204.60	1209.20 ± 229.90	0.05	1043.53 ± 174.67	1196.36 ± 242.72	0.05
L1L4	94.24 ± 19.30	112.81 ± 21.76	0.01	96.24 ± 19.36	108.83 ± 23.26	0.10
L1L4/body mass	1.28 ± 0.28	1.43 ± 0.31	0.16	1.22 ± 0.20	1.45 ± 0.32	0.02
L1L4/BMI	3.88 ± 0.81	4.53 ± 1.00	0.04	3.70 ± 0.63	4.56 ± 0.99	0.01
L2L4	68.34 ± 13.64	80.71 ± 12.07	0.01	72.31 ± 13.80	76.29 ± 14.46	0.42
L2L4/body mass	0.93 ± 0.18	1.03 ± 0.20	0.14	0.92 ± 0.15	1.02 ± 0.22	0.14
L2L4/BMI	2.80 ± 0.48	3.25 ± 0.65	0.03	2.78 ± 0.43	3.20 ± 0.65	0.04
BMD (g/cm^2)						
Whole body	1.27 ± 0.10	1.30 ± 0.09	0.35	1.27 ± 0.09	1.30 ± 0.10	0.34
Arms	1.01 ± 0.09	1.04 ± 0.10	0.25	1.02 ± 0.09	1.03 ± 0.10	0.65
Legs	1.44 ± 0.12	1.48 ± 0.13	0.36	1.43 ± 0.11	1.48 ± 0.14	0.29
Trunk	1.04 ± 0.11	1.09 ± 0.09	0.14	1.03 ± 0.09	1.08 ± 0.10	0.07
Lumbar L1L4	1.04 ± 0.15	1.06 ± 0.12	0.69	1.05 ± 0.15	1.06 ± 0.12	0.80
Lumbar L2L4	1.15 ± 0.14	1.16 ± 0.16	0.80	1.14 ± 0.16	1.17 ± 0.14	0.49

Abbreviations: BMC, body mineral content; BMD, body mineral density; BMI, Body mass index.
[1] T test.

body BMC, height-adjusted whole body BMC, BMI-adjusted whole body BMC, trunk BMC, lumbar L1-L4 BMC, BMI-adjusted lumbar L1-L4 BMC, lumbar L2-L4 BMC and BMI-adjusted lumbar L2-L4 BMC than participants who consumed less than 1000 mg/d of calcium. Participants who expended greater energy had higher levels of body mass adjusted whole body BMC, BMI-adjusted whole body BMC, trunk BMC, body mass adjusted lumbar L1-L4 BMC, BMI-adjusted lumbar L1-L4 BMC, body mass adjusted lumbar L2-L4 BMC and BMI-adjusted lumbar L2-L4 BMC than participants who expended less energy (Table 2).

There were no between-group differences in blood pressure or blood lipids based either on calcium intake level or on energy expenditure engaged in moderate- to vigorous-intensity PA level (Table 3).

Discussion

High intake of calcium and high energy expended engaged in moderate- to vigorous-intensity PA was associated with high bone mass in the young men participating in the current study. Higher BMC was observed in whole body, trunk and lumbar regions but not in legs or arms of young men who consumed more than 1000 mg/d of calcium compared to those who consumed less than 1000 mg/d of calcium. There was no difference in the absolute values of bone mineralization but when these values were adjusted for body mass or BMI, participants who expended more than 20% of the EE engaged in moderate- to vigorous-intensity PA had higher of levels of whole body BMC, trunk BMC, Lumbar L1-L4 BMC, and Lumbar L2-L4 than participants who expended less.

The association between high bone mass and high intake of calcium is similar to other studies [9-12,23] as is the relationship between calcium intake and lumbar spine but not legs or arms [18,32,33]. Lumbar spine consists of primarily cancellous bone which is more metabolically active [18] and therefore more responsive to

dietary intake and, or PA intervention than peripheral cortical bone [5,8,13,18].

Calcium intake had no effect on any of the BMD measurements in the current study, also consistent with other studies [6,8,10,34]. On the other hand, calcium intake was shown to have an effect on BMD in girls. Positive association between calcium intake and bone mass were reported in young women aged 19–35 y [11] and BMD increased from 11 to 17 y in girls with consistently high calcium intake [23]. Bone mineral density does not account effectively for diverse body sizes [10] and BMC has been suggested to be a better indicator of accretion in bone mineralisation than BMD [6].

The finding of the current study that high intake of calcium did not adversely affect blood lipids or blood pressure is also similar to another study [6]. Supplementation with dairy products to at least 1000 mg/d for 12 months in 91 girls aged 15–16 years did not adversely affect blood lipids [6]. High intake of calcium could have been related to high intake of dairy and consequently high intake of fat. However this was not the case in this study. Intake of fat as a percentage of energy was similar in participants who consumed less or more than 1000 mg/d of calcium.

High nutrient density foods such as low-fat dairy foods were the main sources of calcium for participants who consumed more calcium as evidenced by no between-group differences in protein and fat percentage contribution to EI. Further, participants who consumed more than 1000 mg/d of calcium had higher energy adjusted calcium compared to participants who consumed less.

High protein intake has been shown to produce negative calcium balance from increased urinary calcium excretion if phosphorus intake is kept low [6]. Calcium balance does not seem to have been negative in the participants of the current study because intake of protein was within the recommended intake accounting for more than 16% of the energy intake.

Table 3 Serum lipids in the young men having low and high calcium intake and expending low and high percentage of daily energy engaged in moderate- to vigorous- intensity physical activity (PA)

	Low calcium intake	High calcium intake	P values[1]	Low PA	High PA	P values[1]
Diastolic (mmHg)	119.24 ± 10.12	124.56 ± 9.55	0.12	123.29 ± 7.68	121.10 ± 11.46	0.53
Systolic (mmHg)	59.53 ± 7.73	57.50 ± 6.72	0.41	60.36 ± 7.09	57.24 ± 7.16	0.21
TC (mmol/L)	4.46 ± 1.31	4.45 ± 0.54	0.98	4.60 ± 1.30	4.36 ± 0.71	0.48
HDL-C (mmol/L)	1.39 ± 0.28	1.40 ± 0.24	0.92	1.37 ± 0.21	1.41 ± 0.29	0.68
LDL-C (mmol/L)	2.66 ± 1.01	2.66 ± 0.55	0.99	2.77 ± 1.03	2.59 ± 0.61	0.54
Triglycerides (mmol/L)	1.19 ± 1.4	1.01 ± 0.44	0.61	1.39 ± 1.53	0.90 ± 0.36	0.25
TC/HDL-C	3.32 ± 1.10	3.27 ± 0.65	0.87	3.41 ± 0.99	3.22 ± 0.82	0.53
LDL-C/HDL-C	2.00 ± 0.84	1.98 ± 0.59	0.94	2.06 ± 0.77	1.94 ± 0.68	0.60

Abbreviations: TC, Total cholesterol, HDL-C, High density cholesterol, LDL-C, Low density cholesterol.
[1] T test.

A high Ca/P intake ratio in participants who consumed more than 1000 mg/d of calcium compared to participants who consumed less may also have contributed to a higher bone mass. High Ca/P intake ratio has been shown to be positively associated with bone mass [12,35].

Participants of the current study who expended more than 20% of total energy engaged in moderate- to vigorous-intensity PA had higher VO_2 max than participants who expended less. This finding indicates that data are reliable despite using subjective measurements to assess PA.

A significant positive effect of moderate- to vigorous-intensity PA was observed on whole body BMC normalized to either BMI or body mass. Whole body BMC normalized to either BMI or body mass may be a better measurement of bone mass because BMC is known to be heavily influenced by body weight, body height and body lean mass. Bones are mineralized, in part, due to forces they are habitually exposed to and therefore larger individuals necessarily expose their bones to larger forces, resulting in higher BMC and BMD [18].

The effects of moderate- to vigorous-intensity PA in participants of the current study were evident in the lumbar spine. Similar findings were observed in other studies with young adults [36,37]. A 12 y follow-up study with participants aged 20–29 y at baseline showed that increased PA was associated with increased BMD at the lumbar spine [36]. A study with 12 men and 12 women aged between 18 and 23 years participating in a resistance training applying loads to the hip and spine for 24 weeks, on three nonconsecutive days per week showed that males had an increase in BMD of 7.7% in the lateral spine L2-L4 while the change in women was 1.5% [37]. A study with resistance athletes, runners and cyclists found that muscle contraction makes a significant contribution to the lean bone mass-associated increases in BMD [38]. Continued heavy training leads to continuous reactivating remodelling [15,21] by replacing damaged and degraded bone tissue with new tissue [15] and increases bone mineralization [7,11,14,16,18].

A small sample size was a limitation of the current study. Another limitation is that RMR of half of the participants was assessed using different equipment due to technical problems. However the likelihood of measurement bias is small because a similar proportion of lean and overweight participants was assessed using each of the equipments. Nevertheless, the findings contribute to a better understanding of the bone mineralization of young Australian men, an important group which has been under-represented in previous work.

Conclusion

High intake of calcium and high energy expended engaged in moderate- to vigorous- intensity PA were positively associated with bone mineralization particularly in lumbar region of young men.

Competing interests

The authors declare that they have no competing interests.

Authors' contributions

SCL defined the design of the study, undertook data collection, data collation, data analysis and manuscript preparation. JB helped with manuscript writing. APH secured support for this study and helped with manuscript writing. All authors read and approved the manuscript.

Acknowledgements

The authors acknowledge the voluntary participants and the Queensland University of Technology for the use of its Laboratories and facilities. SL acknowledges financial support from the Conselho Nacional de Desenvolvimento Científico e Tecnológico (processo 140931/2001-5) and (processo 201075/03-2).

Author details

[1]Menzies School of Health Research, Charles Darwin University, Darwin, NT, Australia. [2]Departamento de Nutrição e Saúde, Universidade Federal de Viçosa, Viçosa, MG, Brazil. [3]Mater Mother's Hospital/Mater Research Institute, Griffith Health Institute/Griffith University, Brisbane, QLD, Australia.

References

1. Lv L, Claessens AL, Lysens R, Koninckx PR, Beunen G: Association between bone, body composition and strength in premenarcheal girls and postmenopausal women. Ann Hum Biol 2004, 31(2):228–244.
2. Löfgren B, Stenevi-Lundgren S, Dencker M, Karlsson MK: The mode of school transportation in pre- pubertal children does not influence the accrual of bone mineral or the gain in bone size - two year prospective data from the paediatric osteoporosis preventive (POP) study. BMC Musculoskelet Disord 2010, 11:1–7.
3. Guadalupe-Grau A, Fuentes T, Guerra B, Calbet JAL: Exercise and bone mass in adults. Sports Med 2009, 39(6):439–468.
4. Ondrak KS, Morgan DW: Physical activity, calcium intake and bone health in children and adolescents. Sports Med 2007, 37(7):587–601.
5. Alwis G, Linden C, Ahlborg HG, Dencker M, Gardsell P, Karlsson MK: A 2-year school-based exercise programme in pre-pubertal boys induces skeletal benefits in lumbar spine. Acta Paediatr 2008, 97(11):1564–1571.
6. Merrilees MJ, Smart EJ, Gilchrist NL, March RL, Maguire P, Turner JG, Frampton C, Hooke E: Effects of dairy food supplements on bone mineral density in teenage girls. Eur J Nutr 2000, 39(6):256–262.
7. Bratteby LE, Samuelson G, Sandhagen B, Mallmin H, Lantz H, Sjöström L: Whole-body mineral measurements in Swedish adolescents at 17 years compared to 15 years of age. Acta Paediatr 2002, 91(10):1031–1038.
8. Cheng JCY, Maffulli N, Leung SSSF, Lee WTK, Lau JTF, Chan KM: Axial and peripheral bone mineral acquisition: a 3-year longitudinal study in Chinese adolescents. Eur J Pediatr 1999, 158(6):506–512.
9. Beaudoin CM, Blum JW: Calcium knowledge, dietary calcium intake, and bone mineral content and density in young women. N Am J Psychol 2005, 7(2):265–277.
10. McVeigh JA, Norris SA, Pettifor JM: Bone mass accretion rates in pre- and early-pubertal South African black and white children in relation to habitual physical activity and dietary calcium intakes. Acta Paediatr 2007, 96(6):874–880.
11. Bedford JL, Barr SI: The relationship between 24-h urinary cortisol and bone in healthy young women. Int J Behav Med 2010, 17(3):207–215.
12. Brot C, Jørgensen N, Madsen OR, Jensen LB, Sørensen OH: Relationships between bone mineral density, serum vitamin D metabolites and calcium:phosphorus intake in healthy perimenopausal women. J Intern Med 1999, 245(5):509–516.
13. Cornish SM, Chilibeck PD, Paus-Jennsen L, Biem HJ, Khozani T, Senanayake V, Vatanparast H, Little JP, Whiting SJ, Pahwa P: A randomized controlled trial of the effects of flaxseed lignan complex on metabolic syndrome composite score and bone mineral in older adults. Appl Physiol Nutr Metab 2009, 34(2):89–98.

14. Kannus P, Haapasalo H: Effect of starting age of physical activity on bone mass in the dominant arm of tennis and squash. Ann Intern Med 1995, 123(1):27–31.
15. Suominen H: Physical activity and health: musculoskeletal issues. Adv Physiother 2007, 9(2):65–75.
16. Breban S, Chappard C, Jaffre C, Khacef F, Briot K, Benhamou CL: Positive influence of long-lasting and intensive weight-bearing physical activity on hip structure of young adults. J Clin Densitom 2011, 14(2):129–137.
17. Pettersson U, Nilsson M, Sundh V, Mellstrom D, Lorentzon M: Physical activity is the strongest predictor of calcaneal peak bone mass in young Swedish men. Osteoporos Int 2010, 21(3):447–455.
18. Bareither ML, Grabiner MD, Troy KL: Habitual site-specific upper extremity loading is associated with increased bone mineral of the ultradistal radius in young women. J Women's Health (15409996) 2008, 17(10):1577–1581.
19. Nowak A, Straburzyńska-Lupa A, Kusy K, Zieliński J, Felsenberg D, Rittweger J, Karolkiewicz J, Straburzyńska-Migaj E, Pilaczyńska-Szcześniak Ł: Bone mineral density and bone turnover in male masters athletes aged 40–64. Aging Male 2010, 13(2):133–141.
20. Karlsson MK, Nordqvist A, Karlsson C: Sustainability of exercise-induced increases in bone density and skeletal structure. Food Nutr Res 2008, 52:1–6.
21. Chilibeck PD, Davison KS, Whiting SJ, Suzuki Y, Janzen CL, Peloso P: The effect of strength training combined with bisphosphonate (etidronate) therapy on bone mineral, lean tissue, and fat mass in postmenopausal women. Can J Physiol Pharmacol 2002, 80(10):941–950.
22. Bacon L, Stern JS, Keim NL, Van Loan MD: Low bone mass in premenopausal chronic dieting obese women. Eur J Clin Nutr 2004, 58(6):966–971.
23. Magarey AM, Boulton TJC, Chatterton BE, Schultz C, Nordin BEC: Familial and environmental influences on bone growth from 11–17 years. Acta Paediatr 1999, 88(11):1204–1210.
24. NHMRC: Nutrient reference values for Australia and New Zealand. Australian Government National Health and Medical Research Council; 2006.
25. McLennan W, Podger A: National nutrition survey. nutrient intakes and physical measurements. Australia. 1995, ABS Catalogue. Canberra: Commonwealth of Australia; 1998:180.
26. McLennan W, Podger A: National nutrition survey: nutrient intakes and physical measurements, ABS publications. Canberra: Australian Bureau of Statistics and Department of Health and Aged Care; 1995:1–170.
27. Liberato SC, Bressan J, Hills AP: A quantitative analysis of energy intake reported by young men. Nutr Diet 2008, 65(4):259–265.
28. Nauck M, Graziani MS, Bruton D, Cobbaert C, Cole TG, Lefevre F, Riesen W, Bachorik PS, Rifai N: Analytical and clinical performance of a detergent-based homogeneous LDL-cholesterol assay: a multicenter evaluation. Clin Chem 2000, 46(4):506–514.
29. Bouchard C, Tremblay A, Leblanc C, Lortie G, Savard R, Theriault G: A method to assess energy expenditure in children and adults. Am J Clin Nutr 1983, 37(3):461–467.
30. Pate RR, Pratt M, Blair SN, Haskell WL, Macera CA, Bouchard C, Buchner D, Ettinger W, Heath GW, King AC, et al: Physical activity and public health: a recommendation from the centers for disease control and prevention and the American college of sports medicine. J Am Med Assoc 1995, 273(5):402–407.
31. Dionne I, Almeras N, Bouchard C, Tremblay A: The association between vigorous physical activities and fat deposition in male adolescents. Med Sci Sports Exerc 2000, 32(2):392–395.
32. Fulkerson JA, Himes JH, French SA, Jensen S, Petit MA, Stewart C, Story M, Ensrud K, Fillhouer S, Jacobsen K: Bone outcomes and technical measurement issues of bone health among children and adolescents: considerations for nutrition and physical activity intervention trials. Osteoporos Int 2004, 15(12):929–941.
33. Roy BD, Bourgeois J, Rodriguez C, Payne E, Young K, Shaughnessy SG, Tarnopolosky MA: Conjugated linoleic acid prevents growth attenuation induced by corticosteroid administration and increases bone mineral content in young rats. Appl Physiol Nutr Metab 2008, 33(6):1096–1104.
34. Hinton PS, Scott Rector R, Donnelly JE, Smith BK, Bailey B: Total body bone mineral content and density during weight loss and maintenance on a low- or recommended-dairy weight-maintenance diet in obese men and women. Eur J Clin Nutr 2010, 64(4):392–399.
35. Ito S, Ishida H, Uenishi K, Murakami K, Sasaki S: The relationship between habitual dietary phosphorus and calcium intake, and bone mineral density in young Japanese women: a cross-sectional study. Asia Pac J Clin Nutr 2011, 20(3):411–417.
36. Laaksonen MM, Impivaara O, Sievanen H, Viikari JS, Lehtimaki TJ, Lamberg-Allardt CJ, Karkkainen MU, Valimaki M, Heikkinen J, Kroger LM, et al: Associations of genetic lactase non-persistence and sex with bone loss in young adulthood. Bone 2009, 44(5):1003–1009.
37. Almstedt HC, Canepa JA, Ramirez DA, Shoepe TC: Changes in bone mineral density in response to 24 weeks of resistance training in college-age men and women. J Strength Cond Res 2011, 25(4):1098–1103.
38. Rector RS, Rogers R, Ruebel M, Widzer MO, Hinton PS: Lean body mass and weight-bearing activity in the prediction of bone mineral density in physically active men. J Strength Cond Res 2009, 23(2):427–435.

Changes in foot volume, body composition, and hydration status in male and female 24-hour ultra-mountain bikers

Daniela Chlíbková[1†], Beat Knechtle[2*†], Thomas Rosemann[2†], Alena Žákovská[3†], Ivana Tomášková[4†], Marcus Shortall[5†] and Iva Tomášková[6†]

Abstract

Background: The effects of running and cycling on changes in hydration status and body composition during a 24-hour race have been described previously, but data for 24-hour ultra-mountain bikers are missing. The present study investigated changes in foot volume, body composition, and hydration status in male and female 24-hour ultra-mountain bikers.

Methods: We compared in 49 (37 men and 12 women) 24-hour ultra-mountain bikers (ultra-MTBers) changes (Δ) in body mass (BM). Fat mass (FM), percent body fat (%BF) and skeletal muscle mass (SM) were estimated using anthropometric methods. Changes in total body water (TBW), extracellular fluid (ECF) and intracellular fluid (ICF) were determined using bioelectrical impedance and changes in foot volume using plethysmography. Haematocrit, plasma [Na$^+$], plasma urea, plasma osmolality, urine urea, urine specific gravity and urine osmolality were measured in a subgroup of 25 ultra-MTBers (16 men and 9 women).

Results: In male 24-hour ultra-MTBers, BM ($P < 0.001$), FM ($P < 0.001$), %BF ($P < 0.001$) and ECF ($P < 0.05$) decreased whereas SM and TBW did not change ($P > 0.05$). A significant correlation was found between post-race BM and post-race FM (r = 0.63, $P < 0.001$). In female ultra-MTBers, BM ($P < 0.05$), %BF ($P < 0.05$) and FM ($P < 0.001$) decreased, whereas SM, ECF and TBW remained stable ($P > 0.05$). Absolute ranking in the race was related to Δ%BM ($P < 0.001$) and Δ%FM in men ($P < 0.001$) and to Δ%BM ($P < 0.05$) in women. In male ultra-MTBers, increased post-race plasma urea ($P < 0.001$) was negatively related to absolute ranking in the race, Δ%BM, post-race FM and Δ%ECF ($P < 0.05$). Foot volume remained stable in both sexes ($P > 0.05$).

Conclusions: Male and female 24-hour ultra-MTBers experienced a significant loss in BM and FM, whereas SM remained stable. Body weight changes and increases in plasma urea do not reflect a change in body hydration status. No oedema of the lower limbs occurred.

Keywords: Body mass, Fat mass, Hydration, Foot volume

Background

Ultra-endurance races defined as an event exceeding six hours in duration and lasting up to 40 hours or several days [1] pose specific problems for competitors such as a possibility of lack of fluids [2-6], fluid overload and/or an increase in total body water [4,7-17], sleep deprivation [2,18-21], inadequate energy intake [2,15,21-24] or unfavorable conditions like extreme heat or extreme cold [2,5,7,12,16,25,26]. Issues associated with body composition and hydration status include a decrease in body mass in ultra-running [2,9,16,27-29], in road ultra-cycling [21,22,24], in mountain-biking [5,7,30], swimming [12,31], triathlon [6,15,32] and skiing [26].

Within ultra-races, there is a difference between single stage races [30,33-37], multi-stage races [7,22,25,33, 38-40] and time-limited races such as 24-hour races [2,16,18-21,27-29,41]. Little is known about the effects

---

* Correspondence: beat.knechtle@hispeed.ch

†Equal contributors

[2]Institute of General Practise and for Health Services Research, University of Zurich, Zurich, Switzerland

Full list of author information is available at the end of the article

of running or cycling on changes in hydration status [16,28,41] and body composition [2,16,18,20,27,29] during a 24-hour race. Non-stop ultra-endurance races and races lasting for several days without defined breaks lead generally to a decrease in body mass [15,22,24], and there seemed to be differences between cycling and running races. A decrease in fat mass has been rather reported for ultra-cycling [5,21,22,24,36], whereas a decrease in skeletal mass has been more often reported for ultra-running [17,42]. However, a reduction in fat mass has not been confirmed for a 24-hour cycling road race. Knechtle et al. [20] showed that an energy deficit did not always result in a reciprocal loss of adipose subcutaneous tissue or skeletal muscle mass.

A decrease in body mass could also be attributed to dehydration [2,5], but dehydration cannot be established without the determination of plasma sodium concentration [Na$^+$] or osmolality in both plasma and urine [43]. Male ultra-MTBers during a 120-km race suffered a significant decrease in both body mass and skeletal mass, but no dehydration was observed when other determinants of hydration status were assessed [30]. On the contrary, body mass can increase [13,23] or remain stable [25,42] in ultra-endurance races with breaks due to an increase in total body water.

An increase in total body water can occur in several ways such as fluid overload [8,9], plasma [Na$^+$] retention [30] due to an increased aldosterone activity [34], protein catabolism [6], an increased vasopressin activity [44] or an impaired renal function [17,45]. Prolonged strenuous endurance exercise may lead to an increase in extracellular fluid, plasma volume and total body water [8,10,17] and a decrease in haematocrit due to haemodilution [7]. For male 100-km ultra-runners, a loss of both skeletal muscle mass and fat mass with an increase in total body water has been reported [46]. Similar findings were recorded in a Triple Iron ultra-triathlon (i.e. 11.4 km swimming, 540 km cycling, and 126.6 km running) where total body water and plasma volume increased and these changes seemed to be associated with oedema of the feet [10]. Two field studies using plethysmography found a potential association between fluid intake and the formation of peripheral oedema [8,9].

Moreover, only a few studies investigated changes in body composition and hydration status in female ultra-endurance athletes [12,41,47-52], but the reported findings were not consistent. In open-water ultra-distance swimmers, Weitkunat et al. [12] summarized that changes in body composition and hydration status were different in male compared to female athletes. For ultra-marathoners, it has been shown that female runners lost body mass during a 24-hour run [41]. Knechtle et al. [47] observed in 11 female 100-km ultra-runners a loss in body mass despite unchanged total body water and plasma [Na$^+$]. On the contrary, in one female ultra-runner during a 1,200-km multi-stage ultra-marathon, body mass increased, percent body fat decreased, while percent total body water and skeletal mass increased [51].

Additionally, there are no studies showing whether changes in body composition and hydration status were associated with an increased prevalence of peripheral oedema in ultra-endurance mountain bikers such as 24-hour ultra-MTBers. The aim of the present study was therefore to investigate changes in foot volume, body composition and hydration status in male and female 24-hour ultra-MTBers. Based on present literature, we hypothesized to find a loss in body mass as has previously reported for ultra-cycling [21,24,36] and non-stop ultra-endurance races [15,22,24,26]. We hypothesized that this type of MTB races would lead to an increase in foot volume due to peripheral oedema.

Methods

Participants

The present work combines data from two 24-hour races held in the Czech Republic in 2012. Subjects were recruited via pre-race emails and during race registration. A total of 28 (22 men and 6 women) recreational 24-hour ultra-MTBers in the solo category from the 'Czech Championship 24-hour MTB 2012' in Jihlava city in the Czech Republic and 24 (18 men and 6 women) ultra-MTBers from the 'Bike Race Marathon MTB Rohozec 24 hours' in Liberec city in the Czech Republic in the solo category consented to participate in the study. Of those, 37 men and 12 women finished the race successfully. One cyclist had to give up due to technical problems and two athletes because of medical complications. Athletes were informed that participation was voluntary and that the project had received approval in accordance with the law (No. 96/2001 Coll. M. S. on Human Rights and Biomedicine and Act No. 101/2000 Coll. Privacy). The pre-race anthropometry and training data of the participants are presented in Table 1.

Races details

The first measurement was performed at the 3rd edition of the 'Czech Championship 24-hour MTB 2012' in Jihlava. The ultra-MTBers began the race at 12:00 on 19th May 2012 and finished at 12:00 on 20th May 2012. The course comprised a 9.5 km single-track with an elevation of 220 m. A single aid station, located at the start/finish area was provided by the organizer where a variety of food and beverages such as hypotonic sports drinks, tea, soup, caffeinated drinks, water, fruit, vegetables, energy bars, bread, soup, sausages, cheese, bread, chocolate and biscuits were available. The ultra-MTBers could also use their own supplies in their pit stops. Temperature was +16°C at the start, rose to a maximum of +20°C, dropped to +6°C

Table 1 The pre-race experience and training parameters (n = 49)

	Male ultra-MTBers (n = 37)	Female ultra-MTBers (n = 12)
	$M \pm SD$	$M \pm SD$
Years as active biker (yr)	9.2 ± 5.8	8.8 ± 5.9
Number of finished ultra-marathons (n)	8.0 ± 6.5	6.7 ± 5.3
Personal best km in 24 hour (km)	315.5 ± 89.7	279.6 ± 106.7
Total hours weekly (h)	10.5 ± 5.3	10.2 ± 5.5
Weekly cycling kilometers (km)	225.8 ± 149.5	191.8 ± 134.5
Weekly cycling hours (h)	9.9 ± 5.1	9.2 ± 5.2
Mean cycling intensity (beat/min)	133.8** ± 7.6	134.5** ± 22.8
Mean cycling speed (km/h)	23.0** ± 3.6	21.1** ± 5.3
Longest trail (km)	176.8** ± 84.7	141.7** ± 75.5
Amount of km in 2011 (km)	7,107.5 ± 5,782.4	5,696.9 ± 5,037.9

Results are presented as mean ± SD; * = $P < 0.05$, ** = $P < 0.001$.

during the night and rose to +23°C from the morning of the next day till the end of the race. Cloud cover was minimal and no precipitation was recorded during the race. The relative humidity was stable at 43% during the race. The 'Bike Race Marathon MTB Rohozec' in Liberec took place from 9th June to 10th June 2012. The course comprised a 12.6 km track with an elevation of 250 m. The track surface consisted of paved and unpaved roads and paths. There was one aid station located at the start and finish area with food and beverages similar to those mentioned above. The temperature was +19°C at the start, rose to a maximum of +23°C, dropped to +6°C during the night and changed to +11°C until the end of the race. Weather conditions varied from sunny to cloudy with a short shower in the afternoon and relative humidity increased from 44% to 98%.

Procedures, measurements and calculations

Participants were instructed to keep a training diary until the start of the race. The training three months before the race (i.e. training units in hours, cycling units in hours, training distances in kilometers, cycling speed, heart rate during training units, volume of kilometers in the year 2011, and the years of active cycling) was recorded. Participant recruitment and pre-race testing took place during event registration in the morning before the race between 07:00 a.m. and 11:00 a.m. in a private room adjacent to the registration area. The athletes were informed of the procedures and gave their informed written consent. Post-race measurements were taken between 12:00 and 1:00 p.m. immediately upon completion of the race in the same place. No measurements were made during the race. Between the pre- and the post-race measurements, all athletes recorded their fluid intake using a written record.

Anthropometric measurements and plethysmography of the foot

Anthropometric measurements were recorded in all forty-nine ultra-MTBers (37 males and 12 females) (Table 2, also Figure 1) to estimate skeletal muscle mass and fat mass. Body mass, total body water, extracellular fluid and intracellular fluid were measured using a multiple-frequency bioelectrical impedance analyser (InBody 720, Biospace, Seoul, South Korea). Inbody 720 has a tetra polar 8-point tactile electrode system performing at each session 30 impedance measurements by using six different frequencies (i.e. 1 kHz, 5 kHz, 50 kHz, 250 kHz, 500 kHz, and 1,000 kHz) at each five segments (i.e. right arm, left arm, trunk, right leg, and left leg). Subjects were barefoot and generally clothed in cycling attire for both the pre- and post-race measurements and participants were advised to void their urinary bladder prior to the anthropometric measurements. Body height was determined using a stadiometer (TANITA HR 001, Tanita Europe B.V., Amsterdam, The Netherland) to the nearest 0.01 m. Body mass index was calculated using body mass and body height. The circumferences of mid-upper arm, mid-thigh and mid-calf were measured on the right side of the body to the nearest 0.01 cm using a non-elastic tape measure (KaWe CE, Kirchner und Welhelm, Germany). The skin-fold measurements were taken on the right side of the body for all eight skin-folds (i.e. pectoralis, axillar, triceps, subscapular, abdomen, suprailiac, front thigh, and medial calf) using a skin-fold calliper (Harpenden skinfold caliper, Baty International Ltd) and recorded to the nearest 0.2 mm. An anthropometric equation [53] using body stature, corrected upper arm and thigh girth, sex, age and race of the participants was used to estimate skeletal muscle mass in kg. Fat-free mass (kg) was estimated using an equation for male [54] and female [55] athletes. Fat mass (kg) was determined based on subtracting fat-free mass from total body mass. Percent body fat was estimated using a specific equation for men [56] and women [57]. Hydration status was classified according to the criteria established by Noakes et al. [11] with overhydration classified as any weight gain above initial body mass, euhydration as a decrease in body mass of 0.01% to 3.0%, and dehydration as any decrease in body mass greater than 3.0%. The changes of the volume of the right foot were estimated using the principle of plethysmography [8]. We used a Plexiglas vessel, the dimensions were chosen so that any foot size of an ultra-MTBer would fit in the vessel. Outside the vessel, a scale in mm was fixed on the front window to measure changes in the level of water

Table 2 Age and anthropometric characteristics of the ultra-MTBers (n = 49)

Parameter	Pre-race M ± SD	Post- race M ± SD	Absolute change	Change (%)
Male ultra-MTBers (n = 37)				
Body height (cm)	180.4 ± 0.1			
Age (yr)	36.6 ± 8.4			
Body mass (kg)	77.9 ± 9.6	75.9 ± 9.8	−2.0 ± 1.6**	−2.6 ± 2.1**
Skeletal muscle mass (kg)	38.4 ± 4.9	38.1 ± 4.9	−0.3 ± 1.1	−0.6 ± 2.7
Fat mass (kg)	10.6 ± 5.3	9.2 ± 4.9	−1.4 ± 1.2**	−14.9 ± 14.5**
Percent body fat (%)	13.2 ± 5.7	11.8 ± 5.4	−1.4 ± 1.4**	−12.7 ± 14.6**
Total body water (L)	49.3 ± 5.5	48.9 ± 5.7	−0.4 ± 1.4	−0.9 ± 2.8
Extracellular fluid (L)	18.3 ± 2.0	18.1 ± 2.1	−0.2 ± 0.6*	−1.2 ± 3.2*
Intracellular fluid (L)	31.0 ± 3.5	30.8 ± 3.6	−0.2 ± 0.8	−0.7 ± 2.6
Volume of the foot (L)	1.132 ± 1.502	1.145 ± 1.302	0.013 ± 0.097	1.8 ± 9.6
Female ultra-MTBers (n = 12)				
Body height (cm)	167.8 ± 29.3			
Age (yr)	36.8 ± 8.9			
Body mass (kg)	60.6 ± 4.9	59.7 ± 4.9	−0.9 ± 1.2*	−1.5 ± 1.9*
Skeletal muscle mass (kg)	26.7 ± 3.3	26.8 ± 3.2	0.1 ± 0.7	0.4 ± 2.7
Fat mass (kg)	10.9 ± 3.9	9.7 ± 3.9	−1.2 ± 1.0**	−8.2 ± 10.8**
Percent body fat (%)	15.4 ± 6.5	13.7 ± 6.2	−2.7 ± 3.6*	−11.0 ± 15.5*
Total body water (L)	35.3 ± 4.4	35.4 ± 4.5	0.1 ± 0.9	0.2 ± 2.7
Extracellular fluid (L)	13.3 ± 1.7	13.3 ± 1.7	0.0 ± 0.5	0.0 ± 3.6
Intracellular fluid (L)	22.0 ± 2.7	22.1 ± 2.8	0.1 ± 0.5	0.4 ± 2.3
Volume of the foot (L)	0.858 ± 1.205	0.908 ± 1.100	0.050 ± 0.116	6.9 ± 14.4

Results are presented as mean ± SD; * = $P < 0.05$, ** = $P < 0.001$.

from the bottom to the top. The vessel was filled to the level of 100 mm with tap water. The right foot was immersed in the water and the upper limit of the water was at the middle of *malleolus medialis*. After immersion of the foot, the new water level was recorded to the nearest 1 mm and the volume of the foot was calculated. The corresponding calculated volume in ml using the length, width and height in mm of the displaced water was defined as the volume of the right foot. No measurements were made during the race.

Haematological and biochemical measurements

Haematocrit (HCT), plasma sodium [Na^+], plasma urea, plasma osmolality, urine urea, urine specific gravity (USG) and urine osmolality pre- and post-race measurements were determined in a subgroup of twenty-five athletes (16 men and 9 women) to investigate changes in hydration status (Table 3). These procedures were performed at the same time as the anthropometric measurements, before the start and directly after finishing the race. The recording procedure for pre- and post-race measurements was identical. After venipuncture of an antecubital vein, one Sarstedt S-Monovette (plasma gel, 7.5 mL) for chemical and one Sarstedt S-Monovette (EDTA, 2.7 mL) for haematological analysis were cooled and sent to the laboratory and were analysed within six hours. Haematocrit was determined using Sysmex XE 2100 (Sysmex Corporation, Japan), plasma [Na^+] and plasma urea

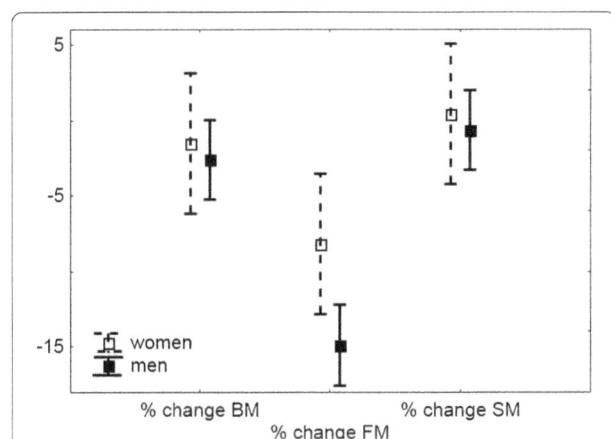

Figure 1 Absolute ranking related to %ΔBM and fluid intake in men (n = 37) and women (n = 12). Absolute ranking – according to the number of achieved kilometers during 24 hours, %ΔBM – percent change in body mass.

Table 3 Haematological and urinary parameters (n = 25)

Parameter	Pre-race M ± SD	Post-race M ± SD	Absolute change	Change (%)
Male ultra-MTBers(n = 16)				
Haematocrit (%)	43.1 ± 3.3	42.6 ± 3.1	−0.5 ± 3.7	−0.7 ± 8.8
Plasma sodium (mmol/L)	138.2 ± 1.4	137.8 ± 2.3	−0.4 ± 2.9**	−0.3 ± 2.1
Plasma urea (mmol/L)	6.1 ± 1.3	13.5 ± 4.1	7.4 ± 3.8**	124.0 ± 67.2
Plasma osmolality (mosmol/kg H_2O)	289.4 ± 4.1	293.6 ± 4.4	4.2 ± 4.5**	1.5 ± 1.6
Urine urea (mmol/L)	239.3 ± 172.1	576.0 ± 78.0	336.7 ± 174.8**	298.0 ± 315.5
Urine osmolality (mosmol/kg H_2O)	415.7 ± 190.3	776.7 ± 133.4	361.0 ± 184.4**	132.0 ± 132.4
Urine specific gravity (g/mL)	1.013 ± 0.002	1.022 ± 0.004	0.009 ± 0.004**	0.8 ± 0.3
Female ultra-MTBers (n = 9)				
Haematocrit (%)	42.0 ± 2.7	40.0 ± 2.8	−2.0 ± 4.1	−4.5 ± 10.0
Plasma sodium (mmol/L)	137.4 ± 2.8	137.1 ± 1.8	−0.3 ± 3.0	−0.2 ± 2.2
Plasma urea (mmol/L)	5.8 ± 1.5	8.7 ± 2.5	2.9 ± 1.2**	46.9 ± 18.5
Plasma osmolality (mosmol/kg H_2O)	292.2 ± 2.8	290.6 ± 4.6	−1.7 ± 4.3	−0.6 ± 1.5
Urine urea (mmol/L)	290.5 ± 204.9	463.0 ± 172.5	172.5 ± 246.5	190.6 ± 292.3
Urine osmolality (mosmol/kg H_2O)	724.3 ± 214.0	716,4 ± 329.1	−7.9 ± 276.5	−1.0 ± 36.6
Urine specific gravity (g/mL)	1.000 ± 0.005	1.001 ± 0.005	0.001 ± 0.005	0.1 ± 0.4

Results are presented as mean ± SD; * = $P < 0.05$, ** = $P < 0.001$.

using a biochemical analyzer Modula SWA, Modul P + ISE (Hitachi High Technologies Corporation, Japan, Roche Diagnostic), and plasma osmolality using Arkray Osmotation (Arkray Factory, Inc., Japan). Samples of urine were collected in one Sarstedt monovette for urine (10 mL) and sent to the laboratory. Urine urea was determined using a biochemical analyzer Modula SWA, Modul P + ISE (Hitachi High Technologies Corporation, Japan, Roche Diagnostic), urine specific gravity using Au Max-4030 (Arkray Factory, Inc., Japan), and urine osmolality using Arkray Osmotation (Arkray Factory, Inc., Japan).

Statistical analysis

Results are presented as mean ± standard deviation (SD). The Shapiro-Wilk test was applied to check for normal distribution of data. Differences between men and women in parameters of pre-race experience and training, the average race speed and the total number of kilometers were evaluated using paired t-test. The correlations of the changes in parameters during the race were evaluated using Pearson product–moment in male group and Spearman correlation analysis to assess uni-variate associations in female group. Paired t-tests in male group and the Wilcoxon signed rank tests in female group were used to check for significant changes in the anthropometric and laboratory parameters before and after the race. The critical value for rejecting the null hypothesis was set at 0.05. The data was evaluated in the program Statistic 7.0 (StatSoft, Tulsa, U.S.A.).

Results

Pre-race experience and training parameters

Pre-race results of 37 male and 12 female 24-hour ultra-MTBers are presented in Table 1. Male ultra-MTBers displayed a significantly higher body stature and body mass compared to female ultra-MTBers. Additionally, mean training cycling intensity, mean training cycling speed and session duration during pre-race training were higher in men compared to women. On the contrary, no significant differences between sexes were noted in the years spent as an active MTBer, in the number of finished ultra-cycling marathons, in the personal best performance in a 24-hour cycling race, in total hours spent cycling in training, in the total duration (hour) and the distance (km) of a cycling training in the three months before the race.

Race performance and changes in body composition

Forty-nine ultra-MTBers (37 men and 12 women) finished the race. Significant differences in the average cycling speed during the race were observed between male (16.7 ± 2.2 km/h) and female (14.2 ± 1.7 km/h) ultra-MTBers ($P < 0.001$). Men achieved a mean distance of 282.9 ± 82.9 km during the 24 hours, whereas women achieved 242.4 ± 69.6 km. Despite the differences in the average speed for each sex, men did not achieve a significantly higher number of kilometers during the 24 hours ($P > 0.05$).

In men, the change in body mass was significantly and negatively related to the achieved number of kilometers during the 24 hours (r = −0.41, $P < 0.05$). Their absolute ranking in the race was significantly and positively related to post-race body mass (r = 0.40, $P < 0.05$), the change in body mass (r = 0.46, $P < 0.001$), the percent change in body mass (r = 0.50, $P = 0.001$) (Figure 1) and the percent change in fat mass (r = 0.44, $P < 0.001$) and significantly and negatively related to fluid intake (r = −0.54, $P < 0.05$) (Figure 1) and percent change in plasma urea (r = −0.53, $P < 0.05$). Men's' absolute ranking in the race was not related to changes in plasma [Na$^+$], or percent changes in urine specific gravity ($P > 0.05$).

Changes in body mass were significantly and negatively related to the number of achieved kilometers during the 24 hours also in women (r = −0.80, $P < 0.001$). Their absolute ranking during the race was significantly and positively related to the change in body mass (r = 0.70, $P < 0.05$), the percent change in body mass (r = 0.77, $P < 0.05$) (Figure 1), and significantly and negatively related to fluid intake (r = −0.73, $P < 0.05$) (Figure 1) during the race. Women' absolute ranking in the race was not related to percent change in fat mass, or percent change in urine specific gravity ($P > 0.05$).

Changes in body composition with regard to anthropometric, urine and blood measurements

The correlation matrix of post-race body mass, change in body mass, percent change in body mass, post-race fat mass, percent change in fat mass, percent change in extracellular fluid and percent change in plasma urea for men is shown in Table 4. The correlation matrix of change in body mass, percent change in body mass and percent change in fat mass for women is presented in Table 5.

In male ultra-MTBers (n = 37) body mass decreased significantly during the race by 2.0 ± 1.6 kg, equal to 2.6 ± 2.1% ($P < 0.001$) (Table 2, also Figure 2). Fat mass decreased significantly by 1.4 ± 1.2 kg ($P < 0.001$), percent body fat decreased significantly by 1.4 ± 1.4% ($P < 0.001$), whereas skeletal muscle mass decreased non-significantly by 0.6 ± 2.7% ($P > 0.05$) (Table 2, also Figure 2). In men, post-race body mass was significantly and positively related to post-race fat mass (r = 0.63, $P < 0.001$). Percent changes in body mass were significantly and positively related to post-race fat mass (r = 0.53, $P < 0.05$) and percent changes in skeletal muscle mass (r = 0.73, $P < 0.001$) (Table 4). The change in body mass was neither related to the change in plasma [Na$^+$], nor to the percent change in urine specific gravity ($P > 0.05$).

For men, the percent changes in haematocrit remained stable, and plasma volume increased non-significantly by 3.5% (14.8%). Plasma [Na$^+$] in male ultra-MTBers decreased significantly ($P < 0.001$) by 0.3% from 138.2 mmol/L pre-race to 137.8 mmol/L post-race (Table 3). Urine specific gravity increased significantly ($P < 0.001$) (Table 3).

Table 4 Correlation matrix of PR BM, ΔBM, %ΔBM, PR FM, %ΔFM, %ΔECF and %Δ plasma urea for men (n = 37)

PR BM	0.20	0.33*	0.63**	0.17	0.35*	-0.10
	ΔBM	0.99**	0.19	0.30	0.88**	-0.44
		%ΔBM	0.53*	0.33*	0.83**	-0.50*
			PR FM	0.45**	0.29	-0.53*
				%ΔFM	-0.05	-0.31
					%ΔEXW	-0.52*
						%ΔPU

PR BM – post-race body mass, ΔBM – change in body mass, %ΔBM – percent change in body mass, PR FM – post-race body mass, %ΔFM – percent change in fat mass, %ΔECF – percent change in extracellular fluid, %Δ plasma urea – percent change in plasma urea. Output file contain both the Pearson's r values and the scatter plot, one star (*) above the Pearson value represents significance level $P < 0.05$, two stars (**) $P < 0.001$.

Table 5 The correlation matrix of ΔBM, %ΔBM and %ΔFM for women (n = 12)

ΔBM		0.99**		0.35

ΔBM – change in body mass, %ΔBM – percent change in body mass, %ΔFM – percent change in fat mass. Output file contain both the Spearman's rank correlation coefficient and the scatter plot, one star (*) above the Spearman value represents significance level $P < 0.05$, two stars (**) $P < 0.01$.

Changes in plasma [Na$^+$] were not related to percent changes in urine specific gravity ($P > 0.05$). Post-race plasma osmolality increased significantly ($P < 0.001$) (Table 3), but was not related to the changes in body mass, plasma [Na$^+$], urine osmolality, or urine urea ($P > 0.05$). Percent changes in urine osmolality were not related to percent changes in urine urea. Percent changes in plasma urea were significantly and positively related to post-race plasma osmolality (r = 0.49, $P < 0.05$), and significantly and negatively to percent changes in body mass (r = −0.50, $P < 0.05$), post-race fat mass (r = −0.53, $P < 0.05$) and percent changes in skeletal mass (r = −0.51, $P < 0.05$) (Table 4). Post-race plasma urea or the changes in plasma urea were not related to percent changes in urine specific gravity ($P > 0.05$).

In females ultra-MTBers (n = 12), body mass decreased by 0.9 ± 1.2 kg, equal to 1.5 ± 1.9% ($P < 0.05$) (Table 2, also Figure 2). Fat mass decreased significantly by 1.2 ± 1.2 kg ($P < 0.001$), percent body fat decreased by 2.7 ± 3.6% ($P < 0.05$) whereas skeletal muscle mass remained stable ($P > 0.05$) (Table 2, also Figure 2). The percent changes in body mass were not related to post-race fat mass ($P > 0.05$), or fluid intake ($P > 0.05$).

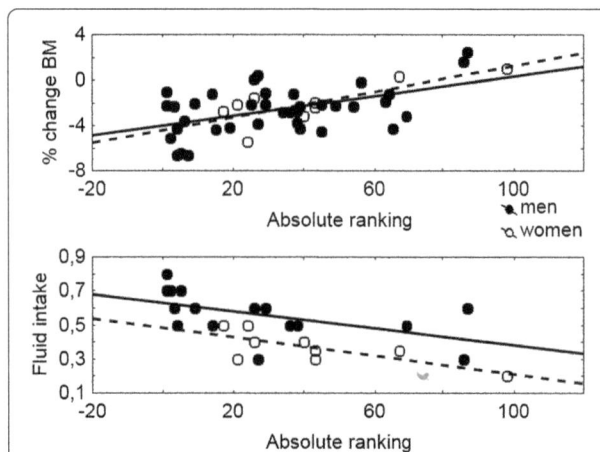

Figure 2 Percentage change of BM, FM, and SM in the 37 men and 12 women during the 24 hour MTB race. BM – body mass, FM – fat mass, SM – skeletal muscle mass.

Percent changes in body mass were significantly and positively related to percent changes in skeletal muscle mass (r = −0.59, $P < 0.05$), however, skeletal muscle mass did not change significantly ($P > 0.05$). The changes in body mass were not related to percent changes in urine specific gravity. The percent change in haematocrit remained stable post-race ($P > 0.05$). Plasma volume increased non-significantly by 5.6% (13.5%) ($P > 0.05$) and was not associated with percent changes in total body water, extracellular fluid or intracellular fluid ($P > 0.05$). Plasma urea increased significantly ($P < 0.001$) (Table 3). The changes in plasma urea were not related to the changes in body mass, fat mass, or in urine specific gravity ($P > 0.05$). Post-race plasma [Na$^+$], plasma and urine osmolality and urine urea remained stable ($P > 0.05$).

Changes in body water, fluid intake, and foot volumes

The correlation matrix of post-race body mass, changes in body mass, percent change in body mass, post-race fat mass, percent change in fat mass, percent change in extracellular fluid and percent change in plasma urea is shown for men in Table 4.

The male group (n = 37) consumed a total of 13.4 L of fluids during the race, equal to 0.6 ± 0.1 L/h. Fluid intake varied between 0.30 L/h and 0.80 L /h. Fluid intake was not related to changes in body mass, fat mass, extracellular fluid, plasma urea or post-race plasma [Na$^+$] ($P > 0.05$). Extracellular fluid decreased by 0.2 ± 0.6 L ($P < 0.05$), whereas total body water and intracellular fluid decreased non-significantly in men ($P > 0.05$) (Table 2). Percent changes in extracellular fluid were significantly and positively related to changes in body mass (r = 0.88, $P < 0.001$), and significantly and negatively to percent changes in plasma urea (r = −0.52, $P < 0.05$). On the contrary, percent changes in extracellular fluid were not associated with percent changes in plasma volume or fluid intake. The volume of the lower leg remained unchanged in men ($P > 0.05$) (Table 2), and was neither related to fluid intake nor to changes in plasma [Na$^+$] ($P > 0.05$). The male 24-hour ultra-MTBers were on average euhydrated post-race (Table 2). Thereof, twenty male ultra-MTBers were euhydrated (54.2%), thirteen were dehydrated (35.1%), and four males were overhydrated (10.7%) following the definition of Noakes et al. [11].

The female group (n = 12) consumed a total of 8.88 L of fluids during the race, equal to 0.37 L/h. Fluid intake varied between 0.20 L/h and 0.50 L/h. Fluid intake was not related to percent changes in body mass, changes in fat mass, or changes in plasma urea ($P > 0.05$). The volume of the lower leg remained unchanged in women ($P > 0.05$) (Table 2), and was neither related to fluid intake nor to changes in plasma [Na$^+$] ($P > 0.05$). The female ultra-MTBers were on average euhydrated (Table 2). Thereof, seven female ultra-MTBers were euhydrated (58.3%), two were dehydrated (16.7%) and three were overhydrated (25.0%) following the definition of Noakes et al. [11].

Discussion

The first important finding of this study was that both male and female 24-hour ultra-MTBers suffered significant losses in body mass and fat mass during the 24-hour MTB race. Skeletal muscle mass showed, however, no significant changes in contrast to fat mass. The second important finding for men was that changes in body mass were related to a decrease in post-race fat mass, and correlated with the changes in extracellular fluid and post-race plasma urea. The third important finding was that the volume of the lower leg remained unchanged in both men and women and was neither related to fluid intake nor to the changes in plasma [Na^+]. And a last finding was that faster men and women drank more than the slower ones and showed higher losses in body mass, in men also higher fat mass losses. However, fluid intake was not correlated to changes in body mass.

Decrease in total body mass

Changes in body mass reached statistical significance ($P < 0.05$) for both male and female 24-hour ultra-MTBers. Compared to women, men's average decrease in body mass was 1.1 percent points (pp) lower. In ultra-endurance settings where athletes race for hours, days, or weeks without a break during the night, a decrease of body mass is a common finding, in which both fat mass and skeletal muscle mass seemed to decrease [2,6,22,24,26].

Changes in fat mass in male and female ultra-MTBers were heterogeneous and did not reach statistical significance ($P > 0.05$). Nevertheless, men's change in fat mass was 6.7 pp lower and was related to a decrease in body mass. A better explanation of the higher changes of body mass and fat mass in men could be the reason that their pre-race values of body mass were higher than in women, men were faster than women and also the substrate utilisation during submaximal exercise in endurance-trained athletes differs between the sexes [23,58], where the contribution of intramyocellular lipids to energy supply during endurance performance could be higher in men compared to women. A decrease in fat mass is expected in an ultra-endurance performance of approximately two days [26]. Studies on ultra-triathletes [59] and ultra-cyclists [36] reported a decrease in fat mass. The 24-hour ultra-MTBers in the present study had to continuously perform for nearly 24 hours, which might explain their great losses in both body mass and fat mass. We assume that adipose subcutaneous tissue was the main energy source for a long-lasting performance such as a 24-hour MTB race and the ability to use body fat as fuel is

important in a such a type of ultra-endurance performance [23,26].

In the present study, skeletal muscle mass showed no statistically significant changes in both male and female ultra-bikers. Skeletal muscle mass decreased in ultra-endurance races without breaks [22,24]. An excessive increase in endurance activities might lead to a reduction in skeletal muscle mass [12,31]. However, a loss in skeletal muscle mass might be dependent upon race intensity and was not reported for all endurance sports [12]. The decrease in skeletal muscle mass has been demonstrated rather in case reports [15,22,24] than in field studies [27,44,60], and a decrease in body mass was mainly due to a decrease in fat mass [22,24,26] than in skeletal muscle mass, such as in the present study.

Furthermore, in a study of an ultra-cycling race over 230 km with 5,500 m of altitude no evidence of exercise-induced skeletal muscle damage was reported [37]. In another study of a 600-km cycling race, again no decrease in skeletal muscle mass was found [36]. Cycling involves predominantly concentric muscle activity which will not lead to skeletal muscle damage, which may explain the lack of skeletal muscle mass loss in cyclists [39,61]. In general, we assume that a 24-hour MTB race may rather lead to a reduction of adipose subcutaneous tissue as has been reported in other studies [23,26], due to the fact that fatty acids of adipose subcutaneous tissue are oxidized in the contracting skeletal muscle [62]. Also low temperatures during night could increase carbohydrate metabolism, especially when shivering [63]. The reduction of glycogen stores along with glycogen-bound water [46,59] would result also in a loss of body mass. It is likely that the present male and female 24-hour ultra-MTBers started the race with full glycogen stores in both skeletal muscles and liver and the stores decreased during the race. We presume that the decrease in body mass could be the result of the metabolic breakdown of fuel, which includes a loss of fat, glycogen and water stored with glycogen. It is possible that the 24-hour race format may lead to a large energy deficit resulting in increased oxidisation of subcutaneous fat stores which coupled a decrease in extracellular fluid would result in the large body mass losses in male ultra-MTBers.

Plasma urea, skeletal muscle damage, and protein catabolism

In male ultra-MTBers, post-race body mass was related to significant losses in post-race fat mass, decreases in extracellular fluid and increases in plasma urea (Table 4). Plasma urea increased in men by 108% (Table 3) and in women by 46.9%. In a 525-km cycling race, plasma urea rose significantly by 97% [37]. In another study investigating body composition and hydration status in one male ultra-endurance swimmer during a 24-hour swim, increases in plasma urea were associated with parameters of skeletal muscle mass damage [16]. We assume for the present male ultra-MTBers that the increase in plasma urea could be associated with skeletal muscle mass damage, because an increased plasma urea was related to changes in skeletal muscle mass in the present subjects. Nevertheless, due to the fact that absolute and percent changes in skeletal muscle mass were non-significantly, we assume that skeletal muscle mass damage was moderate in the present athletes. In contrast to cycling, Fellmann et al. demonstrated that a 24-hour running race caused more muscular lesions than a triathlon, where ultra-cycling was a part of the event [41]. After a Double Iron ultra-triathlon, plasma urea increased significantly [6] and indicated a state of protein catabolism of the organism in the athlete. Faster 24-hour ultra-MTBers in the present study showed increases in plasma urea, therefore a post-race increase in plasma urea may be attributed also to enhanced protein catabolism during ultra-endurance performance as was reported after an ultra-cycling race [39]. We speculate that an increase in plasma urea cannot be solely attributed to skeletal muscle damage and protein catabolism. Increased plasma urea in both sexes suggests an increased metabolic activity [64]. Plasma urea increases also in cases of an impaired renal function [39]. However, there was no association between the change in plasma urea and the change in urine specific gravity in both sexes in the present study.

Race performance, fluid intake, and losses in body mass and fat mass

Despite the differences in the average cycling speed between women and men, men did not achieve a significantly higher number of kilometers during the 24 hours. Women may have on average shorter breaks during their race. Therefore, women were able to achieve a similar amount of kilometers as men. The better performance in the faster male and female ultra-MTBers could be also influenced by numerous reasons like the specific character of 24-hour races or good race tactics [18].

Another interesting finding was that in both male and female ultra-MTBers, faster finishers drank more than the slower ones, similarly as reported for 100-km ultra-marathoners [65]. Faster ultra-MTBers probably could have a higher sweating rate and lost more fluids, however total fluid intake was not related to changes in body mass, only to absolute ranking in the race in both sexes. Faster men and women showed also higher losses in body mass than slower ones, furthermore faster men lost more body fat than slower ones. Zouhal et al. [66] presented an inverse relationship between percent body weight change and finishing times in 643 forty-two-kilometer marathon runners. A decrease in body fat

during an ultra-endurance triathlon was also associated with race intensity in ultra-triathletes [59]. Therefore, we assume that greater decreases in body mass seen here in male and female ultra-MTBers could be attributed to greater race intensity as well as decreases in fat mass in present male ultra-MTBers.

Dehydration or overhydration in ultra-endurance performance?

Another important finding was the fact that foot volume remained stable in both sexes and no oedema of the lower limbs occurred in these ultra-MTBers. Moreover, the volume of the lower leg was neither related to fluid intake nor to changes in plasma [Na^+]. This finding is in contrast with previous studies where an increased fluid intake was related to the formation of peripheral oedema [8,9]. Furthermore, fluid intake in the present study was not associated with changes in body mass, fat mass or plasma urea.

In case of a fluid overload we would expect an increase of solid mass and a decrease in plasma [Na^+]. Fluid homeostasis in both sexes was relatively stable since haematocrit remained unchanged and plasma volume increased non-significantly. An increase in plasma volume in both groups may be due to [Na^+] retention, as a consequence of an increased aldosterone activity [34]. Plasma [Na^+] decreased only in men. Furthermore, the changes in plasma [Na^+] were not related to the changes in plasma osmolality, or urine specific gravity. External factors such as compression socks might have an effect on running performance [67]. A recent study showed that male runners in a stepwise treadmill test improved running performance with the use of compression socks [67]. In the present study, 8 (21%) male 24-hour ultra-MTBers and 2 (17%) female 24-hour ultra-MTBers wore compression socks during the 24-hour race. Changes in total body water were non-significantly in both groups, and there were no differences in foot volume measured by plethysmography, so we did not assume that there was an accumulation of water with a subsequent extra-cellular oedema. On the contrary, during an intense performance in a hot environment, dehydration may occur [2], which may lead to a decrease in body mass [2,31], an increase in urine specific gravity [31], an increase in plasma and urine osmolality, and a decrease in total body water [43].

The present 24-hour ultra-MTBers appeared to have been relatively dehydrated since body mass decreased, however, as per definition of Noakes et al. [11] they were euhydrated. Urine specific gravity significantly increased in men where post-race urine specific gravity was 1.022 mg/L. Urine specific gravity > 1.020 mg/L is indicating significant dehydration according to Kavouras [43]. Urine specific gravity trended toward significance (1.020 mg/L) in women; they were minimally dehydrated according to Kavouras [43].

Urine specific gravity is considered as a reliable marker of hydration status [31,43], however, the change in urine specific gravity was very small and both pre- and post-race measurements were within the normal range limits [68] in both sexes. Moreover, the increase in urine specific gravity was not related to changes in body mass.

In both male and female ultra-MTBers, plasma osmolality did not reach post-race threshold value of 301 ± 5 mmol/kg, which is suggested [69] as a starting point for the estimation of the probability of dehydration. There was no association between percent changes in plasma osmolality and percent changes in plasma [Na^+]; however, male finishers with an increased plasma osmolality had also increased plasma urea levels. The increase in plasma urea might lead to a change in plasma osmolality which might be a trigger for an increased activity of vasopressin [70]. Catabolic products of protein metabolism associated with a physical strain [3] could be also related to an increased urine osmolality, so it limits its potential utility for the assessment of dehydration. Similar limitations apply for urine specific gravity, and fluctuations in the volume of body fluid compartments will also affect plasma osmolality [3].

Prolonged exercise in the heat may cause increased losses of total body water by sweating and respiration [71]. However, total body water was stable in both sexes although extracellular fluid decreased significantly in men. The decrease in extracellular fluid in men was significantly and positively related to the change in body mass and significantly and negatively to the change in plasma urea. On the contrary, the change in extracellular fluid was not correlated to fluid intake or change in plasma volume. We assume that the present ultra-MTBers drank *ad libitum* and their average fluid intake was in line with the recommendation of the International Marathon Medical Directors Association (IMMDA) [72]. In the male ultra-MTBers, the decrease of extracellular fluid could be due to the race intensity accompanied by the reduction of the glycogen stores rather than due to dehydration. Ultra-MTBers in both sexes were not dehydrated, but they suffered a significant loss in solid masses.

Limitations
The limitation was the relatively small number of female ultra-endurance ultra-MTBers. Probably a high energy deficit occurred during 24-hour races and we did not determine energy intake, in future studies it should be recorded.

Practical applications for coaches and ultra-MTBers
Ultra-MTBers in both genders respond individualistically, although they had an equal access to fluid. These data support the finding that change in body mass during exercise may not reflect exact changes in hydration status, and higher losses of body mass did not impair race performance.

Conclusions
To summarize, completing a 24-hour MTB race led to a significant decrease in total body mass and fat mass whereas skeletal muscle mass remained stable in both male and female competitors. The volume of the lower leg remained unchanged both in men and women. Body weight changes and increased plasma urea in both sexes under testing conditions do not reflect a change in body hydration, but rather represent a balance of both fluid and energy losses from both external and internal sources.

Consent
Written informed consent was obtained from all testing subjects for the publication of this report and any accompanying images.

Competing interests
The authors declare that they have no competing interests.

Authors' contributions
DCH, BK and TR developed the objectives of the study and intervention, DCH managed recruitment and data collection, TR supported a laboratory processing of samples, DCH and AZ participated in the practical measurement in all field studies, DCH and IT[4] performed statistical analysis, DCH, BK and IT[4] lead the drafting of the manuscript, interpreted the findings and critically reviewed the manuscript. MS helped with translation and the extensively correction of the whole text. All authors read and approved the final manuscript.

Acknowledgements
The authors gratefully acknowledge the athletes for their splendid cooperation without which this study could not have been done. We thank the organizers and the medical crew of the 'Czech Championship 24-hour MTB race' in Jihlava and the 'Bike Race Marathon Rohozec' in Liberec for their generous support. A special thank goes to the laboratory staff of the University Hospital 'U Svaté Anny' in Brno, Czech Republic, for their efforts in analyzing haematological and biochemical samples even during the night-times.

Author details
[1]Centre of Sports Activities, Brno University of Technology, Brno, Czech Republic. [2]Institute of General Practise and for Health Services Research, University of Zurich, Zurich, Switzerland. [3]Institute of Experimental Biology, Faculty of Science, Masaryk University, Brno, Czech Republic. [4]Faculty of Forestry and Wood Sciences, Czech University of Life Sciences, Prague, Czech Republic. [5]Institute of Technology Tallaght, Dublin, Ireland. [6]SurGal clinic s.r.o., Center for Sports Medicine, Brno, Czech Republic.

References
1. Zaryski C, Smith DJ: **Training principles and issues for ultra-endurance athletes.** *Curr Sports Med Rep* 2005, **4:**165–170.
2. Kao WF, Shyu CL, Yang XW, Hsu TF, Chen JJ, Kao WC, Polun C, Huang YJ, Kuo FC, Huang CI, Lee CH: **Athletic performance and serial weight changes during 12- and 24-hour ultra-marathons.** *Clin J Sport Med* 2008, **18**(2):155–158.
3. Cheuvront SN, Kenefick RW, Charkoudian N, Sawka MN: **Physiologic basis for understanding quantitative dehydration.** *Am J Clin Nutr* 2013, **97:**455–462.
4. American College of Sports Medicine, Sawka MN, Burke LM, Eichner ER, Maughan RJ, Montain SJ, Stachenfeld NS: **American College of Sports Medicine position stand. Exercise and fluid replacement.** *Med Sci Sports Exerc* 2007, **39**(2):377–390.

5.   Linderman J, Demchak T, Dallas J, Buckworth J: **Ultra-endurance cycling: a field study of human performance during a 12-hour mountain bike race.** *JEP Online* 2003, **6**(3):14–23.

6.   Lehmann M, Huonker M, Dimeo F, Heinz N, Gastmann U, Treis N, Steinacker JM, Keul J, Kajewski R, Häussinger D: **Serum amino acid concentrations in nine athletes before and after the 1993 Colmar ultra triathlon.** *Int J Sports Med* 1995, **16**(3):155–159.

7.   Stuempfle KJ, Lehmann DR, Case HS, Hughes SL, Evans D: **Change in serum sodium concentration during a cold weather ultradistance race.** *Clin J Sport Med* 2003, **13**(3):171–175.

8.   Cejka C, Knechtle B, Knechtle P, Rüst CA, Rosemann T: **An increased fluid intake leads to feet swelling in 100-km ultra-marathoners – an observational field study.** *J Int Soc Sports Nutr* 2012, **9**(11):1–10.

9.   Bracher A, Knechtle B, Gnädinger M, Bürge J, Rüst CA, Knechtle P, Rosemann T: **Fluid intake and changes in limb volumes in male ultra-marathoners: does fluid overload lead to peripheral oedema?** *Eur J Appl Physiol* 2011, **112**(3):991–1003.

10. Knechtle B, Vinzent T, Kirby S, Knechtle P, Rosemann T: **The recovery phase following a Triple Iron triathlon.** *J Hum Kinet* 2009, **21**(1):65–74.

11. Noakes TD, Sharwood K, Speedy D, Hew T, Reid S, Dugas J, Almond C, Wharam P, Weschler L: **Three independent biological mechanisms cause exercise-associated hyponatremia:evidence from 2, 135 weighed competitive athletic performances.** *Proc Natl Acad Sci U S A* 2005, **102**(51):18550–18555.

12. Weitkunat T, Knechtle B, Knechtle P, Rüst CA, Rosemann T: **Body composition and hydration status changes in male and female open-water swimmers during an ultra-endurance event.** *J Sports Sci* 2012, **30**(10):1003–1013.

13. Hew-Butler T, Almond C, Ayus JC, Dugas J, Meeuwisse W, Noakes T, Reid S, Siegel A, Speedy D, Stuempfle K, Verbalis J, Weschler L: **Exercise-associated hyponatremia (EAH) consensus panel. Consensus statement of the 1st International Exercise-Associated Hyponatremia Consensus Development Conference, Cape Town, South Africa 2005.** *Clin J Sport Med* 2005, **15**(4):208–213.

14. Speedy DB, Noakes TD, Rogers IR, Thompson JM, Campbell RG, Kuttner JA, Boswell DR, Wright S, Hamlin M: **Hyponatremia in ultradistance triathletes.** *Med Sci Sports Exerc* 1999, **31**:809–815.

15. Knechtle B, Knechtle P, Schück R, Andonie JL, Kohler G: **Effects of a Deca Iron Triathlon on body composition – A case study.** *Int J Sports Med* 2008, **29**(4):343–351.

16. Knechtle B, Wirth A, Knechtle P, Rosemann T, Senn O: **Do ultra-runners in a 24-h run really dehydrate?** *Irish J Med Sci* 2011, **180**(1):129–134.

17. Knechtle B, Duff B, Schulze I, Kohler G: **A multi-stage ultra-endurance run over 1,200 km leads to a continuous accumulation of total body water.** *J Sports Sci Med* 2008, **7**:357–364.

18. Chlíbková D, Tomášková I: **A Field Study of Human Performance During a 24hour Mountain Bike Race.** In *8th International Conference Sport & Quality of Life 2011. Book of Abstracts.* Edited by Zvonař M, Sebera M; 2011:25.

19. Chlíbková D, Žákovská A, Tomášková I: **Predictor variables for 7-day race in ultra-marathoners.** *Procedia Soc Behav Sci* 2012, **46**:2362–2366.

20. Knechtle B, Knechtle P, Müller G, Zwyssig D: **Energieumsatz an einem 24 Stunden Radrennen: Verhalten von Körpergewicht und Subkutanfett.** *Österr J Sportsmed* 2003, **33**(4):11–18.

21. Bescós R, Dodríguez FA, Iglesias X, Benítez A, Marina M, Padullés JM, Torrado P, Vazquez J, Knechtle B: **High energy deficit in an ultraendurance athlete in a 24-hour ultracycling race.** *Proc (Bayl Univ Med Cent)* 2012, **25**(2):124–128.

22. Knechtle B, Enggist A, Jehle T: **Energy turnover at the Race Across America (RAAM)-A case report.** *Int J Sports Med* 2005, **26**:499–503.

23. Raschka C, Plath M: **Body fat compartment and its relationship to food intake and clinical chemical parameters during extreme endurance performance.** *Schweiz Z Sportmed* 1992, **40**(1):13–25.

24. Bircher S, Enggist A, Jehle T, Knechtle B: **Effects of an extreme endurance race on energy balance and body composition - a case study.** *J Sports Sci Med* 2006, **5**:154–162.

25. Rose SP, Futre EM: **Ad libitum adjustements to fluid intake in cool environmental conditions maintain hydration status in a three-day mountain bike race.** *Br J Sports Med* 2010, **44**:430–436.

26. Helge JW, Lundy C, Christensen DL, Langfort J, Messonnier L, Zacho M, Andersen JL, Saltin B: **Skiing across the Greenland icecap: divergent effect on limb muscle adaptations and substrate oxidation.** *J Exp Biol* 2003, **206**:1075–1083.

27. Knechte B, Knechtle P, Rüst CA, Rosemann T: **Leg skinfold thicknesses and race performance in male 24-hour ultra-marathoners.** *Proc (Bayl Univ Med Cent)* 2011, **24**(2):110–114.

28. Knechtle B, Knechtle P, Rosemann T: **No exercise-associated hyponatremia found in an observational field study of male ultra-marathoners participating in a 24-hour ultra-run.** *Phys Sportsmed* 2010, **38**(4):94–100.

29. Knechtle B, Knechtle P, Rosemann T: **No association of skin-fold thicknesses and training with race performance in male ultraendurance runners in a 24-hour run.** *J Hum Sports Exerc* 2011, **6**(1):94–100.

30. Knechtle P, Rosemann T, Senn O: **No dehydration in mountain bike ultra-marathoners.** *Clin J Sport Med* 2009, **19**(5):415–420.

31. Knechtle B, Knechtle P, Kohler G, Rosemann T: **Does a 24-hour ultra-swim lead to dehydration?** *J Hum Sports Exerc* 2011, **6**(1):68–79.

32. Meyer M, Knechtle B, Bürge J, Knechtle P, Mrazek C, Wirth A, Ellenrieder B, Rüst CA, Rosemann T: **Ad libitum fluid intake leads to no leg swelling in male Ironman triathletes – an observational field study.** *J Int Soc Sports Nutr* 2012, **9**(1):1–13.

33. Knechtle B, Gnädinger M, Knechtle P, Imoberdorf R, Kohler G, Ballmer P, Rosemann T, Senn O: **Prevalence of exercise-associated hyponatremia in male ultraendurance athletes.** *Clin J Sport Med* 2011, **21**(3):226–232.

34. Knechtle B, Knechtle P, Roseman T: **No case of exercise-associated hyponatraemia in male ultra-endurance mountain bikers in the 'Swiss Bike Masters'.** *Chin J Physiol* 2011, **54**(6):379–384.

35. Rüst CA, Knechtle B, Knechtle P, Rosemann T: **No case of exercise-associated hyponatraemia in top male ultra-endurance cyclists: the 'Swiss Cycling Marathon'.** *Eur J Appl Physiol* 2012, **112**(2):689–697.

36. Knechtle B, Wirth A, Knechtle P, Rosemann T: **An ultra-cycling race leads to no decrease in skeletal muscle mass.** *Int J Sports Med* 2009, **30**(3):163–167.

37. Neumayr G, Pfister R, Hoertnagl H, Mitterbauer G, Prokop W, Joannidis M: **Renal function and plasma volume following ultramarathon cycling.** *Int J Sports Med* 2005, **26**(1/02):2–8.

38. Schenk K, Gatterer H, Ferrari M, Ferrari P, Cascio VL, Burtscher M: **Bike Transalp 2008: liquid intake and its effect on the body's fluid homeostasis in the course of a multistage, crosscountry, MTB marathon race in the central Alps.** *Clin J Sport Med* 2010, **20**(1):47–52.

39. Knechtle B, Knechtle P, Kohler G: **The effects of 1,000 km nonstop cycling on fat mass and skeletal muscle mass.** *Res Sports Med* 2011, **19**(3):170–185.

40. Bischof M, Knechtle B, Rüst CA, Knechtle P, Rosemann T: **Changes in skinfold thicknesses and body fat in ultra-endurance cyclists.** *Asian J Sports Med* 2013, **4**(1):15–22.

41. Fellmann N, Sagnol M, Bedu M, Falgairette G, Van Praagh E, Gaillard G, Jouanel P, Coudert J: **Enzymatic and hormonal responses following a 24 h endurance run and a 10 h triathlon race.** *Eur J Appl Physiol* 1988, **57**:545–553.

42. Knechtle B, Kohler G: **Running 338 kilometres within five days has no effect on body mass and body fat but reduces skeletal muscle mass – the Isarrun 2006.** *J Sports Sci Med* 2007, **6**:401–407.

43. Kavouras SA: **Assessing hydration status.** *Curr Opin Clin Nutr Metab Care* 2002, **5**(5):519–524.

44. Hew-Butler T, Jordaan E, Stuempfle KJ, Speedy DB, Siegel AJ, Noakes TD, Soldin SJ, Verbalis JG: **Osmotic and nonosmotic regulativ of arginine vasopressin during prolonged endurance exercise.** *J Clin Endocrinol Metab* 2008, **93**(6):2072–2078.

45. Skenderi KP, Kavouras SA, Anastasiou CA, Yiannakouris N, Matalas AL: **Exertional rhabdomyolysis during a 246-km continuous running race.** *Med Sci Sports Exerc* 2006, **38**(6):1054–1057.

46. Knechtle B, Wirth A, Knechtle P, Rosemann T: **Increase of total body water with decrease of body mass while running 100 km nonstop – formation of edema?** *Res Q Exerc Sport* 2009, **80**(3):593–603.

47. Knechtle B, Senn O, Imoberdorf R, Joleska I, Wirth A, Knechtle P, Rosemann T: **Maintained total body water content and serum sodium concentrations despite body mass loss in female ultra-runners drinking ad libitum during a 100 km race.** *Asia Pac J Clin Nutr* 2010, **19**(1):83–90.

48. Frisch RE, Hall GM, Aoki TT, Birnholz J, Jacob R, Landsberg L, Munro H, Parker-Jones K, Tulchinsky D, Young J: **Metabolic, endocrine, and reproductive changes of woman channel swimmer.** *Metabolism* 1984, **33**:1106–1111.

49. Mertens DJ, Rhind S, Berkhoff F, Dugmore D, Shek PN, Shephard RJ: **Nutritional, immunologic and psychological responses to a 7250 km run.** *J Sports Med Phys Fitness* 1996, **36**:132–138.

50. Clark N, Tobin J, Ellis C: Feeding the ultraendurance athlete:practical tips and a case study. *J Am Diet Assoc* 1992, **92**:1258–1262.

51. Knechtle B, Duff B, Schulze I, Kohler G: The effects of running 1,200 km within 17 days on body composition in a female ultrarunner – Deutschlandlauf 2007. *Res Sports Med* 2008, **16**:167–188.

52. Knechtle B, Salas Fraire O, Andonie JL, Kohler G: Effect of a multistage ultra-endurance triathlon on body composition: World Challenge Deca Iron Triathlon 2006. *Br J Sports Med* 2008, **2**:121–125.

53. Lee RC, Wang Z, Heo M, Ross R, Janssen I, Heymsfield SB: Total-body skeletal muscle mass: development and cross-validation of anthropometric prediction models. *Am J Clin Nutr* 2000, **72**(3):796–803.

54. Stewart AD, Hannan WJ: Prediction of fat and fat-free mass in male athletes using dual X-ray absorptiometry as the reference method. *J Sports Sci* 2000, **18**(4):263–274.

55. Warner ER, Fornetti WC, Jallo JJ, Pivarnik JM: A skinfold model to predict fat-free mass in female athletes. *J Athl Train* 2004, **39**(3):259–262.

56. Ball SD, Altena TS, Stan PD: Comparison of anthropometry to DXA: a new prediction equation for men. *Eur J Clin Nutr* 2004, **58**:1525–1531.

57. Ball SD, Stan P, Desimone R: Accuracy of anthropometry compared to dual energy X-ray absorptiometry. A new generalizable equation for women. *Res Q Exerc Sport* 2004, **75**(3):248–258.

58. Zehnder M, Ith M, Kreis R, Saris W, Boutellier U, Boesch D: Gender-specific usage of intramyocellular lipids and glycogen during exercise. *Med Sci Sports Exer* 2005, **37**(9):1517–1524.

59. Knechtle B, Schwanke M, Knechtle P, Kohler G: Decrease in body fat during an ultra-endurance triathlon is associated with race intensity. *Br J Sports Med* 2008, **42**:609–613.

60. Mueller SM, Anliker E, Knechtle P, Knechtle B, Toigo M: Changes in body composition in triathletes during an Ironman race. *Eur J Appl Physiol* 2013, **113**:2343–2352.

61. Vissing K, Overgaard K, Nedergaard A, Fredsted A, Schjerling P: Effects of concentric and repeated eccentric exercise on muscle damage and calpain-calpastatin gene expression in human skeletal muscle. *Eur J Appl Physiol* 2008, **103**:323–332.

62. Romijn JA, Coyle EF, Sidossis LS, Gastaldelli A, Horowitz JF, Endert E, Wolfe RR: Regulation of endogenous fat and carbohydrate metabolism in relation to exercise intensity and duration. *Am J Physiol* 1993, **265**:E380–E391.

63. Jeukendrup AE: Modulation of carbohydrate and fat utilization by diet, exercise and environment. *Biochem Soc Trans* 2003, **31**(6):1270–1273.

64. Riley WJ, Pyke FS, Roberts AD, England JF: The effects of long-distance running on some biochemical variables. *Clin Chim Acta* 1975, **65**:83–89.

65. Knechtle B, Knechtle P, Wirth A, Rüst CA, Rosemann T: A faster running speed is associated with a greater body weight loss in 100-km ultra-marathoners. *J Sports Sci* 2012, **30**(11):1131–1140.

66. Zouhal H, Groussard C, Minter G, Vincent S, Cretual A, Gratas-Delamarche A, Delamarche P, Noakes TD: Inverse relationship between percentage body weight change and finishing time in 643 forty-two kilometer marathon runners. *Br J Sports Med* 2011, **45**(14):1101–1105.

67. Kemmler W, von Stengel S, Köckritz C, Mayhew J, Wassermann A, Zapf J: Effects of compression stockings on running performance in men runners. *J Strength Cond Res* 2009, **23**:101–103.

68. Kratz A, Lewandrowski KB: Normal reference laboratory values. *N Engl J Med* 1998, **339**:1063–1072.

69. Cheuvront SN, Ely BR, Kenefick RW, Sawka MN: Biological variation and diagnostic accuracy of dehydration assessment markers. *Am J Clin Nutr* 2010, **92**:565–573.

70. Bürge J, Knechtle B, Knechtle P, Gnädinger M, Rüst CA, Rosemann T: Maintained serum sodium in male ultra-marathoners – the role of fluid intake, vasopressin, and aldosterone in fluid and electrolyte regulation. *Horm Metab Res* 2011, **43**(9):646–652.

71. Greenleaf JE, Convertino VA, Mangseth GR: Plasma volume during stress in man: Osmolality and red cell volume. *J Appl Physiol* 1979, **47**:1031–1038.

72. Hew-Butler T, Verbalis JG, Noakes TD: Updated fluid recommendation: position statement from The International Marathon Medical Directors Association (IMMDA). *Clin J Sport Med* 2006, **16**(4):283–292.

The effects of a multi-ingredient dietary supplement on body composition, adipokines, blood lipids, and metabolic health in overweight and obese men and women: a randomized controlled trial

Michael J Ormsbee[1,2,3]*, Shweta R Rawal[1], Daniel A Baur[1], Amber W Kinsey[1], Marcus L Elam[1], Maria T Spicer[1], Nicholas T Fischer[1], Takudzwa A Madzima[1] and D David Thomas[1]

Abstract

Background: The present study investigated the effects of a multi-ingredient dietary supplement (MIDS) containing caffeine, conjugated linoleic acid (CLA), green tea, and branched-chain amino acids (BCAA) taken for 8 weeks on body composition, blood lipid profile, glucose, insulin, adiponectin, leptin, and high-sensitivity C-reactive protein (hs-CRP) in overweight and obese men and women.

Methods: Twenty-two participants completed the study (PL, n = 11; 7 women, 4 men; age, 34 ± 3.5 years; height, 169.2 ± 3.3 cm; body mass, 96.9 ± 6.8 kg; BMI, 34.1 ± 1.8 kg/m^2; MIDS, n = 11; 9 women, 2 men; age, 36 ± 3.4 years; height, 173.2 ± 2.9 cm; body mass, 91.9 ± 5.6 kg; BMI, 30.0 ± 1.5 kg/m^2). Participants were randomly assigned and stratified by body fat percentage to two groups: 1) a soybean oil placebo (PL) or 2) MIDS. Each group consumed two pills with breakfast and two pills with lunch. Body composition and android fat, waist and hip circumferences, blood pressure and heart rate were measured at baseline and after 8 weeks of supplementation.

Results: There were no significant changes for any of the variables of body composition. Feelings of hunger were significantly higher in MIDS versus PL with no changes observed in satiety or desire to eat. Heart rate and blood pressure were unaltered in MIDS after 8 weeks of supplementation. Furthermore, lipid profile, food intake, mood state variables, fasting blood glucose, and endocrine markers did not significantly change regardless of group.

Conclusion: MIDS intake does not appear to alter body composition or markers of cardiovascular health versus PL. Moreover, MIDS may actually increase feelings of hunger versus PL.

Keywords: Green tea, Caffeine, Conjugated linoleic acid, Branched chain amino acids, Body composition, Obesity

Background

Obesity is a growing trend in the United States with current estimates suggesting prevalence as high as 35% among adults [1]. These high rates potentiate a severe health crisis as obesity increases the likelihood of developing chronic diseases which include hypertension, insulin resistance, type 2 diabetes mellitus (T2DM), arteriosclerosis, coronary heart disease, and metabolic syndrome [2]. Therefore, finding safe and effective methods for reducing body weight in obese individuals is essential.

Reducing body weight requires manipulation of the energy balance equation to produce energy deficits. This can be accomplished through diet and exercise, pharmacological interventions, or surgical means. However, each of these methods comes with disadvantages. For instance, many diet and exercise lifestyle interventions suffer from a lack of long-term (≥1 yr) adherence [3]. Furthermore,

* Correspondence: mormsbee@fsu.edu
[1]Department of Nutrition, Food and Exercise Sciences, Florida State University, Tallahassee, FL 32306, USA
[2]University of KwaZulu-Natal, Durban, South Africa
Full list of author information is available at the end of the article

pharmacological and/or surgical means to reduce body weight are typically expensive and are sometimes accompanied by potentially unpleasant and/or dangerous side effects [4,5]. As such, consideration of alternative weight loss methods is warranted.

The consumption of natural ingredients and/or dietary supplements may provide a safe and effective means to induce weight loss and improve overall health. Indeed, recent evidence suggests that consumption of certain multi-ingredient dietary supplements may improve body composition and mood state [6,7]. The supplements utilized in these studies contained unique proprietary blends containing such ingredients as caffeine and green tea extract. These ingredients have been studied extensively and are now recognized as potential modulators of body weight, composition, adipokines, and metabolic health [8,9]. Beneficial effects of consuming green tea or caffeine, respectively, are likely a result of inhibited degradation of catecholamines (epinephrine and norepinephrine) or cyclic amino monophospates (cAMP) thereby enhancing thermogenesis and promoting lipolysis [10,11]. Of interest, the lipolytic effects reported with green tea and caffeine consumption may be the result of a synergistic effect as noted in a recent meta-analysis [12].

Supplementation with conjugated-linoleic acid (CLA) and branched-chain amino acids (BCAA) may also provide weight loss benefits [13,14]. These CLA-derived effects may be a result of enhanced β-oxidation via stimulation of enzymes responsible for transport of lipids into the mitochondria (i.e. carnitine palmitoyl transferase [CPT1]) [15], or through inhibition of adipocyte differentiation [16]. BCAA may improve body composition by enhancing protein synthesis, which maintains or increases lean mass [17]. While the efficacy of these ingredients has been extensively studied individually, there is a lack of research on the impact of combining these ingredients on body weight, composition and other markers of health. Furthermore, combining CLA and BCAA with green tea extracts and caffeine has also yet to be studied.

Therefore, the purpose of the present study was to examine the effects of a multi-ingredient dietary supplement (MIDS) containing a proprietary blend of green tea extracts, caffeine, CLA, and BCAA on body composition, blood lipid profile, glucose, insulin, adiponectin, leptin, and high-sensitivity C-reactive protein (hs-CRP) concentrations in overweight and obese men and women.

Methods

Participants
Thirty-four inactive (<2 times/week of planned physical activity for no more than 60 minutes per session) overweight or obese (BMI of 25 to 47 kg/m^2) but otherwise healthy men and women, ages 18–50 years old were recruited from Tallahassee, Florida and surrounding areas.

Prior to participation, each participant provided a written consent and completed a brief questionnaire regarding his or her medical and exercise training history. Participants were excluded if they were physically active (>2 times/week of planned physical activity for > 60 minutes), if they had uncontrolled hypertension (BP >140/90 mmHg), if they had high low-density lipoprotein cholesterol (LDL >160 mg/dL) or if they took cholesterol medication. In addition, those diagnosed with cardiovascular disease, stroke, diabetes, thyroid or kidney dysfunction, and smokers (>5 cigarettes per week) were excluded. Those who consumed any dietary supplements intended to alter body composition and body weight were excluded. In addition, those who had any allergies to soy, wheat, and grain products that would cause a health problem were excluded. This study was approved by Florida State University Institutional Review Board.

Study design
This was a randomized, double-blinded, placebo-controlled study with two treatment groups. The participants were stratified based on body fat percentage and assigned to a placebo group (PL; soybean oil) or an isocaloric multi-ingredient dietary supplement group (MIDS; Suarez Corporation Industries, Canton, Ohio; 10 calories; 1 g fat, 99 mg caffeine, 1510 mg of a proprietary blend of: green tea, CLA, and BCAA per 2-pill serving [2 servings = 4 pills/day]). The green tea was standardized for 45% epigallocatechin gallate and 90% polyphenols. Both groups ingested 2 identical pills with both breakfast and lunch 7 days per week for 8 weeks.

All laboratory procedures were conducted following an 8 – 10 h overnight fast and a 24 h abstinence from caffeine, alcohol intake and any intense physical activity. Additionally, participants abstained from consuming their assigned treatment on testing days. Every visit was completed between 7 am and 10 am.

Anthropometrics
Height and body mass were measured using a wall-mounted stadiometer and a digital scale (SECA, Birmingham, UK) every 2 weeks under identical conditions (shorts, t-shirt) for each subject. Waist and hip circumferences were obtained at baseline and after 8 weeks using a standard tape measure (with strain gauge) at the maximum area around the waist line and around the largest component of the gluteus maximus. All circumference measurements were conducted by the same researcher.

Total and regional body composition was determined by dual energy X-ray absorptiometry (iDXA; GE Lunar, Madison, WI) with participants in the supine position. Total body adiposity was expressed as percent body fat (% BF). Abdominal adiposity was determined by creating regions of interest (ROI) for the abdomen (region 1) using the ROI option within the manual analysis menu of the iDXA software and included the area just below the last rib to just above the iliac crest, as described previously [18]. Abdominal adiposity was expressed as percent android fat (% android fat). A certified radiologist technician performed all iDXA analyses.

Waist circumferences were measured at the maximum circumference around the umbilical point. Although this is not the standard measurement method for waist circumference, the abdominal obesity of many of the participants prevented the use of standard waist measurement techniques (i.e. 1–2 cm below the last rib typically corresponding with the narrowest part of the waist). Measurements were taken by the same researcher to minimize errors.

Heart rate and blood pressure

Resting heart rate and blood pressure were measured at 0, 2, 4, 6, and 8 weeks. The participants were instructed to rest in a seated position, with both feet flat on the floor for 5 minutes before measurements were taken. Resting blood pressures were obtained by the same investigator on the same arm using an appropriately sized cuff and a sphygmomanometer (American Diagnostic Corp., Hauppauge, NY). Resting heart rate was obtained from a radial pulse. Two readings were taken for blood pressures and resting heart rate with 1 min intervals between each reading. The mean of the two readings were used for statistical analysis.

Questionnaires: dietary intake, physical activity, hunger, and mood-state

Two-day diet logs were completed at weeks 0, 4, and 8 to quantify calorie and macronutrient intake. The participants were asked to maintain their food intake throughout the duration of the study. The Food Processor software (version 10.9 ESHA Research Salem, OR, USA) was used to analyze the food logs.

Participants were asked to not change their physical activity during intervention period. Physical activity logs completed by each participant were collected at weeks 0, 4 and 8. Adverse events forms were collected and recorded at weeks 2, 4, 6 and 8 by research staff.

Mood state was accessed via the completion of a 65-question mood state questionnaire which assessed mood state at weeks 0, 4 and 8. This was a simple likert scale (0, very – 4, not at all) questionnaire. Hunger was assessed at the same time points using a simple visual analog scale (VAS) (1 to 100 mm). Participants were instructed to place a mark on the 100 mm line to indicate their levels of hunger, satiety, and desire to eat. A mark at 0 indicated a complete lack of hunger, satiety, or desire to eat and a mark at 100 indicated extreme hunger, satiety, or desire to eat for each VAS, respectively. For each of the three measures (hunger, satiety, and desire to eat), the degree in which each sensation was felt was quantified by measuring

how far the mark was from the 0 mm mark. For this measurement, a standard millimeter ruler was used and all scores were computed by the same investigator. VAS scales were completed at baseline (week 0) and post-intervention (week 8) in a fasted state.

Hormones, blood lipids and blood glucose

A venous blood sample (20 ml) was obtained from the antecubital vein at baseline and after 8 weeks of supplementation (post). Whole blood was used to measure total cholesterol (TC), high-density lipoprotein cholesterol (HDL-C), low density lipoprotein cholesterol (LDL-C), triglycerides (TRG), and glucose concentrations using the Cholestech LDX blood analysis system (Hayward, CA). Inter-assay coefficients of variation were 2.1%, 4.0%, 4.1%, 4.7%, and 2.3% for TC, HDL, LDL, TRG, and glucose, respectively. Remaining samples were centrifuged (IEC CL3R Multispeed Centrifuge, ThermoElectron Corporation, Needham Heights, MA) for 15 minutes at 3500 rpm at 4°C. Serum aliquots of 300 μL were transferred into microtubes and stored at –80°C for later analysis of insulin, leptin, adiponectin, and hs-CRP. All assays were performed in duplicate in a single assay using commercially available ELISA kits according to the manufacturer's instructions (leptin and adiponectin: R&D Systems Inc., Minneapolis, MN, USA; hs-CRP and insulin: IBL International, Inc., Hamburg, Germany). The mean of duplicate samples were used for statistical analysis. Inter-assay coefficients of variation were 1.3%, 6.2%, and 5.2% for leptin, adiponectin, and hs-CRP, respectively. Inter-assay data were missing for insulin due to technical errors. Intra-assay coefficients of variation were 5.6%, 13.8%, 3.8%, and 8.1% for insulin, leptin, adiponectin, and hs-CRP respectively. Insulin resistance was assessed using the homeostatic model of assessment, as described previously [19].

Compliance

Compliance was checked by asking participants to bring supplement containers every 4 weeks. Weekly calls or emails were sent to remind participants to take the supplement and maintain their food and physical activity logs for the duration of the study.

Statistical analysis

An *a priori* power analysis was performed which revealed a need for a minimum of 6 participants per group to achieve a power of 0.80, $\alpha = 0.05$, standard deviation = 1.1, difference = 6 (41). One way analysis of variance (ANOVA) was performed to examine possible group differences at baseline. Data were analyzed using a 2X5 repeated measures ANOVA ([PL × MIDS]) × ([week 0 × week 2 × week 4 × week 6 × week 8]). Data were analyzed using JMP PRO 9 software (Cary, NC). If significant main effects were identified by ANOVA, a Tukey post hoc comparison test was performed to locate differences.

Results

Participant demographics

A total of 160 individuals were pre-screened for participation in this study. Of the 68 individuals eligible for the study, 34 decided to participate. Out of these 34 participants, 5 participants withdrew from the study due to personal reasons. A total of 29 participants completed the study, however, data from 7 participants was excluded due to low compliance (<80% of total supplement intake). Therefore, 22 participants with 11 in each group were included in the statistical analysis. Aside from fat mass (p<0.05), there were no statistical differences between groups at baseline (Table 1).

Body composition

Body composition and anthropometric data is presented in Figure 1 and Table 2. There were no main time or group × time interactions observed for the following variables: body mass, body mass index, percent body fat, % android fat, percent gynoid fat, fat mass, fat free mass, waist and hip circumference, and waist to hip ratio. However, a significant time effect was observed for BMI (+1.2 and +1.0%) and FM (+1.7 and +1.9%) for PL and MIDS, respectively (Table 2). Additionally, post hoc analyses revealed no differences between genders.

Lipid profile, heart rate, and blood pressure

The lipid profile variables measured were total cholesterol, high density lipoprotein, low density lipoprotein and triglycerides. There was no significant main time or group × time interactions observed for any variables of the lipid profile or fasting blood glucose (Table 3). We observed a main time and group × time effect for heart rate. Specifically, heart rate increased in PL and was unchanged in MIDS (PL, Δ + 4.0 bpm vs. MIDS, Δ 0 bpm, p = 0.005). There was also a main time and group × time effect for diastolic blood pressure (PL, Δ + 2 mmHg vs. MIDS, Δ -1 mmHg, p = 0.04) with no changes in systolic blood pressure (Figure 2).

Food intake

Dietary intake of total calories, carbohydrates, proteins, and fats was not different at baseline and did not change

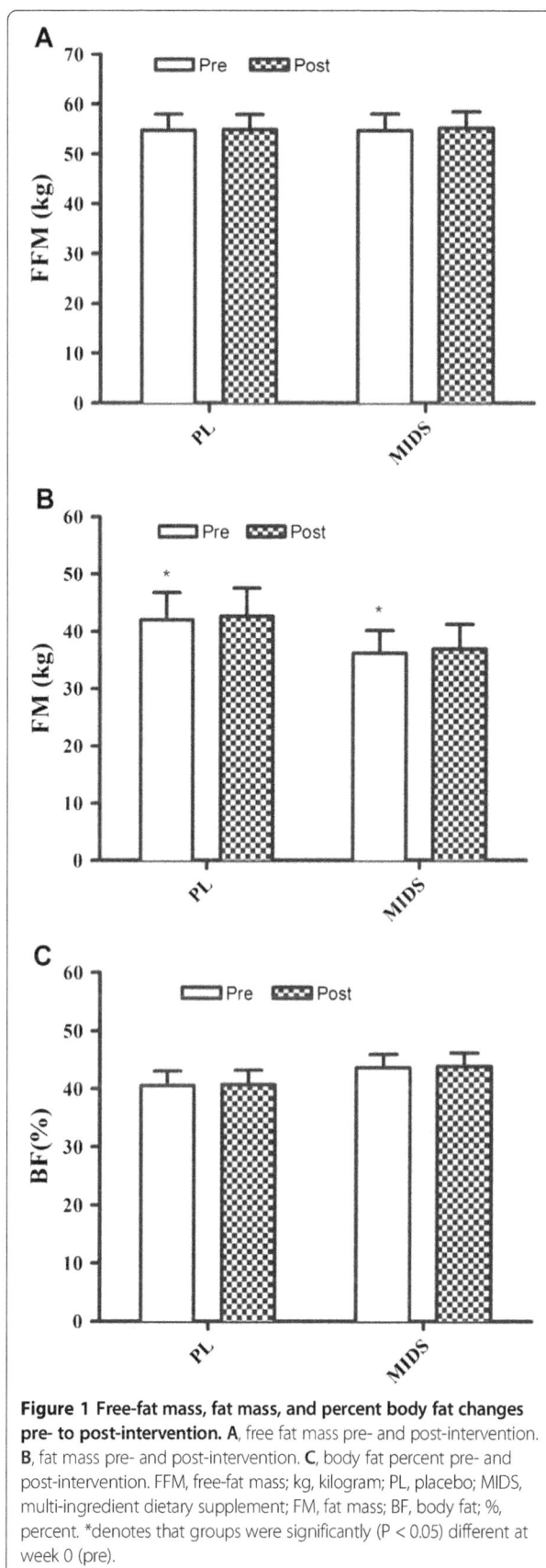

Figure 1 Free-fat mass, fat mass, and percent body fat changes pre- to post-intervention. A, free fat mass pre- and post-intervention. **B,** fat mass pre- and post-intervention. **C,** body fat percent pre- and post-intervention. FFM, free-fat mass; kg, kilogram; PL, placebo; MIDS, multi-ingredient dietary supplement; FM, fat mass; BF, body fat; %, percent. *denotes that groups were significantly (P < 0.05) different at week 0 (pre).

Table 1 Participant demographics at week 0 (N = 22)

Variables	PL [n = 11 (7 women, 4 men)]	MIDS [n = 11 (9 women, 2 men)]	p
Age (years)	33. 8 ± 3.5	35.9 ± 3.4	0.67
Height (cm)	169.2 ± 3.3	173.2 ± 2.9	0.36
BM (Kg)	96.9 ± 6.8	91.9 ± 5.6	0.57
% BF	43.6 ± 2.5	40.5 ± 2.4	0.45

Data are mean ± SEM. PL, Placebo; MIDS, multi-ingredient dietary supplement; BM, body mass; BMI, body mass index; %BF, percent body fat; FM, fat mass; FFM, fat free mass; W/H ratio, wait to hip ratio.

Table 2 Body composition and anthropometrics at week 0 and week 8

Variables	Group	n	Week 0	Week 8	Δ	Time p	Time × group p
BM (kg)	PL	11	96.9 ± 6.8	97.9 ± 7.1	+1.0	0.24	0.70
	MIDS	11	91.9 ± 5.6	92.4 ± 5.9	+0.5		
BMI (kg/m²)	PL	11	34.1 ± 1.8	34.5 ± 1.9	+0.4	0.02	0.62
	MIDS	11	30.0 ± 1.5	30.3 ± 1.5	+0.3		
% BF	PL	11	43.6 ± 2.5	43.8 ± 2.4	+0.2	0.38	0.91
	MIDS	11	40.5 ± 2.4	40.7 ± 2.6	+0.2		
% Android fat	PL	11	49.9 ± 3.2	49.2 ± 2.8	−0.7	0.85	0.07
	MIDS	11	44.8 ± 2.8	45.5 ± 3.1	+0.7		
% Gynoid fat	PL	11	46.5 ± 2.9	46.7 ± 2.7	+0.2	0.63	0.23
	MIDS	11	43.0 ± 2.6	42.6 ± 2.8	−0.5		
FM (kg)	PL	11	41.9 ± 4.8	42.6 ± 4.9	+0.7	0.04	0.84
	MIDS	11	36.2 ± 4.0	36.9 ± 4.3	+0.7		
FFM (kg)	PL	11	54.7 ± 3.2	54.9 ± 3.0	+0.2	0.24	0.50
	MIDS	11	54.7 ± 3.3	55.2 ± 3.3	+0.5		
Waist (cm)	PL	11	107.0 ± 4.3	105.2 ± 3.9	−1.8	0.32	0.69
	MIDS	11	99.9 ± 3.2	99.1 ± 3.3	−0.8		
Hip (cm)	PL	11	121.0 ± 4.9	120.6 ± 4.7	−0.5	0.59	0.90
	MIDS	11	114.0 ± 3.3	113.7 ± 3.6	−0.2		
Waist to hip ratio	PL	11	0.89 ± 0.02	0.88 ± 0.02	−0.01	0.48	0.73
	MIDS	11	0.88 ± 0.02	0.87 ± 0.03	−0.01		

Data are mean ± SEM; PL, Placebo; MIDS, multi-ingredient dietary supplement; BM, body mass; BMI, body mass index; % BF, percent body fat; % Android fat, percent Android fat; % Gynoid fat, percent gynoid fat; waist, waist circumference; hip, hip circumference.
Δ change from week 0 to week 8.

after 8 weeks of supplementation regardless of group. Data are presented in Table 4.

Hunger scale
Ratings of hunger, satiety, and desire to eat are presented in Figure 3. No significant group × time interactions or time effects were observed for satiety or desire to eat. However, a significant group × time interaction was

observed for hunger (PL, Δ - 15.8 mm vs. MIDS, Δ + 10.3 mm, p = 0.04).

Mood state
No significant group × time interactions or time effects were observed for any of the mood state variables. However, a main time effect (p = 0.02) was observed for tension

Table 3 Lipid profile at week 0 and week 8

Variables	Group	n	Week 0	Week 8	Δ	Time p	Time × group p
TC (mg/dl)	PL	11	179.7 ± 7.9	183.8 ± 8.8	+4.0	0.39	0.91
	MIDS	11	178.9 ± 8.6	184.2 ± 14.2	+5.0		
TRG (mg/dl)	PL	10	119.5 ± 18.7	129.7 ± 23.4	+9.0	0.99	0.19
	MIDS	11	107.0 ± 19.3	96.9 ± 21.1	−10		
HDL (mg/dl)	PL	11	56.1 ± 5.1	50.6 ± 5.1	−5.0	0.39	0.27
	MIDS	11	52.4 ± 3.6	53.1 ± 3.9	+1.0		
LDL (mg/dl)	PL	10	102.1 ± 10.7	109.3 ± 7.4	+7.0	0.12	0.96
	MIDS	11	105.1 ± 8.6	111.8 ± 12.1	+7.0		
LDL/HDL	PL	10	2.2 ± 0.4	2.4 ± 0.3	+0.2	0.14	0.68
	MIDS	11	2.1 ± 0.3	2.3 ± 0.4	+0.1		

Data are mean ± SEM; PL, Placebo; MIDS, multi-ingredient dietary supplement; TC, total cholesterol; TRG, triglycerides; HDL, high density lipoprotein; LDL, low density lipoprotein; HR, heart rate; SBP, systolic blood pressure; DBP, diastolic blood pressure; n is different for TRG, LDL, LDL/HDL as a result of insufficient data.
Δ change from week 0 to week 8.

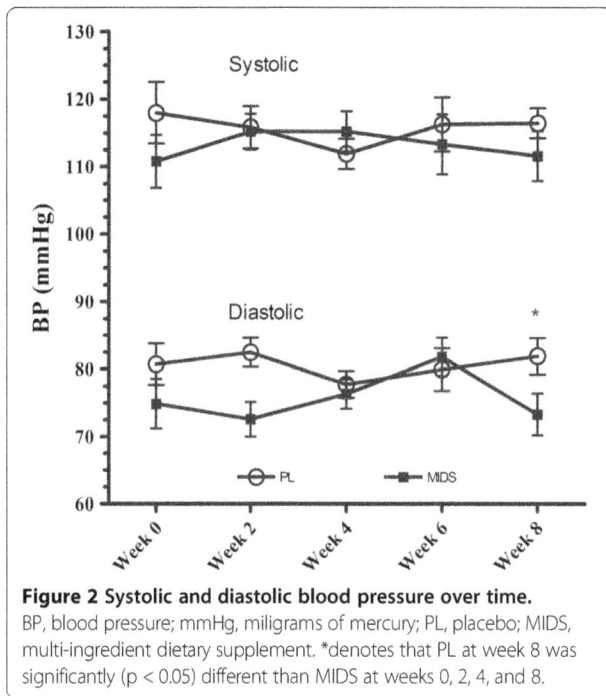

Figure 2 Systolic and diastolic blood pressure over time.
BP, blood pressure; mmHg, miligrams of mercury; PL, placebo; MIDS, multi-ingredient dietary supplement. *denotes that PL at week 8 was significantly (p < 0.05) different than MIDS at weeks 0, 2, 4, and 8.

(PL, Δ - 3.78 vs. MIDS, Δ − 2.2) and confusion (PL, Δ -3.2; vs. MIDS, Δ -1.2).

Hormones

Fasting concentrations of insulin, leptin, adiponectin, and hs-CRP are presented in Table 5. No significant time effects or group by time interactions were observed for any of the measured hormones. Additionally, insulin resistance was not different between groups over time and

no significant changes were observed in either group after 8 weeks of treatment.

No significant group by time interactions or time effects were observed for adiponectin to leptin (A/L) ratio for either group (Table 5). However, A/L ratios were significantly higher in MIDS at baseline and post-intervention compared to PL.

Reported side effects
In PL, there was a report of insomnia (n = 1) and bloating (n = 1). Side effects reported for MIDS were acne (n = 1), jitteriness (n = 1), nausea (n = 1), weight gain (n = 1), and loss of appetite (n = 1). No other side effects were reported in either group.

Discussion
The primary findings of this study were that 8 weeks of MIDS supplementation in overweight/obese men and women did not reduce body mass or improve body composition versus PL. Furthermore, endocrine markers (insulin, leptin, adiponectin, and hs-CRP), blood lipids, satiety, food intake, and mood state variables were not significantly different or after 8 weeks regardless of group.

The results of the present study are in opposition to recent reports of enhanced body composition, mood state, and mental focus with the consumption of other multi-ingredient dietary supplements [6,7]. In these studies, supplements were consumed which contained green tea extracts and caffeine among other ingredients. As MIDS shared these ingredients in common with the supplements used in these studies, the lack of improvement in body composition was unexpected.

Table 4 Food intake at week 0 and week 8

Variables	Group	n	Week 0	Week 8	Δ	Time p	Time × group p
Calories (kcal)	PL	10	2666.2 ± 283.1	2366.9 ± 343.1	−299.3	0.36	0.41
	MIDS	11	2846.0 ± 244.6	2478.5 ± 377.8	−367.5		
Carbohydrate (g)	PL	10	335.2 ± 37.1	271.35 ± 39.8	−63.85	0.27	0.63
	MIDS	11	333.5 ± 37.3	299.0 ± 55.1	−34.53		
Carbohydrate (%)	PL	10	50.9 ± 2.8	46.3 ± 3.3	−4.6	0.31	0.54
	MIDS	11	46.9 ± 3.2	47.9 ± 2.5	+1.0		
Protein (g)	PL	10	93.0 ± 10.6	97.2 ± 16.2	+4.2	0.27	0.60
	MIDS	11	112.3 ± 10.0	95.4 ± 12.1	−16.9		
Protein (%)	PL	10	14.8 ± 1.7	16.6 ± 1.4	+1.8	0.88	0.55
	MIDS	11	16.8 ± 2.1	16.3 ± 1.5	−0.5		
Fat (g)	PL	10	101.9 ± 14.7	91.9 ± 18.0	−10	0.55	0.06
	MIDS	11	119.9 ± 15.8	101.6 ± 16.6	−18.3		
Fat (%)	PL	10	33.1 ± 2.1	34.4 ± 3.2	+1.8	0.13	0.08
	MIDS	11	37.1 ± 2.5	36.6 ± 2.3	−0.5		

Data are mean ± SEM; PL, Placebo; MIDS, multi-ingredient dietary supplement.
Δ change from week 0 to week 8.

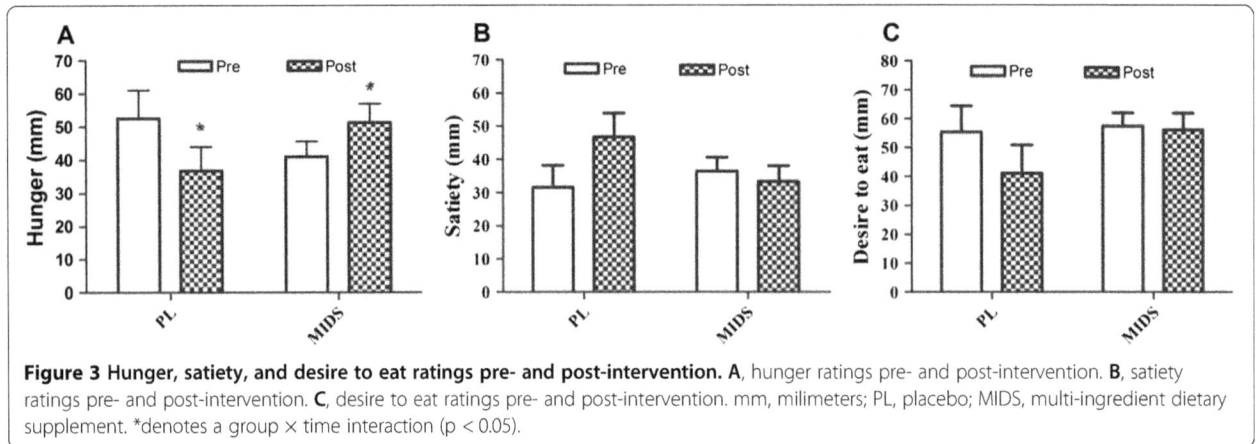

Figure 3 Hunger, satiety, and desire to eat ratings pre- and post-intervention. **A**, hunger ratings pre- and post-intervention. **B**, satiety ratings pre- and post-intervention. **C**, desire to eat ratings pre- and post-intervention. mm, milimeters; PL, placebo; MIDS, multi-ingredient dietary supplement. *denotes a group × time interaction ($p < 0.05$).

Indeed, research examining green tea and caffeine either alone or in combination have consistently reported these ingredients to reduce body mass and fat mass in overweight or obese individuals [8,20-22]. Moreover, the mechanisms for these effects are also well-researched. Caffeine stimulates the release of catecholamines and inhibits degradation of cAMP, which enhances sympathetic stimulation [11,23]. Similarly, green tea can also increase thermogenesis as it contains caffeine and numerous polyphenols (catechins, epicatechin, epigallocatechin, and their gallates). Epigallo Catechin Gallate (EGCG), the most abundant polyphenol in GT, prevents catecholamine degradation via inhibition of catechol-o-methyltransferase (COMT) enzyme activity [10]. This, similar to the effects of caffeine, can effectively prolong norepinephrine-induced sympathetic stimulation thereby enhancing thermogenesis [10].

The lack of significant change in body mass or composition can be explained by a number of factors. Interestingly the impact of caffeine may be attenuated by the development of tolerance. Robertson et al. [24] demonstrated that caffeine (250 mg/day) increased plasma catecholamines after 3 days of ingestion in healthy men and women. However, after 14 days of continuous supplementation the plasma catecholamine concentrations decreased and were comparable to the placebo [24]. The participants in our study were moderate consumers of caffeine (~137 mg/day as self-reported; range: 0 to ~618 mg/day), possibly resulting in attenuated sensitivity to caffeine supplementation during the trial period. The lack of change in heart rate and blood pressure in MIDS appears to confirm this. The ineffectiveness of caffeine in the current study may also be related to genetic factors. Indeed, Womack et al. [25] noted a genetic polymorphism which influences one's

Table 5 Endocrine changes at week 0 and week 8

Variables	Group	n	Pre	Post	Δ	Time p	Time × group p
Insulin (μIU/mL)	PL	11	18.8 ± 3.6	17.2 ± 1.5	−1.6	0.57	0.16
	MIDS	10	11.4 ± 1.2	15.1 ± 2.0	+3.7		
Leptin (pg/mL)	PL	11	52.2 ± 11.4	42.0 ± 8.1	−10.2	0.13	0.58
	MIDS	11	30.7 ± 7.6	25.9 ± 7.5	−4.8		
Adiponectin (μg/mL)	PL	11	5.9 ± 0.8	6.5 ± 1.2	+0.6	0.73	0.12
	MIDS	11	9.8 ± 1.7	8.9 ± 1.5	−0.9		
hs – CRP (mg/L)	PL	11	4.4 ± 1.1	4.6 ± 1.3	+0.2	0.89	0.37
	MIDS	10	2.8 ± 0.9	2.5 ± 0.6	−0.3		
Glucose (mg/dl)	PL	11	99.0 ± 3.3	98.2 ± 4.4	- 0.8	0.94	0.78
	MIDS	11	96.3 ± 4.3	96.9 ± 5.0	+0.6		
HOMA-IR	PL	11	4.66 ± 0.98	4.19 ± 0.42	−0.47	0.73	0.19
	MIDS	10	2.82 ± 0.44	3.61 ± 0.52	+0.81		
A/L	PL	11	0.36 ± 0.1	0.44 ± 0.1	+0.08	0.13	0.39
	MIDS	11	1.1 ± 0.2	1.3 ± 0.23	+0.2		

Data are mean ± SEM; PL, Placebo; MIDS, multi-ingredient dietary supplement; hs-CRP, high sensitivity C reactive protein; HOMA-IR, homeostatic model assessment insulin resistance; A, Adiponectin; L, Leptin; n is different for insulin and hs-CRP as data was missing due to technical errors.
Δ change from week 0 to week 8.

responsiveness to caffeine in terms of exercise performance. Perhaps the majority of subjects in our study were 'non-responders' to caffeine although this is purely speculation. Additionally, a meta-analysis on the body mass and composition effects of caffeine and GT noted ethnicity to be a significant factor [26]. Indeed, caffeine and GT may have more pronounced effects on Asians versus Caucasians. This may be due to genetic differences in COMT activity [27]. As our study was composed of various ethnicities (e.g. Caucasian, African American, and Asian), this may have increased variability resulting in the observed non-significant effects. Finally, the composition of the multi-ingredient dietary supplements utilized in other studies [6,7] is significantly different from MIDS. Thus, the influence of other ingredients may explain the benefits reported in these studies. Another possibility is that the ingredients in these other supplements may synergistically enhance body composition. Alternatively, the potential benefits of the green tea and caffeine in MIDS may have been counteracted by some of its other ingredients, but the experimental design did not allow for examination of the weighted-effects of the various ingredients.

Our findings of a lack of change in body mass or composition is also somewhat unexpected based on reported benefits of CLA ingestion. CLA, a fatty acid abundant in seed oils, may aid in the regulation of lipid metabolism. Specifically, CLA has been reported to reduce uptake of lipids into adipocytes by inhibiting gene expression and activity of stearoyl-CoA desaturase and lipoprotein lipase [28,29]. Additionally, CLA seems to increase the activity of CPT1 thereby increasing fatty acid oxidation. These mechanisms may explain improvements in body composition that have been consistently reported with CLA supplementation in animals [28,30].

There is some evidence to suggest that CLA improves body composition in humans. Blankson et al. [31], studied overweight/obese participants that consumed various amounts of CLA (1.7, 3.4, 5.1, 6.8 g/day) following exercise for 12 wks. As a result of the intervention, participants who received the highest dose of CLA (6.8 g/day) increased lean mass to a greater degree than the other groups. In addition, decreases in fat mass were reported in the groups receiving 3.4 and 6.8 g/day CLA, (but not 5.1 g/day). Others have also reported enhanced lean mass regain following weight loss in overweight participants with 1.8 to 3.4 g/day of CLA [32] and reduced % BF in healthy, normal weight, individuals with 4.2 g/day of CLA [33]. With this in mind, our findings of no change in body mass or composition could be the result of sub-optimal doses of CLA. In the current study, the proprietary blend consumed in MIDS combined the dose of CLA with BCAA (2.52 g/day composed of CLA and BCAAs). Thus, even if the majority of the proprietary blend was composed of CLA, the dose would still likely fall at the low-end of reported effective dosages (1.8-6.8 g/day).

Alternatively, it is also possible that the benefits of CLA are only realized when combined with exercise [31]. Participants in our study were inactive prior to and during the study, which may have influenced the effectiveness of CLA. Whatever the case may be, our findings are in line with numerous others reporting that CLA supplementation has no effect on body mass or composition [34-36]. Further study on the true effects of CLA on body mass and composition in humans in clearly warranted.

In the present study, body composition was not improved despite the BCAA content of MIDS. Increasing dietary protein helps to reduce weight, and preserve lean body mass in healthy adults [37], and some of the benefits may be attributable to BCAA [38]. These effects may be a function of the stimulatory effect that certain BCAA (e.g. leucine) have on muscle protein synthesis [17]. Positive effects from BCAA consumption on body composition are often reported when combined with exercise [39]. However, the influence of BCAA on body composition in inactive individuals is relatively unknown. Our findings suggest that consuming additional BCAA (<2.52 g/day) in combination with the other ingredients in MIDS has no effect on body composition. Alternatively, perhaps a higher dose is required to realize potential benefits. Indeed, many animal studies reporting BCAA-induced losses in fat mass utilize >5 g/day [40].

Maintaining low levels of LDL, TC, and TRG and high levels of HDL may help to prevent cardiovascular disease [41]. Our findings do not support MIDS as being cardioprotective as we observed no changes in blood lipids. Some studies have reported caffeine, green tea, and/or CLA to reduce LDL, TC, and TRG while maintaining or increasing HDL [22,31,42]. However, the doses used in these studies were typically higher than in the current study and/or were combined with exercise or dietary interventions. Perhaps more robust dietary and/or physical activity changes are required to see significant changes in blood lipids.

Endocrine biomarkers were similarly unaffected by MIDS or PL. This was not altogether unexpected as the ingredients in MIDS may have opposing effects on the hormones measured. For instance, caffeine and CLA are known to reduce insulin sensitivity [43,44]. However, caffeine and green tea have also been reported to increase adiponectin, a hormone produced in adipose that may prevent insulin resistance [45,46]. These opposing effects may explain why insulin and fasting glucose were unchanged with MIDS. Leptin, a hormone that may regulate energy intake, and hs-CRP, a proinflammatory cytokine implicated in atherogenesis, were similarly unchanged following MIDS supplementation. Although there is some evidence suggesting that CLA may reduce leptin levels [47], the effects of the other ingredients on leptin and hs-CRP are relatively unknown. The results of the current study suggest that MIDS consumption does not alter leptin, hs-CRP, or hormones related to insulin sensitivity.

Satiety was also unaffected by MIDS supplementation. When attempting to lose weight, increasing satiety may help to reduce energy intake. Previous studies have reported enhanced satiety with increased dietary protein intake [37]. Additionally, caffeine supplementation may reduce spontaneous energy intake [48]. Nevertheless, we observed no changed in satiety or food intake. As mentioned, our subjects were moderate caffeine consumers, which likely attenuated any caffeine-mediated effects on satiety. Moreover, participants in the current study did not increase dietary protein intake, but rather supplemented with a relatively small dose of BCAA. Perhaps BCAAs-alone may have minimal effects on satiety, or the dose was too small to elicit any changes in satiety. It is worth noting that participants consuming MIDS reported an increase in hunger. A study by Chiou et al. [49] reported that participants taking a purported dietary supplement, which was actually a non-caloric placebo, showed a preference for a buffet meal rather than an organic meal. Furthermore, subjects receiving the sham supplement also showed reduced desire to exercise [49]. In the current study, it is possible that participants that believed they were receiving a dietary supplement felt increased license for hedonic behavior possibly contributing to the increased hunger ratings. However, it should be noted that in the present study participants in either group did not increase food intake. Thus, further study on the true effects of MIDS on satiety and hunger are warranted.

In conclusion, consumption of MIDS for 8 wks in overweight and obese, but otherwise healthy, men and women resulted in no changes in body mass or composition, blood lipids, endocrine biomarkers, mood state, or satiety. In future studies, larger doses of MIDS should be administered, and the effects of MIDS in combination with diet and/or exercise should be investigated.

Abbreviations
MIDS: Multi-ingredient dietary supplement; PL: Placebo; GT: Green tea; CLA: Conjugated linoleic acid; BCAA: Branched chain amino acids.

Competing interests
The authors declare that they have no competing interests.

Authors' contributions
MJO designed and managed the study, secured funding, analyzed the data and drafted the manuscript. SRR carried out all practical aspects of the study and assisted with data analysis, and manuscript preparation. MTS assisted with study design and manuscript preparation. DAB, AWK, MEE, NF, TAM, and DT assisted data collection and analysis and manuscript preparation. All authors read and approved the final manuscript.

Acknowledgements
This study was supported by a grant from the International Society of Sports Nutrition to MJO. We would like to thank Emery Ward and Wyatt Eddy for their help with data collection. We would also like to thank all of the volunteers for this study.

Author details
[1]Department of Nutrition, Food and Exercise Sciences, Florida State University, Tallahassee, FL 32306, USA. [2]University of KwaZulu-Natal, Durban, South Africa. [3]Institute of Sports Science & Medicine, Florida State University, Tallahassee, FL, USA.

References
1.   Ogden CL, Carroll MD, Kit BK, Flegal KM: **Prevalence of obesity in the United States, 2009-2010.** *NCHS Data Brief* 2012, **82:**1–8.
2.   Must A, Spadano J, Coakley EH, Field AE, Colditz G, Dietz WH: **The disease burden associated with overweight and obesity.** *JAMA* 1999, **282:**1523–1529.
3.   Barte JCM, ter Bogt NCW, Bogers RP, Teixeira PJ, Blissmer B, Mori TA, Bemelmans WJE: **Maintenance of weight loss after lifestyle interventions for overweight and obesity, a systematic review.** *Obes Rev* 2010, **11:**899–906.
4.   Kernan WN, Viscoli CM, Brass LM, Broderick JP, Brott T, Feldmann E, Morgenstern LB, Wilterdink JL, Horwitz RI: **Phenylpropanolamine and the risk of hemorrhagic stroke.** *N Engl J Med* 2000, **343:**1826–1832.
5.   McEwen LN, Coelho RB, Baumann LM, Bilik D, Nota-Kirby B, Herman WH: **The cost, quality of life impact, and cost-utility of bariatric surgery in a managed care population.** *Obes Surg* 2010, **20:**919–928.
6.   Outlaw J, Wilborn C, Smith A, Urbina S, Hayward S, Foster C, Wells S, Wildman R, Taylor L: **Effects of ingestion of a commercially available thermogenic dietary supplement on resting energy expenditure, mood state and cardiovascular measures.** *J Int Soc Sport Nutr* 2013, **10:**25.
7.   Lopez HL, Ziegenfuss TN, Hofheins JE, Habowski SM, Arent SM, Weir JP, Ferrando A a: **Eight weeks of supplementation with a multi-ingredient weight loss product enhances body composition, reduces hip and waist girth, and increases energy levels in overweight men and women.** *J Int Soc Sport Nutr* 2013, **10:**22.
8.   Nagao T, Hase T, Tokimitsu I: **A green tea extract high in catechins reduces body fat and cardiovascular risks in humans.** *Obes (Silver Spring)* 2007, **15:**1473–1483.
9.   Superko HR, Bortz W, Williams PT, Albers JJ, Wood PD: **Caffeinated and decaffeinated coffee effects on plasma lipoprotein cholesterol, apolipoproteins, and lipase activity: a controlled, randomized trial.** *Am J Clin Nutr* 1991, **54:**599–605.
10. Dulloo AG, Duret C, Rohrer D, Girardier L, Mensi N, Fathi M, Chantre P, Vandermander J: **Efficacy of a green tea extract rich in catechin polyphenols and caffeine in increasing 24-h energy expenditure and fat oxidation in humans.** *Am J Clin Nutr* 1999, **70:**1040–1045.
11. Acheson KJ, Zahorska-Markiewicz B, Pittet P, Anantharaman K, Jéquier E: **Caffeine and coffee: their influence on metabolic rate and substrate utilization in normal weight and obese individuals.** *Am J Clin Nutr* 1980, **33:**989–997.
12. Hursel R, Viechtbauer W, Dulloo AG, Tremblay A, Tappy L, Rumpler W, Westerterp-Plantenga MS: **The effects of catechin rich teas and caffeine on energy expenditure and fat oxidation: a meta-analysis.** *Obes Rev* 2011, **12:**e573–e581.
13. Moloney F, Yeow T-P, Mullen A, Nolan JJ, Roche HM: **Conjugated linoleic acid supplementation, insulin sensitivity, and lipoprotein metabolism in patients with type 2 diabetes mellitus.** *Am J Clin Nutr* 2004, **80:**887–895.
14. Zhang Y, Guo K, LeBlanc RE, Loh D, Schwartz GJ, Yu Y-H: **Increasing dietary leucine intake reduces diet-induced obesity and improves glucose and cholesterol metabolism in mice via multimechanisms.** *Diabetes* 2007, **56:**1647–1654.
15. Evans M, Lin X, Odle J, McIntosh M: **Trans-10, cis-12 conjugated linoleic acid increases fatty acid oxidation in 3 T3-L1 preadipocytes.** *J Nutr* 2002, **132:**450–455.
16. Granlund L, Juvet LK, Pedersen JI, Nebb HI: **Trans10, cis12-conjugated linoleic acid prevents triacylglycerol accumulation in adipocytes by acting as a PPARgamma modulator.** *J Lip Res* 2003, **44:**1441–1452.
17. Rieu I, Balage M, Sornet C, Giraudet C, Pujos E, Grizard J, Mosoni L, Dardevet D: **Leucine supplementation improves muscle protein synthesis in elderly men independently of hyperaminoacidaemia.** *J Physiol* 2006, **575:**305–315.
18. Arciero P, Gentile C, Martin-Pressman R, Ormsbee M, Everett M, Zwicky L, Steele C: **Increased dietary protein and combined high intensity aerobic and resistance exercise improves body fat distribution and cardiovascular risk factors.** *Int J Sport Nutr Exerc Metab* 2006, **16:**373–392.

19. Matthews DR, Hosker JP, Rudenski AS, Naylor BA, Treacher DF, Turner RC: Homeostasis model assessment: insulin resistance and beta-cell function from fasting plasma glucose and insulin concentrations in man. *Diabetologia* 1985, 28:412–419.

20. Wang H, Wen Y, Du Y, Yan X, Guo H, Rycroft JA, Boon N, Kovacs EMR, Mela DJ: Effects of catechin enriched green tea on body composition. *Obesity (Silver Spring)* 2010, 18:773–779.

21. Chantre P, Lairon D: Recent findings of green tea extract AR25 (Exolise) and its activity for the treatment of obesity. *Phytomedicine* 2002, 9:3–8.

22. Kajimoto O, Kajimoto Y, Yabune M, Nakamura T, Kotani K, Suzuki Y, Nozawa A, Nagata K, Unno T, Sagesaka YM, Kakuda T, Yoshikawa T: Tea catechins with a galloyl moiety reduce body weight and Fat. *J Health Sci* 2005, 51:161–171.

23. Astrup A, Toubro S, Cannon S, Hein P, Breum L, Madsen J: Caffeine: a double-blind, placebo-controlled study of its thermogenic, metabolic, and cardiovascular effects in healthy volunteers. *Am J Clin Nutr* 1990, 51:759–767.

24. Robertson D, Wade D, Workman R, Woosley RL, Oates JA: Tolerance to the humoral and hemodynamic effects of caffeine in man. *J Clin Invest* 1981, 67:1111–1117.

25. Womack CJ, Saunders MJ, Bechtel MK, Bolton DJ, Martin M, Luden ND, Dunham W, Hancock M: The influence of a CYP1A2 polymorphism on the ergogenic effects of caffeine. *J Int Soc Sport Nutr* 2012, 9:7.

26. Hursel R, Viechtbauer W, Westerterp-Plantenga MS: The effects of green tea on weight loss and weight maintenance: a meta-analysis. *Int J Obes* 2009, 33:956–961.

27. Palmatier MA, Kang AM, Kidd KK: Global variation in the frequencies of functionally different catechol-O-methyltransferase alleles. *Biol Psych* 1999, 46:557–567.

28. Park Y, Albright KJ, Liu W, Storkson JM, Cook ME, Pariza MW: Effect of conjugated linoleic acid on body composition in mice. *Lipids* 1997, 32:853–858.

29. Choi Y, Kim YC, Han YB, Park Y, Pariza MW, Ntambi JM: The trans-10, cis-12 isomer of conjugated linoleic acid downregulates stearoyl-CoA desaturase 1 gene expression in 3 T3–L1 adipocytes. *J Nutr* 2000, 130:1920–1924.

30. West DB, Delany JP, Camet PM, Blohm F, Truett AA, Scimeca J: Effects of conjugated linoleic acid on body fat and energy metabolism in the mouse. *Am J Physiol* 1998, 275:R667–R672.

31. Blankson H, Stakkestad JA, Fagertun H, Thom E, Wadstein J, Gudmundsen O: Conjugated linoleic acid reduces body fat mass in overweight and obese humans. *J Nutr* 2000, 130:2943–2948.

32. Kamphuis MMJW, Lejeune MPGM, Saris WHM, Westerterp-Plantenga MS: The effect of conjugated linoleic acid supplementation after weight loss on body weight regain, body composition, and resting metabolic rate in overweight subjects. *Int J Obes Relat Metab Disord* 2003, 27:840–847.

33. Smedman A, Vessby B: Conjugated linoleic acid supplementation in humans - Metabolic effects. *Lipids* 2001, 36:773–781.

34. Nazare J-A, de la Perrière AB, Bonnet F, Desage M, Peyrat J, Maitrepierre C, Louche-Pelissier C, Bruzeau J, Goudable J, Lassel T, Vidal H, Laville M: Daily intake of conjugated linoleic acid-enriched yoghurts: effects on energy metabolism and adipose tissue gene expression in healthy subjects. *Br J Nutr* 2007, 97:273–280.

35. Tricon S, Burdge GC, Kew S, Banerjee T, Russell JJ, Jones EL, Grimble RF, Williams CM, Yaqoob P, Calder PC: Opposing effects of cis-9, trans-11 and trans-10, cis-12 conjugated linoleic acid on blood lipids in healthy humans. *Am J Clin Nutr* 2004, 80:614–620.

36. House RL, Cassady JP, Eisen EJ, McIntosh MK, Odle J: Conjugated linoleic acid evokes de-lipidation through the regulation of genes controlling lipid metabolism in adipose and liver tissue. *Obes Rev* 2005, 6:247–258.

37. Arciero PJ, Gentile CL, Pressman R, Everett M, Ormsbee MJ, Martin J, Santamore J, Gorman L, Fehling PC, Vukovich MD, Nindl BC: Moderate protein intake improves total and regional body composition and insulin sensitivity in overweight adults. *Metabolism* 2008, 57:757–765.

38. Qin L-Q, Xun P, Bujnowski D, Daviglus ML, Van Horn L, Stamler J, He K: Higher branched-chain amino acid intake is associated with a lower prevalence of being overweight or obese in middle-aged East Asian and Western adults. *J Nutr* 2011, 141:249–254.

39. Manders RGF, Wagenmakers AJM, Koopman R, Zorenc AHG, Menheere PPCA, Schaper NC, Saris WHM, van Loon LJC: Co-ingestion of a protein hydrolysate and amino acid mixture with carbohydrate improves plasma glucose disposal in patients with type 2 diabetes. *Am J Clin Nutr* 2005, 82:76–83.

40. Donato J, Pedrosa RG, Cruzat VF, Pires IS d O, Tirapegui J: Effects of leucine supplementation on the body composition and protein status of rats submitted to food restriction. *Nutrition* 2006, 22:520–527.

41. Gordon DJ, Probstfield JL, Garrison RJ, Neaton JD, Castelli WP, Knoke JD, Jacobs DR, Bangdiwala S, Tyroler HA: High-density lipoprotein cholesterol and cardiovascular disease. Four prospective American studies. *Circulation* 1989, 79:8–15.

42. Astrup A, Breum L, Toubro S, Hein P, Quaade F: The effect and safety of an ephedrine/caffeine compound compared to ephedrine, caffeine and placebo in obese subjects on an energy restricted diet. A double blind trial. *Int J Obes Relat Metab Disord* 1992, 16:269–277.

43. Keijzers GB, De Galan BE, Tack CJ, Smits P: Caffeine can decrease insulin sensitivity in humans. *Diabetes Care* 2002, 25:364–369.

44. Thrush AB, Chabowski A, Heigenhauser GJ, McBride BW, Or-Rashid M, Dyck DJ: Conjugated linoleic acid increases skeletal muscle ceramide content and decreases insulin sensitivity in overweight, non-diabetic humans. *Appl Physiol Nutr Metab* 2007, 32:372–382.

45. Williams CJ, Fargnoli JL, Hwang JJ, van Dam RM, Blackburn GL, Hu FB, Mantzoros CS: Coffee consumption is associated with higher plasma adiponectin concentrations in women with or without type 2 diabetes: a prospective cohort study. *Diabetes Care* 2008, 31:504–507.

46. Hsu C-H, Tsai T-H, Kao Y-H, Hwang K-C, Tseng T-Y, Chou P: Effect of green tea extract on obese women: a randomized, double-blind, placebo-controlled clinical trial. *Clin Nutr* 2008, 27:363–370.

47. Poirier H, Rouault C, Clément L, Niot I, Monnot M-C, Guerre-Millo M, Besnard P: Hyperinsulinaemia triggered by dietary conjugated linoleic acid is associated with a decrease in leptin and adiponectin plasma levels and pancreatic beta cell hyperplasia in the mouse. *Diabetologia* 2005, 48:1059–1065.

48. Tremblay A, Masson E, Leduc S, Houde A, Després J-P: Caffeine reduces spontaneous energy intake in men but not in women. *Nutr Res* 1988, 8:553–558.

49. Chiou W-B, Yang C-C, Wan C-S: Ironic effects of dietary supplementation: illusory invulnerability created by taking dietary supplements licenses health-risk behaviors. *Psychol Sci* 2011, 22:1081–1086.

4

Changes induced by diet and nutritional intake in the lipid profile of female professional volleyball players after 11 weeks of training

Juan Mielgo-Ayuso[1*], Pilar S Collado[2,3], Aritz Urdampilleta[4], José Miguel Martínez-Sanz[5] and Jesús Seco[3,6]

Abstract

Background: The relationship between cardiovascular disease and lipid profile is well known. Apart from a heart-healthy diet, exercise is the primary factor that can modify this lipid-associated cardiovascular risk. The aim of the study was to evaluate potential changes in the levels of triglycerides, total cholesterol (TC), low-density lipoprotein-cholesterol (LDLc), and high-density lipoprotein-cholesterol (HDLc), as well as atherogenic indices (TC/HDLc and LDLc/HDLc), and also to analyse the diet over 11 weeks of training in female professional volleyball players.

Methods: The lipid profile of 22 female professional volleyball players was analysed on Day T0 (pre-preseason) and Day T11 (after 11 weeks of training). The consumption of fats by the players was estimated using a food frequency questionnaire, confirmed by seven days of full dietary records.

Results: By the end of the study, the LDLc levels and both atherogenic indices of the players had decreased ($p < 0.05$) compared to the values obtained at baseline. In addition, the diet of the players contained $35.5 \pm 3.2\%$ of fats (saturated fatty acid: $11.1 \pm 1.2\%$, monounsaturated fatty acid: $14.3 \pm 1.9\%$, and polyunsaturated fatty acid: $7.0 \pm 1.1\%$) and 465 ± 57 mg of dietary cholesterol. Their score for the (monounsaturated + polyunsaturated fatty acid)/saturated fatty acid ratio was 1.9 ± 0.4, less than the recommended ≥ 2.

Conclusion: These data indicate that the activity of the female professional volleyball players during the first 11 weeks of training in the season was heart healthy, because their lipid profile improved, despite an inadequate intake of fats.

Keywords: Lipids, Atherogenic indices, Sports nutrition, Team sports, Elite athletes, Dietary intake, Female athletes

Background

Physical activity and a heart-healthy diet, such as the Mediterranean diet [1], have been highlighted as major factors in preventing cardiovascular disease (CVD) [2]. Therapeutic lifestyle changes, including nutrition and exercise, are recommended as the front-line strategy for addressing cardiovascular risk factors. Moreover, the positive relationship between CVD and concentrations of low-density lipoprotein cholesterol (LDLc) and the negative relationship between concentrations of high-density lipoprotein cholesterol (HDLc) and cardiovascular risk have been clearly established in numerous clinical trials [3]. Extensive physical activity is one of the factors that have been shown to be associated with high concentrations of HDLc, which may in part explain the lower risk of coronary heart disease in physically active people [4]. Furthermore, the influence of diet on plasma lipid levels is well known, in particular, the fact that the impact on cardiovascular risk is dependent on the saturated or unsaturated nature, as well as on the number of carbon atoms in the chain, of the fatty acids consumed [5]. In a recent meta-analysis, Kelley et al. [6] concluded that a proper diet along with a programme of aerobic exercise (brisk walking, swimming, cycling, aerobics, or racquet sports) improved the lipid profile (LP), thanks to decreased levels of LDLc, triglycerides (TG), and total cholesterol (TC).

In women's volleyball, as in other sports, the first part of the season is a period of heavy training loads that aim

* Correspondence: juankaya@msn.com
[1]Department of Nutrition and Dietetics, Haro Volleyball Club, Nutrition Centre of La Rioja, C/ Donantes de sangre, 14.26200 Haro, La Rioja, Spain
Full list of author information is available at the end of the article

to develop technical and tactical skills, as well as achieve adequate physical fitness for the competition period [7]. It is difficult to establish the effects of training on the LP of professional volleyball players. This is because, apart from the personal characteristics of each player, particular features of their training, especially those focused on competition, can substantially modify the LP [8], but we have found no studies that analyse the interaction of these factors. Ruiz et al. [9] commented that volleyball is a sport with a strong component of physical stress, so that playing it leads to lower levels of undesirable plasma lipids and lipoproteins than in the case of other less stressful sports. Witek et al. [10] suggested that changes in the LP over the course of a season could be regarded as transient, with no impact on CVD risk, because the lipid levels remained within normal physiological ranges. Both these studies were, however, conducted in men [9,10].

Thus, the primary aim of this study was to evaluate potential changes in the LP (TG, TC, LDLc, HDLc and atherogenic indices, TC/HDLc and LDLc/HDLc) that might be induced by 11 weeks of training in female volleyball players (FVPs). The secondary aim was to collect baseline data on nutrient intake, in order to advise FVPs from the Spanish Super League concerning the fat content and quality of their diet during this period.

Methods

The study was designed in compliance with the recommendations for clinical research of the World Medical Association Declaration of Helsinki [11]. The protocol was reviewed and approved by the clinical research ethics committees University of León and the University of Basque Country. The experimental procedures, associated risks, and benefits were explained to eligible players before they gave written informed consent to participate.

Subjects

The study group consisted of 22 FVPs, undertaking 25 hours per week of performance training (Table 1). All

the participants were required to attend the laboratory at two specific points: (a) Day T0 (baseline, prior to their general preparation phase of training); and (b) Day T11 (11 weeks later, after 6 weeks of general preparation and 5 weeks of the specific preparation, as well as 6 matches in the regular women's volleyball season).

All the participating players also completed a diet record to record their food intake during the study and had two sets of anthropometric measurements taken (detailed below).

Anthropometric measurements

All anthropometric measurements were conducted on Days T0 and T11 by the same Level 2 certified anthropometrist following the protocol of the International Society for the Advancement of Kinanthropometry (ISAK) [12]. Body weight (BW) was measured in kilograms using a SECA® scale, to the nearest 0.1 kg., and height using a stadiometer to the nearest 0.5 cm. Body mass index (BMI) was then calculated using the formula $BW/height^2$ (kg/m^2). A total of six (triceps, abdominal, supra-iliac, sub-scapular, front thigh and calf) skin-fold measurements were taken in millimetres with a Harpenden® skin-fold calliper, to the nearest 0.2 mm and their sum ($\Sigma 6SF$) calculated. Body Fat mass (FM) was calculated using the Faulkner equation [13].

Blood collection and analysis

Venous blood samples were drawn after 12 hours of fasting from the ante-cubital fossa of the forearm, between 8.00 and 9.00 a.m. on days T0 and T11. None of the players trained the day before the samples were taken. The TG, TC, and HDLc levels were measured by an enzymatic spectrophotometric technique with an auto-analyser (COBAS FARA; Roche Diagnostics, Basel, Switzerland). These values were then used to calculate the LDLc with the Friedewald equation [14]: LDLc = (TC - HDLc) - TG/5; and the atherogenic indices (TC/HDLc and LDLc/HDLc).

Table 1 Example of a week of training

		Morning		Afternoon
MONDAY	10:00	STRENGH WORKOUTS All players (1)	18:30	TECH-TAC
TUESDAY		FREE TIME	18:30	TECH-TAC
WEDNESDAY	9:30	STRENGH WORKOUTS Hitters and Libero (2)	15:30	STRENGH WORKOUTS Setters and middle blockers (2)
	10:30	Specific TECH-TAC Setters and middle blockers	18:30	Specific TECH- TAC Hitters and Libero
THURSDAY		FREE TIME	18:30	TECH-TAC
FRIDAY	9:30	13:00	18:30	TECH-TAC
	TECH-TAC	Video		
SATURDAY		OFFICIAL TRAINING		MATCH
SUNDAY		FREE TIME		FREE TIME

TECH-TAC: Technical/Tactical training; (1): Basic strength training (maximal strength through hypertrophy); (2): Specific strength training (explosive strength and plyometrics).

Dietary control

The participating players were taught how to accurately assess their food intake by dieticians. First, after the T11 anthropometric measurements, the participants where requested to complete a validated food frequency questionnaire (FFQ) for the female Spanish population [15], previously used in other studies conducted in Spain [16,17]. This FFQ, which asked the subjects to recall their average consumption over the previous 11 weeks, included 139 different foods and drinks, arranged by food type and meal pattern. Frequency categories were based on the number of times that items were consumed per day, week or month. Daily consumption in grams was determined by dividing the reported intake by the frequency in days.

Second, as a check on the answers to the FFQ, the participants completed a 7-day dietary record the week prior to starting training (T0) and during week 11 (T11), these questionnaires being distributed on the day the anthropometric measurements were taken. The results obtained by the FFQ were found to be highly reproducible regarding the frequency and amount foods consumed compared to the data from the 7-day dietary records. When it was not possible to weigh food, serving sizes consumed were estimated from either product names, the place of food consumption, standard weights of food items or the portion size indicated in a picture booklet of 500 photographs of foods. Food values were converted into intakes of total energy, fats, different fatty acids, and cholesterol by a validated software package developed by the Spanish Centre for Higher Studies in Nutrition and Dietetics (CESNID), which is based on Spanish tables of food composition [18].

Third, on Day T11, the participants completed a validated 14-point Mediterranean Diet Adherence Screener (MEDAS) [19]. This included 10 items to measure the frequency of consumption of beneficial foods pertaining to the typical Mediterranean diet (virgin olive oil, vegetables, fresh fruits, legumes and pulses, fish, nuts, white meat, and wine in moderate quantities). It also had four items to measure the consumption of foods that should be limited in or eliminated from the diet (red and processed meats; cream, butter, and margarine; carbonated and/or sugary beverages; and commercial bakery products such as cakes or pastries). One point was assigned to each of the 14 items, so that the total MEDAS score ranged from 0 to 14 points, as a continuous measure, and scores above 9 were considered to indicate good adherence to the Mediterranean diet.

Statistical analysis

All data are reported as means ± standard deviations. Statistical analysis was performed using SPSS, version 19.0 (SPSS, Chicago). A comparison was made of anthropometric characteristics (BW, BMI, Σ6SF, and FM) and their LP parameters (TG, TC, HDLc, and LDLc, as well as the atherogenic indices) on Days T0 and T11, using the Student's t-test or Mann–Whitney U-test, after normality of the data had been confirmed with the Shapiro-Wilk test. The percentage of change in the outcome variables after 11 weeks was calculated as Δ (%): [(T11 − T0)/T0] × 100. The differences were considered statistically significant when $p < 0.05$.

Results

The mean characteristics of the players are summarised in Table 2. Regarding the anthropometric parameters, significant decreases ($p = 0.027$) in Σ6SF were observed over the 11 weeks of the study.

The levels of serum lipids and associated indices are listed in Table 3. There were significant decreases in the levels of LDLc ($p = 0.034$), TC/HDLc ($p = 0.027$) and LDLc/HDLc ($p = 0.030$) after the 11 weeks of training.

Table 4 compares energy and fat intakes and the recommended allowances for each of these nutrients. Total fat intake, SFA, W6 and cholesterol intakes were above, and MUFAs were below the recommended allowances for adults in the general population, whilst PUFAs and W3 intakes were adequate.

With regard to the diet quality of the players (Table 5), the MEDAS score, and W6/W3 and (MUFA + PUFA)/SFA ratios indicated that they consumed a healthy diet, but the MUFA/SFA ratio was below the recommended figure.

Finally, Table 6 shows the daily food intake by the players over the 11-week study and the recommended amounts for the general population and for athletes. Relative to the recommended allowances for athletes, the FVPs consumed smaller quantities of cereals, potatoes, legumes and pulses, and larger amounts of pastries, margarine, fatty meat and cold meats.

Discussion

The data collected in this study are of interest because, although the FVPs had a diet rich in fats, cholesterol and SFAs, it was found that their LP did improve. Specifically, LDLc and the atherogenic indices declined, whilst HDLc increased, after 11 weeks of training.

Table 2 The anthropometric characteristics of the female volleyball players at T0 and T11 and the percentage changes

	T0 (n = 22)	T11 (n = 22)	% Change	p T0-T11
Weight (kg)	69.6 ± 9.4	70.1 ± 9.2	0.8 ± 3.1	0.274
BMI	21.8 ± 2.0	21.9 ± 1.8	0.8 ± 3.1	0.311
Σ6SF (mm)	93.2 ± 26.7	87.5 ± 24.4	−5.2 ± 6.4	**0.027**
Fat mass (kg)	14.3 ± 4.3	13.9 ± 3.9	−2.0 ± 10.1	0.240

Data are expressed as mean ± standard deviation. BMI: body mass index; Σ6SF: Sum of 6 skinfolds.
% Change calculated as: ((T11-T0) x 100/T0).
p T0-T11: baseline vs. after 11 weeks of training.

Table 3 The lipid profile in the female volleyball players at T0 and T11 and the percentage changes

		% Change	p T0-T11
TG (mg/dL)			
T0	71 ± 35	0.3 ± 29.3	0.329
T11	65 ± 16		
TC (mg/dL)			
T0	182 ± 36	−2.7 ± 15.2	0.284
T11	175 ± 18		
HDLc (mg/dL)			
T0	65 ± 16	7.3 ± 22.6	0.089
T11	71 ± 20		
LDLc (mg/dL)			
T0	102 ± 38	−7.0 ± 18.1	**0.034**
T11	91 ± 23		
TC/HDLc			
T0	3.0 ± 1.0	−9.5 ± 11.4	**0.004**
T11	2.7 ± 0.9		
LDLc/HDLc			
T0	1.7 ± 0.9	−13.2 ± 15.4	**0.011**
T11	1.5 ± 0.7		

Data are expressed as mean ± SD. TG: triglycerides; TC: total cholesterol; HDLc: HDL cholesterol; LDLc: LDL cholesterol. % change calculated as: (T11 − T0)/T0 x 100. p T0-T11: baseline vs. after 11 weeks of training.

There is strong evidence that aerobic exercise is associated with favourable shifts in blood triglycerides and HDLc; further, data from intervention studies [20] and numerous meta-analyses [21,22] also support the view that there is an LDLc lowering response to exercise training, though this is a less well-characterized and seems to be variable. Furthermore, independent of diet, exercise was found to have beneficial effects on the concentration and size of low-density lipoprotein cholesterol particles, concentration of high-density lipoprotein cholesterol, size of high-density lipoprotein cholesterol particles, and triglycerides [23].

Table 5 Quality indices for the diet of the female volleyball players (n = 22)

	Per day	Recommended healthy diet
W6/W3	6.6 ± 6.4	5-10:1[a]
MUFA/SFA	1.4 ± 0.2	≥ 0.5[a]
(MUFA + PUFA)/SFA	1.9 ± 0.4	≥ 2[a]
Mediterranean diet adherence	9.3 ± 2.3	≥ 9[b]

Data are expressed as mean ± standard deviation. SFA: saturated fatty acids; MUFA: monounsaturated fatty acids; PUFA: polyunsaturated fatty acids; W3: omega-3 fatty acids; W6: omega-6 fatty acids. [a]Recommended healthy diet [41]; [b]Recommended good Mediterranean diet adherence [19].

A recent meta-analysis [24] showed that continuous exercise (training) produces a 5 to 8% increase in HDLc levels. This is attributable to an increase in the activity of lecithin-cholesterol acyltransferase (LCAT), which increases the synthesis of HDLc, and a reduction in the activity of hepatic lipase, which is involved in the catabolism of these lipids. The effects of physical activity on LCAT and hepatic lipase depend on the type, intensity, frequency, and duration of the physical activity [25]. Paraoxonases are also associated with HDLc because they induce the hydrolysis of lipid peroxide and they provide protection against atherosclerosis [25]. Additionally, a reduction of up to 20% in paraoxonase levels has been reported in sedentary people [26]. HDLc serum levels are inversely associated with the risk of CVD [8]. In the present study, a slight increase of 7.3 ± 22.6% ($p > 0.05$) was observed in the levels of HDLc in the FVPs after 11 weeks of training. Though the change was not significant, it is interesting to note that an increase of this order of magnitude would decrease their risk of CVD by 16 to 24% [24].

In contrast to HDLc, high levels of LDLc favour the onset and development of CVD [8]. This is why many studies have been conducted to determine which factors lower LDLc levels [6,24,27]. Tambalis et al. [8], in a recent systematic review, pointed out striking evidence that resistance and combined exercise both lower LDLc levels.

Table 4 Energy and macronutrient intake by female volleyball players (n = 22) during the study and the dietary reference recommendations

Nutrient	Per day	Per kg BW	% total energy	Dietary reference recommendations
Energy (kcal)	2840 ± 268	41 ± 6	100	45-50 g/kg BM/day[a]
Fat (g)	113 ± 20	1.6 ± 0.4	35.6 ± 4.8	15-30%[b]
SFA (g)	35.4 ± 9.8	0.5 ± 0.2	11.1 ± 2.3	< 10%[b]
MUFA (g)	46.9 ± 4.7	0.7 ± 0.1	14.9 ± 2.0	15-20%[b]
PUFA (g)	21.0 ± 7.5	0.3 ± 0.1	6.6 ± 2.0	5-8%[b]
W3 (g)	1.6 ± 0.6	0.04 ± 0.01	0.5 ± 2.0	1-2%[b]
W6 (g)	10.4 ± 3.7	0.4 ± 0.2	4.7 ± 10.0	5-8%[b]
Cholesterol (mg)	443 ± 72	6.6 ± 1.5		< 300 mg/day[b]

Data are expressed as mean ± standard deviation. BW: body weight; SFA: saturated fatty acids; MUFA: monounsaturated fatty acids; PUFA: polyunsaturated fatty acids; W3: omega-3 fatty acids; W6: omega-6 fatty acids; [a]Recommended energy and carbohydrate intakes [31]; [b]Recommended lipid intake in the adult population to reduce cardiovascular diseases [2].

Table 6 Servings consumed daily by the female volleyball players (n = 22) during the study and the reference recommendations

Food groups	Daily ingested servings	Recommended servings ATHLETES[a]
Cereals and potatoes	3.3 ± 0.4	6-11/day
Dairy products	3.1 ± 0.9	3-4/day
Fruits	3.1 ± 0.9	2-4/day
Vegetables	3.8 ± 0.6	3-5/day
Olive oil	1.2 ± 0.4	2-4/day
Other oils	0.3 ± 0.1	Not mentioned
Legumes and pulses	0.5 ± 0.2	2-3/week or frequently (1/day)
Dried fruits	0.4 ± 0.2	2-3/week or frequently (1/day)
Fish	0.9 ± 0.2	2-3/day and alternating these food groups
Lean meats and poultry	1.8 ± 0.4	
Eggs	0.5 ± 0.1	
Fatty meat and cold meats	0.5 ± 0.1	A few times per month
Pastries and margarines	2.1 ± 0.5	
Wine and beer	0.3 ± 0.2	Not mentioned

Data are expressed as mean ± standard deviation of the number of ingested servings for each food group per person per day. [a]Proposal to adapt the food pyramid to an athlete's diet [31].

Likewise, the *Lipid Research Clinics Program* [28] revealed that long-term physical activity, undertaken in a frequent and continuous manner, could decrease LDLc and TC levels. In the FVPs, we observed a slight decrease (by 2.7 ± 15.2%; $p > 0.05$) in TC and a significant decrease (by 7.0 ± 18.1%; $p = 0.034$) in LDLc, changes which add up to an improvement in the LP. The fall in LDLc in the players is attributable to their physical activity having the effect on skeletal muscles of increasing the amount and activity of lipoprotein lipase (LPL). This is an enzyme responsible for hydrolysing TG-rich lipoprotein, thereby reducing VLDL (very low-density lipoprotein) cholesterol and LDLc [29].

Furthermore, it appears that the number of weekly workouts is correlated with increased levels of HDLc and decreased LDLc/HDLc and TC/HDLc atherogenic indices [30]. Specifically, the positive effects of exercise on lipid metabolism were found to last 48 hours [30]. Consistent with this, in our study, the FVPs did two workouts a day, six days a week and significant decreases were observed in their LDLc/HDLc ($p = 0.011$) and TC/HDLc ($p = 0.004$) indices, of 13.2 ± 15.4 and 9.5 ± 11.4 respectively. Theses decreases in their atherogenic indices can be considered a useful outcome, since high values are strongly associated with the risk of CVD [10].

The daily energy intake of the FVPs during the 11 weeks of study was 41 ± 6 kcal/kg of BW per day. González-Gross et al. [31] advocated an intake of 45 to 50 kcal/kg/day for athletes who train for more than 75 to 90 min/day, as was the case of the FVPs in our study. However, the 39 to 44 kcal/kg/day recommended by Volek et al. [32] for women who engage predominately in resistance exercise

training seems more adequate for the first 11 weeks of training in the season in the case of women's volleyball, because the subjects' BW remained stable while their FM fell (kg). This was indicated by a significant reduction ($p = 0.027$) in the Σ6SF, skin-fold thicknesses being used as indicators of body FM [33].

It is worth mentioning that total energy intake may also be directly related to the levels of TG, TC, HDLc, and LDLc, especially the amount and type of fat ingested [4]. Fat accounted for 35.5 ± 3.2% of total energy intake by the FVPs, in line with what has been reported by several other authors [34-38], but higher than the data reported by Beals et al. [39] and also higher than the 20 to 35% of the total energy consumed that is recommended for team athletes and for the general adult population [33].

Additionally, the amount of cholesterol and SFA intake was found to be positively correlated with the TC and LDLc [40]. The amount of cholesterol ingested by the FVPs was high (465 ± 57 mg) compared to the 300 mg recommended for the general population [2], similar to the 460 mg reported by Anderson et al. in 15 FVPs at the start of the season after a dietary and nutritional intervention [35] and lower than the 104 mg found by Papadopoulou et al. in teenage FVPs [34]. In addition to these data, we note that the intake of SFAs by the FVPs was also high (11.1 ± 1.2%) compared to the < 10% that has been suggested to be appropriate the general adult population to reduce cardiovascular diseases [2].

This high cholesterol and SFA intake may be due to the players drinking full-fat milk (3.1 ± 0.9 servings/day), even though their daily number of servings was within the recommendations for athletes [31]. In addition, the

FVPs consumed relatively large amounts of pastries and butter, foods containing a considerable quantity of SFAs [18], whose consumption is not recommended more often than a few times per month [31] and particularly not more than once daily, as was the case for the players in this study (2.1 ± 0.5 servings/day). For athletes' nutrition, semi-skimmed or skimmed milk is considered preferable, so as to reduce the intake of cholesterol and calories from SFAs. It is known that the cholesterol metabolism has some negative feedback, in the sense that if large amounts of cholesterol are ingested, the body produces less (in a normal physiological situation). However, an increase in the consumption of SFAs would cause activation of the cholesterol metabolism, with a possible increase in TC [3].

Additionally, the intake of MUFAs ($14.3 \pm 1.9\%$) was below the ideal recommended allowance (15 to 20%) [41]. MUFAs have healthy effects on the heart by increasing HDLc levels [5]. It was also established that the ratios between different fatty acids, as measured by the PUFA/SFA (1.4 ± 0.2) and W6/W3 (6.6 ± 6.4) ratios, were within the recommendations (≥ 0.5 and 5–10:1, respectively), while the PUFA + (MUFA/SFA) intake was below the recommended level (1.9 ± 0.4 vs. ≥ 2) for a healthy diet [41].

An inappropriate dietary intake jeopardizes sports performance and the benefits of training. It is crucial to plan a diet education programme to optimise the pattern of food and drink consumed (in this case, increasing the consumption of carbohydrates while decreasing that of fats and proteins) and hence improve athletes' sporting performance and health.

Future studies should aim to explore LP, as a function of sex, the sport played and the phase of the season (with respect to pre-season, specific preparatory periods, and competitions) and whether there are changes in the profile with diet programmes or supplementation, and in addition should involve hyperlipidaemic subjects.

The limiting factor in this study is the small sample size. For results in future research to be significant, the samples should be larger, or the period of the study should be extended. On the other hand, this study is the first in which the LP of professional sportswomen has been compared with their dietary intake and even these provisional data have allowed us to identify some significant trends that motivate future research.

Conclusions

According to the data recorded, physical activity during the first 11 weeks of training in the professional women's volleyball season is heart-healthy because it improves the LP (with a decrease in the LDLc and TC/HDLc and LDLc/HDLc indices). This was true despite the intakes of fats by the players being inadequate, in terms of both quality and quantity. In addition, the exercise carried out by the players during the 11-week study seemed to improve their HDL levels.

Competing interests
The authors declare that they have no competing interests.

Authors' contributions
All authors read and extensively reviewed and contributed to the final manuscript as follows MAJ: Conception and design, analysis and interpretation of the data, drafting and critically reviewing the manuscript. SCP: Interpretation of the data, drafting and critically reviewing the manuscript. UA: Drafting and critically reviewing the manuscript. MSJ: Drafting and critically reviewing the manuscript. SJ: Conception, interpretation of the data, drafting and critically reviewing the manuscript. All authors read and approved the final version of the manuscript.

Acknowledgements
The authors wish to thank the players involved for their participation in the study and Dr. Juan Miguel Orta Costea for his help in the collection of blood samples.

Author details
[1]Department of Nutrition and Dietetics, Haro Volleyball Club, Nutrition Centre of La Rioja, C/ Donantes de sangre, 14.26200 Haro, La Rioja, Spain. [2]Department of Biomedical Sciences, University of Leon, Leon, Spain. [3]Institute of Biomedicine (IBIOMED), University of Leon, Leon, Spain. [4]Public Sports Education Center, Kirolene, Basque Government, Scientific-Technical Planning for Sports, Nutriaktive, Vitoria-Gasteiz, Spain. [5]Department of Nursing, Faculty of Health Sciences, University of Alicante, Alicante, Spain. [6]Visiting Researcher at the University of the Basque Country, Leioa, Bizkaia, Spain.

References
1. Giacosa A, Barale R, Bavaresco L, Gatenby P, Gerbi V, Janssens J, Johnston B, Kas K, La Vecchia C, Mainguet P: **Cancer prevention in Europe: the Mediterranean diet as a protective choice.** *Eur J Cancer Prev* 2013, **22**(1):90–95.
2. Nishida C, Uauy R, Kumanyika S, Shetty P: **The joint WHO/FAO expert consultation on diet, nutrition and the prevention of chronic diseases: process, product and policy implications.** *Public Health Nutr* 2004, **7**(1A):245–250.
3. Badimon JJ, Santos-Gallego CG, Badimon L: **Importance of HDL cholesterol in atherothrombosis: how did we get here? Where are we going?** *Rev Esp Cardiol* 2010, **63**(Suppl 2):20–35.
4. Katcher HI, Hill AM, Lanford JL, Yoo JS, Kris-Etherton PM: **Lifestyle approaches and dietary strategies to lower LDL-cholesterol and triglycerides and raise HDL-cholesterol.** *Endocrinol Metab Clin North Am* 2009, **38**(1):45–78.
5. Schaefer EJ: **Lipoproteins, nutrition, and heart disease.** *Am J Clin Nutr* 2002, **75**(2):191–212.
6. Kelley GA, Kelley KS, Roberts S, Haskell W: **Combined effects of aerobic exercise and diet on lipids and lipoproteins in overweight and obese adults: a meta-analysis.** *J Obes* 2012, **2012**:985902.
7. Mielgo-Ayuso J, Urdampilleta A, Martinez-Sanz JM, Seco J: **Dietary iron intake and deficiency in elite women volleyball players.** *Nutr Hosp* 2012, **27**(5):1592–1597.
8. Tambalis K, Panagiotakos DB, Kavouras SA, Sidossis LS: **Responses of blood lipids to aerobic, resistance, and combined aerobic with resistance exercise training: a systematic review of current evidence.** *Angiology* 2009, **60**(5):614–632.
9. Ruiz JR, Mesa JL, Mingorance I, Rodriguez-Cuartero A, Castillo MJ: **Sports requiring stressful physical exertion cause abnormalities in plasma lipid profile.** *Rev Esp Cardiol* 2004, **57**(6):499–506.
10. Witek K: **Changes in serum lipid profile of elite volleyball players in the competition period.** *Biomed Hum Kinet* 2009, **1**:63–66.
11. World Medical Association: **Declaration of Helsinki: ethical principles for medical research involving human subjects.** *JAMA* 2000, **284**(23):3043–3045.
12. Stewart A, Marfell-Jones M, Olds T, de Ridder H: *International standards for anthropometric assessment.* ISAK: Lower Hutt, New Zealand; 2011.

13. Faulkner J: Physiology of swimming and diving. In Exercise Physiology. Edited by Fall. New York: Academic press; 1968:415–446.
14. Friedewald WT, Levy RI, Fredrickson DS: Estimation of the concentration of low-density lipoprotein cholesterol in plasma, without use of the preparative ultracentrifuge. Clin Chem 1972, 18(6):499–502.
15. Martin-Moreno JM, Boyle P, Gorgojo L, Maisonneuve P, Fernandez-Rodriguez JC, Salvini S, Willett WC: Development and validation of a food frequency questionnaire in Spain. Int J Epidemiol 1993, 22(3):512–519.
16. Mariscal-Arcas M, Romaguera D, Rivas A, Feriche B, Pons A, Tur JA, Olea-Serrano F: Diet quality of young people in southern Spain evaluated by a Mediterranean adaptation of the Diet Quality Index-International (DQI-I). Br J Nutr 2007, 98(6):1267–1273.
17. Bondia-Pons I, Mayneris-Perxachs J, Serra-Majem L, Castellote AI, Marine A, Lopez-Sabater MC: Diet quality of a population sample from coastal north-east Spain evaluated by a Mediterranean adaptation of the diet quality index (DQI). Public Health Nutr 2010, 13(1):12–24.
18. Farran A, Zamora R, Cervera P: Tablas de composición de alimentos del CESNID. Madrid: McGraw-Hill-Interamericana; 2003.
19. Schroder H, Fito M, Estruch R, Martinez-Gonzalez MA, Corella D, Salas-Salvado J, Lamuela-Raventos R, Ros E, Salaverria I, Fiol M, Lapetra J, Vinyoles E, Gomez-Gracia E, Lahoz C, Serra-Majem L, Pinto X, Ruiz-Gutierrez V, Covas MI: A short screener is valid for assessing Mediterranean diet adherence among older Spanish men and women. J Nutr 2011, 141(6):1140–1145.
20. Ronnemaa T, Marniemi J, Puukka P, Kuusi T: Effects of long-term physical exercise on serum lipids, lipoproteins and lipid metabolizing enzymes in type 2 (non-insulin-dependent) diabetic patients. Diab Res 1988, 7(2):79–84.
21. Halbert JA, Silagy CA, Finucane P, Withers RT, Hamdorf PA: Exercise training and blood lipids in hyperlipidemic and normolipidemic adults: a meta-analysis of randomized, controlled trials. Eur J Clin Nutr 1999, 53(7):514–522.
22. Kelley G, Kelley K: Effects of aerobic exercise on lipids and lipoproteins in adults with type 2 diabetes: a meta-analysis of randomized-controlled trials. Public Health 2007, 121(9):643–655.
23. Huffman KM, Hawk VH, Henes ST, Ocampo CI, Orenduff MC, Slentz CA, Johnson JL, Houmard JA, Samsa GP, Kraus WE, Bales CW: Exercise effects on lipids in persons with varying dietary patterns-does diet matter if they exercise? Responses in Studies of a Targeted Risk Reduction Intervention through Defined Exercise I. Am Heart J 2012, 164(1):117–124.
24. Pattyn N, Cornelissen VA, Eshghi SR, Vanhees L: The effect of exercise on the cardiovascular risk factors constituting the metabolic syndrome: a meta-analysis of controlled trials. Sports Med 2013, 43(2):121–133.
25. Berg A, Frey I, Baumstark MW, Halle M, Keul J: Physical activity and lipoprotein lipid disorders. Sports Med 1994, 17(1):6–21.
26. Cabrera de Leon A, Rodriguez-Perez Mdel C, Rodriguez-Benjumeda LM, Ania-Lafuente B, Brito-Diaz B, Muros de Fuentes M, Almeida-Gonzalez D, Batista-Medina M, Aguirre-Jaime A: Sedentary lifestyle: physical activity duration versus percentage of energy expenditure. Rev Esp Cardiol 2007, 60(3):244–250.
27. Stefanutti C, Mazza F: Multiple lipid-lowering treatment in pediatric patients with hyperlipidemia. Med Chem 2012, 8(6):1171–1181.
28. Green PP, Namboodiri KK, Hannan P, Martin J, Owen AR, Chase GA, Kaplan EB, Williams L, Elston RC: The Collaborative Lipid Research Clinics Program Family Study. III. Transformations and covariate adjustments of lipid and lipoprotein levels. Am J Epidemiol 1984, 119(6):959–974.
29. Kiens B: Skeletal muscle lipid metabolism in exercise and insulin resistance. Physiol Rev 2006, 86(1):205–243.
30. Boraita A: La práctica deportiva mejora el perfil lipídico plasmático, pero ¿a cualquier intensidad? Rev Esp Cardiol 2004, 57(6):495–498.
31. Gonzalez-Gross M, Gutierrez A, Mesa JL, Ruiz-Ruiz J, Castillo MJ: Nutrition in the sport practice: adaptation of the food guide pyramid to the characteristics of athletes diet. Arch Latinoam Nutr 2001, 51(4):321–331.
32. Volek JS, Forsythe CE, Kraemer WJ: Nutritional aspects of women strength athletes. Br J Sports Med 2006, 40(9):742–748.
33. American Dietetic Association, Dietitians of Canada, American College of Sports Medicine, Rodriguez NR, Di Marco NM, Langley S: American College of Sports Medicine position stand. Nutrition and athletic performance. Med Sci Sports Exerc 2009, 41(3):709–731.
34. Papadopoulou SK, Papadopoulou SD, Gallos GK: Macro- and micro-nutrient intake of adolescent Greek female volleyball players. Int J Sport Nutr Exerc Metab 2002, 12(1):73–80.
35. Anderson DE: The impact of feedback on dietary intake and body composition of college women volleyball players over a competitive season. J Strength Cond Res 2010, 24(8):2220–2226.
36. Papadopoulou SK, Papadopoulou SD: Nutritional status of top team-sport athletes according to body fat. Nutrition & Food Science 2010, 40(1):64–73.
37. Gabbett T, Georgieff B: Physiological and anthropometric characteristics of Australian junior national, state, and novice volleyball players. J Strength Cond Res 2007, 21(3):902–908.
38. Hassapidou MN, Manstrantoni A: Dietary intakes of elite female athletes in Greece. J Hum Nutr Diet 2001, 14(5):391–396.
39. Beals KA: Eating behaviors, nutritional status, and menstrual function in elite female adolescent volleyball players. J Am Diet Assoc 2002, 102(9):1293–1296.
40. Mensink RP, Zock PL, Kester AD, Katan MB: Effects of dietary fatty acids and carbohydrates on the ratio of serum total to HDL cholesterol and on serum lipids and apolipoproteins: a meta-analysis of 60 controlled trials. Am J Clin Nutr 2003, 77(5):1146–1155.
41. Moreiras Tuni O, Carbajal Azcona Á, Cabrera L: Tablas de composición de alimentos. Madrid: Ediciones Pirámide; 2005.

5

Effects of 28 days of beta-alanine and creatine supplementation on muscle carnosine, body composition and exercise performance in recreationally active females

Julie Y Kresta[1†], Jonathan M Oliver[2†], Andrew R Jagim[3†], James Fluckey[4], Steven Riechman[5], Katherine Kelly[6], Cynthia Meininger[6], Susanne U Mertens-Talcott[7], Christopher Rasmussen[8] and Richard B Kreider[8*]

Abstract

Background: The purpose of this study was to examine the short-term and chronic effects of β-ALA supplementation with and without creatine monohydrate on body composition, aerobic and anaerobic exercise performance, and muscle carnosine and creatine levels in college-aged recreationally active females.

Methods: Thirty-two females were randomized in a double-blind, placebo-controlled manner into one of four supplementation groups: β-ALA only (BA, n = 8), creatine only (CRE, n = 8), β-ALA and creatine combined (BAC, n = 9) and placebo (PLA, n = 7). Participants supplemented for four weeks included a loading phase for the creatine for week 1 of 0.3 g/kg of body weight and a maintenance phase for weeks 2–4 of 0.1 g/kg of body weight, with or without a continuous dose of β-ALA of 0.1 g/kg of body weight with doses rounded to the nearest 800 mg capsule providing an average of 6.1 ± 0.7 g/day of β-ALA. Participants reported for testing at baseline, day 7 and day 28. Testing sessions consisted of obtaining a resting muscle biopsy of the vastus lateralis, body composition measurements, performing a graded exercise test on the cycle ergometer for VO_{2peak} with lactate threshold determination, and multiple Wingate anaerobic capacity tests.

Results: Although mean changes were consistent with prior studies and large effect sizes were noted, no significant differences were observed among groups in changes in muscle carnosine levels (BA 35.3 ± 45; BAC 42.5 ± 99; CRE 0.72 ± 27; PLA 13.9 ± 44%, p = 0.59). Similarly, although changes in muscle phosphagen levels after one week of supplementation were consistent with prior reports and large effect sizes were seen, no statistically significant effects were observed among groups in changes in muscle phosphagen levels and the impact of CRE supplementation appeared to diminish during the maintenance phase. Additionally, significant time × group × Wingate interactions were observed among groups for repeated sprint peak power normalized to bodyweight (p = 0.02) and rate of fatigue (p = 0.04).

Conclusions: Results of the present study did not reveal any consistent additive benefits of BA and CRE supplementation in recreationally active women.

---

* Correspondence: rkreider@hlkn.tamu.edu
†Equal contributors
[8]Department of Health and Kinesiology, Exercise and Sport Nutrition Lab,
Texas A&M University, College Station, TX 77843-4243, USA
Full list of author information is available at the end of the article

Background

Prior research has shown that beta-alanine (β-ALA) supplementation (e.g., 3.2 g/day to 6.4 g/day for 2 to 10-weeks) increases in muscle carnosine levels, with greater increases observed when larger total dosages have been consumed over time [1-8]. It has been suggested that an increase in intramuscular carnosine levels may lead to an enhanced muscle buffering capacity therefore improving performance by limiting the accumulation of hydrogen ions (H^+) [2,4,6,7,9,10]. The amount of carnosine elevation ranges from around 10% after two weeks [8] to around 80% after ten weeks [10]. A recent review on the ergogenic benefits of β-ALA supplementation suggested bouts of exercise lasting 1–3 minutes seemed to provide the most benefit with mixed results seen during shorter bouts of exercise [11]. There is also some evidence suggesting that β-ALA supplementation may positively affect body composition when combined with training [12], time to exhaustion [5,11], anaerobic exercise markers such as ventilatory threshold (VT) [13], as well as blood lactate levels [14,15]. The effects of creatine monohydrate have been extensively researched over recent years with respects to the effects on anaerobic exercise performance [16]. High intensity exercise bouts require a faster rate of ATP resynthesis, which is most quickly attained by breaking down phosphocreatine (PCr) [17,18]. Creatine monohydrate supplementation (e.g., 20 g/day for 5 to 7-days and 3–5 g/day thereafter) has been shown to increase the muscle creatine and PCr stores to assist in ATP resynthesis during high intensity exercise [19-21].

Given the reported ergogenic value of β-ALA and creatine supplementation, recent studies have begun to examine the combined effects of β-ALA and creatine monohydrate supplementation on anaerobic exercise performance and muscle carnosine and creatine levels. Results have shown improvements in exercise performance variables such as peak oxygen uptake (VO_{2peak}), lactate threshold (LT), and time to exhaustion with a combined supplementation strategy [15]. Similarly, Hoffman and colleagues [22] reported that 10-weeks of β-ALA and creatine monohydrate supplementation during resistance-training had both independent and potentially synergistic ergogenic benefits in male strength/power athletes. However, more research is needed to determine whether there may be additive benefit of co-supplementation of β-ALA and creatine monohydrate supplementation during training. Additionally, the majority of beta-alanine and creatine supplementation studies have used males as participants. Therefore, while it is generally understood how beta-alanine supplementation can affect muscle carnosine levels as well as exercise performance in men, less is known how females will respond to beta-alanine supplementation during training [9,13,14,22-24]. Studies that have examined the effects of β-ALA supplementation in

women have reported mixed results [25,26]. Therefore, the purpose of this study was to examine the short-term (7-days) and chronic effects (28-days) of β-ALA supplementation with and without creatine monohydrate on body composition, aerobic and anaerobic exercise performance, and muscle carnosine and muscle creatine levels in college-aged, recreationally-active females. We theorized that co-supplementation of β-ALA and creatine monohydrate may lead to greater ergogenic and performance adaptations by synergistically enhancing anaerobic and/or aerobic capacity.

Methods

Experimental design

The present study was a randomized double-blind, placebo-controlled trial that recruited apparently healthy, moderately active females between the ages of 18 and 35 years to participate in the study. Moderately active was defined as having a consistent recent history of participating in exercise (e.g., running, cycling, swimming, resistance training, fitness classes, etc.) for at least 30 minutes per day for 3-days per-week for at least 3 months. Participants were not allowed to participate if they had taken ergogenic levels of nutritional supplements that may have affected muscle mass or anaerobic exercise capacity (i.e. creatine, β-ALA, ergogenic levels of nutritional caffeine, etc.) for at least three months prior to the start of the study. Those who met entrance criteria attended a familiarization session during which time they were familiarized to the study protocol with verbal and written explanations of the study requirements. Participants still interested and meeting the entrance criteria signed informed consent statements in compliance with the Human Participants Guidelines of Texas A&M University and the American College of Sports Medicine. During the familiarization session, participants were also weighed using a standing scale and asked to perform a practice Wingate exercise test on the cycle ergometer at 75% maximal effort. Participants were instructed to find a comfortable seat height and handle bar position which was recorded for subsequent testing sessions. Following the practice Wingate test they were given guidelines to follow for maintaining and recording physical activity during their involvement in the study and scheduled for all subsequent testing sessions and randomly assigned to one of four supplementation groups. Figure 1 shows a consort diagram of those found eligible, initiated, and completed the study protocol. Individuals who did not complete the study did so for reasons unrelated to the study protocol.

Resting and exercise testing

Resting and exercise testing was performed at baseline prior to any supplementation, at one week of supplementation, and after four weeks at the completion of the

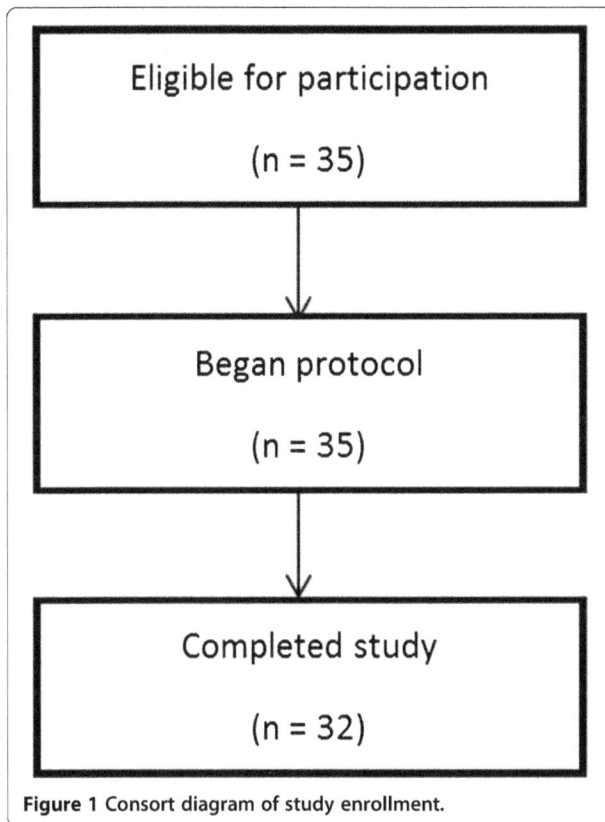

Figure 1 Consort diagram of study enrollment.

study. Figure 2 outlines the events of the testing sessions. Participants were asked to abstain from exercise for 24 hours and fast for at least eight hours prior to baseline testing. One day prior to exercise testing, participants received a percutaneous muscle biopsy from the vastus lateralis muscle of the right leg using standard procedures

for the Bergstrom method [27]. Muscle samples were immediately frozen at −80° until analyzed.

The morning after the biopsy, participants were asked to fast for at least eight hours before being asked to consume a standard meal replacement drink (*Boost® Original, Nestlé S.A., Vevey, Switzerland*) four hours before reporting to the lab in order to standardize nutritional intake prior to exercise testing. Once reporting to the lab, they were weighed using a free standing scale (*Cardinal Detecto Scale Model 8430, Webb City, Missouri*) and had body composition determined using a Dual Energy X-Ray Absorptiometer (DEXA) [*Discovery QDR Series, Hologic Inc., Waltham, MA*]. Quality control calibration procedures were performed on a spine phantom (*Hologic-X-CLAIBER Model DPA/QDR-1 anthropometric spine phantom*) and a density step calibration phantom prior to each testing session. Mean test-retest reliability studies performed on athletes in the lab had yielded mean coefficients of variation for total bone mineral content and total fat free/soft tissue mass of 0.31% to 0.45% with a mean intra-class correlation of 0.985 [28]. They then had their total body water (TBW) measured using bioelectrical impedance analysis (*ImpediMed DF50, San Diego, CA*). Following the resting measures, participants began exercise testing starting with a maximal graded exercise test (GXT) using an incremental protocol on the Lode Excaliber Sport 925900 cycle ergometer (*Lode BV, Groningen, The Netherlands*) with metabolic measurements recorded on the ParvoMedics True One 2400 Metabolic System (*ParvoMedics, Sandy, Utah*). The protocol began at 50 W maintaining 70 rpm and the intensity was increased by 25 W every three minutes until a pedaling rate of 70 rpm was no longer maintained. Previous research has indicated

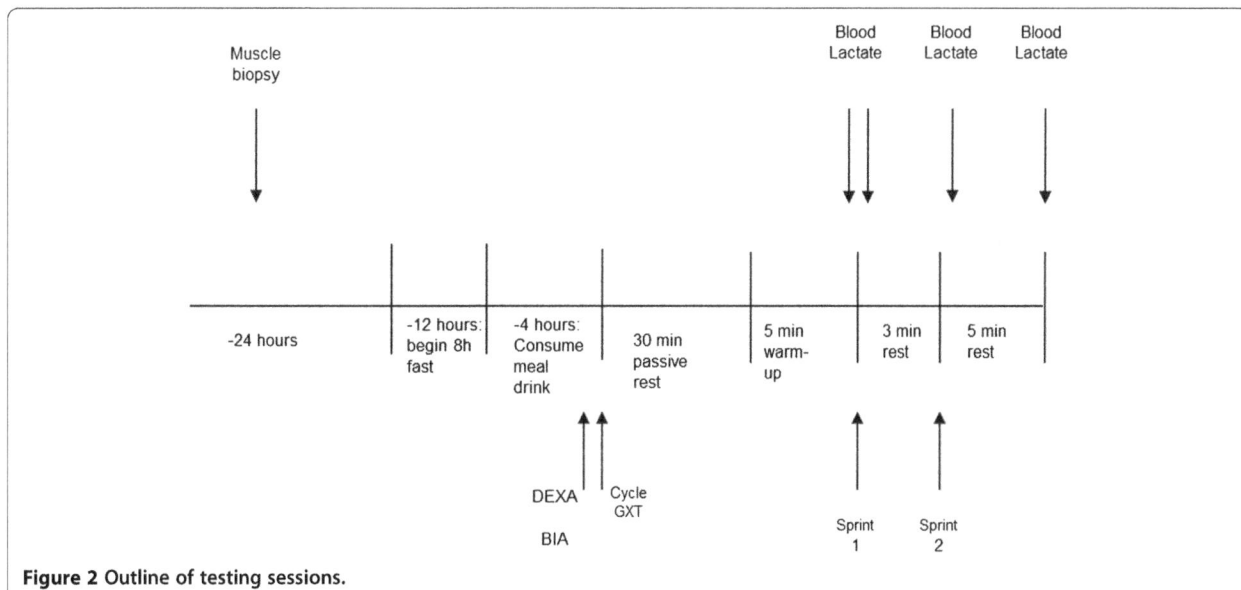

Figure 2 Outline of testing sessions.

a mean intra-class correlation of 0.994 and a mean intra-class coefficient of variation of 4.7% when using the ParvoMedics True One 2400 Metabolic system [29]. Calibration procedures were completed prior to each testing session.

Blood samples were taken from the fingertips in the final minute of each stage of exercise and five minutes into the recovery to determine LT. Lactate was determined using a Lactate Scout (*Sports Resource Group, USA*) handheld analysis device. Previous research has yielded a mean intra-class correlation of 0.91 and a mean intra-class coefficient of variation of 10.2% [30]. Calibration procedures were completed prior to each testing session. The LT was calculated two different ways including the point at which blood lactate concentrations rises more than 1.0 mM/l from the previously recorded value LT and the point at which blood lactate level was greater than or equal to 4.0 (also termed the onset of blood lactate, OBLA). All values were reported as a percent of VO_{2peak}. The ventilatory threshold (VT) was determined as the point during the GXT where pulmonary ventilation increased at a disproportional rate with VO_2, and was also recorded as a percent of VO_{2peak}. Following the GXT, participants rested passively for 30 minutes and then performed two 30-sec Wingate Anaerobic Capacity Tests at a standardized work rate of 7.5 J/kg/rev. The seat position was standardized between trials and the participant was asked to pedal as fast as possible prior to application of the workload and sprint at all-out maximal capacity during the 30-second test with 3 minutes of passive rest in between. Blood was taken from the fingertips before the start of Wingate 1, immediately following Wingate 2, and after 5 minutes of passive recovery following the completion of both Wingate tests. Test-to-test variability in performing repeated Wingate anaerobic capacity tests in our laboratory yielded a coefficient of variation (CV) of ±15% with a test retest correlation of $r = 0.98$ for mean power [31]. Participants practiced the anaerobic capacity test during the familiarization session to minimize learning effects.

Supplementation protocol

The supplementation protocol was modified from those used by Hoffman et al. in 2006 [22] and Zoeller et al. in 2007 [15]. The creatine monohydrate (*Creapure*, *AlzChem Trostberg GmbH, Germany*) supplementation was provided in the form of a powder that the participants were instructed to mix with water (6–10 oz.). The β-ALA used in this study (*CarnoSyn*, *Natural Alternatives International, Inc., San Marcos, CA*) was a sustained release form of β-ALA that was provide in 800 mg capsules. In a double blinded manner, participants were matched to body mass and randomly assigned to either ingest β-ALA (BA, n = 8), creatine monohydrate (CRE,

n = 8), a combination of β-ALA and creatine monohydrate (BAC, n = 9), or a placebo (PLA, n = 7). The β-ALA only group received a dose of 0.1 g/kg body weight per day for the entire 28 days with 0.3 g/kg/day of dextrose for week 1 and 0.1 g/kg/day of dextrose for weeks 2–4. The creatine only group was given a dose of 0.3 g/kg/day of creatine for week 1 and 0.1 g/kg/day for weeks 2–4, with 0.1 g/kg/day maltodextrin for the 28 days. The β-ALA and creatine combined group consumed a 0.1 g/kg/day of β-ALA for the entire 28 days (about 6.1 ± 0.7 g/day) with 0.3 g/kg/day of creatine for week 1 (about 18 ± 1.8 g/day) and 0.1 g/kg/day of creatine for weeks 2–4 (about 6.1 ± 0.7 g/day). Finally, the placebo group was given 0.1 g/kg/day of maltodextrin capsules for all 28 days with 0.3 g/kg/day of dextrose powder for week 1 and 0.1 g/kg/day for weeks 2–4 which served as the placebo for creatine monohydrate. The β-ALA and matched placebo doses were rounded to the nearest 800 mg capsule while the creatine monohydrate and matched placebo doses were rounded to the nearest 0.1 g. The rationale in providing more of a relative dosage of β-ALA was an attempt to help normalize the administration β-ALA to body mass to doses that are commercially available. Participants were instructed to take divided doses of the supplements at 4 intervals throughout the day with water and/or food, as close to 8:00 am, 12:00 pm, 4:00 pm and 8:00 pm as possible. Participants were given supplements one week at a time and were asked to return the empty containers to ensure compliance. They also completed supplementation logs each week to monitor compliance of supplementation.

Muscle analysis

The muscle samples were obtained using a modified Bergstrom muscle biopsy technique and were analyzed for phosphocreatine (PCr) and creatine (Cr) content based on methods from previous studies [32-34]. Percutaneous muscle biopsies (50–70 mg) were obtained from the middle portion of the vastus lateralis muscle of the thigh at the midpoint between the patella and greater trochanter of the femur. The biopsy needle was inserted 1–2 cm into the muscle prior to tissue extraction. Once the biopsy was taken, adipose tissue was trimmed from the muscle specimens and then the muscle sample was immediately frozen in liquid nitrogen and stored at –80°C for later analysis. A total of three muscle samples were obtained, two from one leg and one from the opposite leg (Day 0, 6, & 27). The left leg was used for pre and post biopsies with the right leg being used for the mid biopsy.

Muscle tissue samples were analyzed spectrophotometrically in duplicate to determine PCr and Cr content using methods developed by Harris and colleagues [20,21,32]. Briefly, approximately 50–70 mg of muscle tissue was cut and placed in a microfuge tube, and then placed in a vacuum centrifuge (*Savant ISS110 SpeedVac Concentrator,*

Thermo Scientific, Milford, MA) and centrifuged for 18–24 hours. Connective tissue was removed from the dried samples which were then ground into a powder in a porcelain plate and placed into pre-weighed microfuge tubes. Muscle metabolites were extracted in a 0.5 M perchloric acid/1 mM EDTA solution on ice for 15 minutes, while periodically vortexing. Samples were then centrifuged at 7,000 rpm for 5 minutes. The supernatant was transferred into a pre-weighed microfuge tube and neutralized with 2.1 M $KHCO_3$/0.3 M MOPS solution. The samples were then centrifuged again at 7,000 rpm for 5 minutes and the supernatant was removed and placed into microfuge tubes and frozen at −80°C.

Extracts were assayed for PCr in the presence of 50 mM Tris buffer, pH 7.4; 1 mM magnesium chloride, 0.5 mM dithiothreitol, 100 µM glucose, 50 µM $NADP^+$, 350 U/mL glucose-6-phosphate dehydrogenase. The assay was carried out in 13×75 glass screw-top tubes using 10 µL of sample to 1 mL of reagent. The reactant solution was vortexed and read using a fluorometer (*Shimadzu RFMini 150, Japan*) with an excitation wavelength of 360 nm and an emission wavelength of 460 nm. Twenty five mL of hexokinase solution was added to 1 mL of reagent and stabilized. For PCr, 20 µL of creatine kinase/ sulfodichlorophenol (CK/SDP) solution was added to the tubes, which were vortexed and incubated in a dark at room temperature for 60 minutes when samples were read again for post-reaction absorbance values.

Extracts were assayed for Cr in the presence of 50 mM imidazole buffer, pH 7.4; 5 mM magnesium chloride; 20 mM potassium chloride; 25 µM phosphoenolpyruvate; 200 µM ATP; 45 µM NADH; 1250 U/mL lactate dehydrogenase; 2000 U/mL pyruvate kinase. The assay was carried out in a standard fluorescence microplate reader using 10 µL of sample to 1 mL of reagent. The reactant solution was vortexed and read using a fluorometer (*Shimadzu RFMini 150, Japan*) with an excitation wavelength of 340 nm and an emission wavelength of 460 nm for baseline absorbance values. Five µL of CK (25 µ/mg) was added to 1 mL of the above buffer and stabilized using 1 mL of reagent. After 10 minutes the plate was read again for post-reaction absorbance values. Test to test reliability of duplicate muscle creatine assays was 0.22 ± 2.4% (r = 0.90) with a coefficient of variation of 6.8%. Creatine and PCr were analyzed using a SpectraMax 250 (*Molecular Devices, Sunnyvale, CA*). All results were expressed as mmol/kg dry weight (DW). Total muscle creatine content was calculated by adding the resulting amounts of PCr and Cr content together.

Muscle carnosine was analyzed using the HPLC procedures developed by Dunnett and Harris [35]. The muscle samples were prepared using the same drying methods as before. Muscle samples were analyzed using an Aquity-UPLC system (*Waters, Milford, MA*). Chromatography

was performed using a Thermo Scientific Hypersil ODS (150 mm × 4.6 mm ID) analytical column protected by a Hypersil ODS guard column. Solvents were filtered to 0.45 µm. Compounds were eluted using a solvent gradient at ambient temperature with the following mobile phases: LINE A: Solvent A:20 mM phosphate buffer [(20 mM Na_2HPO_4 (2.84 g/l) + 20 mM $NaH_2PO_4.2H_2O$ (3.12 g/l)], pH 6.8 – tetrahydrofuran (995:5 v/v); LINE B: Solvent B: 20 mM phosphate buffer, pH 6.8 – methanol - acetonitrile (500:350:150, v/v); LINE C: 100% methanol; LINE D: 100% water; 2 liters 20 mM Na_2HPO_4 = 5.68 g; 2 liters 20 mM $NaH_2PO_4.2H_2O$ = 6.24 g.

Statistical analysis

Data were analyzed using SPSS 20.0 software (*IBM, Chicago, IL*). Missing data, if any, were replaced using the last observed value or series mean [36]. One-way Analysis of Variance (ANOVA) was used to analyze baseline demographic data. Multivariate Analysis of Variance (MANOVA) with repeated measures was used to analyze logically-related variables. The Wilks' Lambda time and group × time p-levels were used to assess the overall MANOVA effects. Univariate tests from the MANOVA are presented to show individual variable results. In some instances, quadratic interaction p-levels are reported indicating that non-linear but significant differences were observed among groups over time. On select variables, delta values or percent change values were calculated and analyzed by ANOVA with repeated measures in order to evaluate the change in values from baseline. Data were considered statistically significant when the p-value was less than 0.05 while trends were considered when p-values ranged between 0.05 and 0.10. Tukey's least significant difference (LSD) post hoc analyses were used to determine where the significance was obtained. Cohen's *d* calculations for effect size were performed to assess magnitude of effect. Non-significant data that showed moderate to large effects sizes were also noted as trends for follow-up with larger sample populations. Data are presented as means ± standard deviation, except group means were presented ± standard error of the mean.

Results

A total of 32 apparently healthy, recreationally active females completed the protocol for the present study. Participants were 21.5 ± 2.8 years, 60.5 ± 6.1 kg, 40.2 ± 3.8 kg fat free mass, and 26.7 ± 5.8% body fat. One-way ANOVA analysis revealed no significant differences (p > 0.05) between groups at baseline for age, weight, fat free mass, body fat percentage, muscle carnosine, or muscle phosphagen levels.

Muscle carnosine and phosphagen levels

Table 1 presents muscle carnosine and phosphagen levels observed in the present study. Muscle samples were

Table 1 Muscle carnosine, creatine, phosphocreatine, and total creatine over 4 weeks

	BA	BAC	CRE	PLA	Time	P value
Carnosine (µmol/g)						
Baseline	19.74 ± 8.69	20.81 ± 7.66	20.80 ± 2.81	15.70 ± 4.70	19.27 ± 6.50	T = 0.22
4 Weeks	23.68 ± 1.56	24.23 ± 4.09	21.04 ± 7.00	16.53 ± 4.80	21.37 ± 5.31	G = 0.04
Group	21.71 ± 1.44[d]	22.52 ± 1.34[d]	20.92 ± 1.44[d]	16.12 ± 1.70[abc]		T × G = 0.82
Creatine (mmol/kg DW)						
Baseline	47.13 ± 19.88	59.82 ± 37.7	72.96 ± 29.59	59.85 ± 7.79	59.92 ± 27.6	$T_q = 0.07$
1 Week	50.73 ± 26.83	65.49 ± 15.25	88.55 ± 38.72	68.17 ± 7.74	67.80 ± 24.9	G = 0.14
4 Weeks	42.33 ± 16.24	59.90 ± 9.77	67.72 ± 15.94	57.19 ± 8.07	57.28 ± 14.3	T × G = 0.99
Group	46.73 ± 8.26	61.74 ± 6.24	76.4 ± 8.26	61.74 ± 8.26		
Phosphocreatine (mmol/kg DW)						
Baseline	22.18 ± 4.28	22.94 ± 18.02	31.69 ± 16.54	21.35 ± 4.44	24.29 ± 13.3	T = 0.10
1 Week	25.91 ± 9.88	32.61 ± 19.62	23.43 ± 4.40	24.08 ± 4.23	27.47 ± 13.0	G = 0.98
4 Weeks	34.75 ± 7.38†[b]	26.87 ± 7.04[a]	30.51 ± 6.26	31.43 ± 9.39	30.25 ± 7.49	$T × G_q = 0.05$
Group	27.61 ± 4.69	27.47 ± 3.54	28.55 ± 4.69	25.62 ± 4.69		
Total creatine (mmol/kg DW)						
Baseline	63.04 ± 23.30	82.75 ± 37.19	105.11 ± 26.57	80.76 ± 11.18	82.89 ± 29.8	T = 0.76
1 Week	59.47 ± 27.07	94.79 ± 8.30	111.98 ± 37.99	85.53 ± 4.39	89.02 ± 26.8	G = 0.02
4 Weeks	74.28 ± 11.40	82.89 ± 5.32	96.89 ± 14.61	85.91 ± 18.07	84.66 ± 13.4	T × G = 0.79
Group	65.60 ± 7.65[bc]	86.81 ± 5.78[a]	104.66 ± 7.65[a]	84.07 ± 7.65		

Repeated measures ANOVA was performed on n = 27 (muscle carnosine) and a repeated measures MANOVA was performed on n = 19 (muscle phosphagen) samples. Individual group and time data are presented as means ± SD while time and group effects are presented as means ± SEM. MANOVA analysis on muscle creatine and phosphocreatine levels revealed an overall Wilks' Lambda time (p = 0.22) and group × time (p = 0.80) effects. Univariate ANOVA p-levels from MANOVA analysis are presented for each variable. BA signifies beta-alanine only group; BAC represents beta-alanine and creatine combined group; CRE represents the creatine only group; PLA represents the placebo group; T represents time p-level; G represents group p-level, and T × G represents interaction. $_q$represents quadratic p-level. † represents p < 0.05 difference from baseline. [a]represents p < 0.05 difference from BA group. [b]represents p < 0.05 difference from BAC group. [c]represents p < 0.05 difference from CRE group. [d]represents p < 0.05 difference from PLA group.

obtained from 31 total participants. There was sufficient sample to analyze 27 samples for carnosine and 19 samples for phosphagen levels. Repeated measures ANOVA analysis revealed no significant time (p = 0.22) or time × group (p = 0.82) effects among groups in muscle carnosine levels while a significant group effect (p = 0.04) was observed with supplementation. Post hoc analysis revealed that mean muscle carnosine levels in the PLA group were significantly lower than all other groups. One-way ANOVA of percent changes in muscle carnosine levels suggested that those in the BA and BAC groups observed the greatest increase in muscle carnosine levels; however, these apparent differences were not significantly different among groups (BA 35.3 ± 45; BAC 42.5 ± 99; CRE 0.72 ± 27; PLA 13.9 ± 44%, p = 0.59). Repeated measures MANOVA analysis on muscle creatine (Cr), phosphocreatine (PCr), and total creatine (Cr$_{tot}$) content revealed no overall Wilks' Lamda time (p = 0.22) or time by group (0.80) effects among groups. Univariate repeated measures ANOVA revealed significant quadratic differences among groups in changes in PCr ($p_q = 0.05$). However, differences observed could not be attributed to creatine supplementation. Delta analysis revealed that Cr$_{tot}$ levels increased to a greater degree after one week of loading (BA −3.57 ± 31; BAC 12.04 ± 36; CRE 6.86 ± 26; PLA −3.57 ± 31 mmol/kg DW) but these changes were not maintained during the maintenance period (BA 11.2 ± 17; BAC 0.13 ± 36; CRE −8.23 ± 29; PLA 11.2 ± 17 mmol/kg DW) and no time × group effects were observed among groups (p = 0.79).

Body composition

Table 2 presents changes in body composition and body water. A MANOVA was run on body weight and DEXA determined fat mass, fat free mass, and percent body fat. An overall Wilks' Lamda time effect was observed (p < 0.001) with no significant Wilks' Lamda time by group effects (p = 0.57). Repeated measures univariate ANOVA analysis revealed significant time effects in changes in body weight (p < 0.01), fat mass (p = 0.05), fat free mass (p < 0.001), and body fat (p = 0.02). However, no significant time × group effects were observed. No significant time (p = 0.79) or time × group (p = 0.36) effects were observed in percent total body water.

Table 2 Changes in body weight, body composition, and body water

	BA (n = 8)	BAC (n = 9)	CRE (n = 8)	PLA (n =7)	Time	P value
Body weight (kg)						
Baseline	63.16 ± 7.48	59.18 ± 5.42	61.15 ± 5.68	58.60 ± 5.81	60.54 ± 6.10	T = 0.01
1 Week	63.32 ± 7.30	59.33 ± 5.32	61.38 ± 5.94	59.22 ± 6.07	60.82 ± 6.11	G = 0.50
4 Weeks	63.60 ± 7.28	60.16 ± 5.02	61.26 ± 5.65	59.44 ± 5.88	61.14 ± 5.91†	T × G = 0.49
Group	63.36 ± 2.14	59.56 ± 2.02	61.26 ± 2.14	59.09 ± 2.29		
Fat mass (kg)						
Baseline	16.49 ± 4.93	14.10 ± 3.27	14.30 ± 4.88	14.76 ± 3.94	14.89 ± 4.19	T = 0.05
1 Week	15.52 ± 4.30	13.17 ± 2.57	13.86 ± 4.79	13.84 ± 4.07	14.08 ± 3.88†	G = 0.50
4 Weeks	16.59 ± 4.67	12.99 ± 3.01	13.44 ± 3.00	14.02 ± 4.39	14.23 ± 3.88	T × G = 0.57
Group	16.20 ± 1.38	13.42 ± 1.30	13.89 ± 1.38	14.21 ± 1.47		
Fat free mass (kg)						
Baseline	41.08 ± 4.20	39.77 ± 4.42	41.36 ± 3.33	38.40 ± 3.18	40.19 ± 3.35	T = 0.000
1 Week	42.05 ± 3.78	40.86 ± 4.65	42.06 ± 3.17	39.86 ± 3.38	41.23 ± 3.76†	G = 0.59
4 Weeks	41.40 ± 4.35	41.72 ± 4.44	42.55 ± 3.85	39.92 ± 3.09	41.45 ± 3.93†	T × G = 0.17
Group	41.51 ± 1.35	40.78 ± 1.27	41.99 ± 1.35	39.40 ± 1.44		
Percent fat (%)						
Baseline	28.23 ± 6.72	26.03 ± 5.25	25.25 ± 6.62	27.51 ± 5.34	26.71 ± 5.84	T = 0.02
1 Week	26.51 ± 5.08	24.40 ± 4.56	24.34 ± 6.52	25.46 ± 5.23	25.14 ± 5.19†	G = 0.62
4 Weeks	28.25 ± 6.34	23.76 ± 5.14	23.88 ± 4.11	25.60 ± 5.94	25.32 ± 5.48†	T × G = 0.45
Group	27.66 ± 1.88	24.73 ± 1.78	24.49 ± 1.88	26.19 ± 2.02		
Total body water (%)						
Baseline	51.31 ± 4.09	53.79 ± 6.56	48.86 ± 5.48	50.90 ± 4.48	51.30 ± 5.33	T = 0.66
1 Week	51.27 ± 3.83	52.56 ± 4.22	50.53 ± 3.61	50.01 ± 3.39	51.15 ± 3.72	G = 0.44
4 Weeks	50.61 ± 3.06	53.33 ± 3.96	51.66 ± 3.66	50.53 ± 3.08	51.59 ± 3.66	T × G = 0.30
Group	51.07 ± 1.45	53.23 ± 1.35	50.35 ± 1.47	50.48 ± 1.45		

Individual group and time data are presented as means ± SD while time and group effects are presented as means ± SEM. MANOVA analysis on DEXA body composition revealed overall Wilks' Lambda time (p < 0.001) and group × time (p = 0.57) effects. Univariate ANOVA p-levels from MANOVA analysis are presented for each body composition variable. BA signifies beta-alanine only group; BAC represents beta-alanine and creatine combined group; CRE represents the creatine only group; PLA represents the placebo group; T represents time p-level; G represents group p-level, and T × G represents interaction. † represents p < 0.05 difference from baseline.

Aerobic exercise performance

Table 3 presents changes observed among groups in VO_{2peak}, time to exhaustion, metabolic equivalents (METS), and ventilatory anaerobic threshold (VANT). MANOVA analysis revealed an overall Wilks' Lamda time effect (p = 0.049) and time × group effects (p = 0.017). Univariate ANOVA analysis revealed significant time effects in VANT (p < 0.001) with no significant time effects observed VO_{2peak} (p = 0.54), time to exhaustion (p = 0.30), and METS (p = 0.35). Interaction trends were observed among groups in VO_{2peak} ($p_q = 0.07$) and METS ($p_q = 0.07$) with no significant time × group differences observed among groups in time to exhaustion ($p_q = 0.13$) of VANT (p = 0.19). However, post-hoc analysis did not reveal any meaningful changes over time among or between groups.

Blood lactate and lactate threshold

Blood lactate levels observed during aerobic capacity testing is presented in Table 4. No significant differences were observed among groups in pre-exercise lactate levels. MANOVA analysis revealed no overall Wilks' Lamda time (p = 0.33) or group × time (p = 0.34) effects. ANOVA univariate analysis revealed a significant time × group interaction (p = 0.05) was observed in peak lactate among groups. Post-hoc analysis revealed that participants in the BA group had a significantly higher baseline peak lactate response than other groups and that peak lactate levels decreased after 4-weeks of supplementation after BA supplementation despite performing similar amounts of work. Participants in the BA group also experienced significantly less change in resting to maximal lactate levels despite performing similar amounts of work after

Table 3 Aerobic exercise capacity results observed among groups

	BA (n = 8)	BAC (n = 8)	CRE (n = 8)	PLA (n =6)	Time	P value
VO$_{2peak}$ (ml/kg/min)						
Baseline	41.50 ± 5.60	40.85 ± 6.98	34.20 ± 5.73	35.88 ± 9.65	38.26 ± 7.33	T = 0.54
1 Week	41.58 ± 5.96	39.89 ± 7.62	36.10 ± 6.04	33.75 ± 10.5	38.10 ± 7.72	G = 0.20
4 Weeks	41.53 ± 6.12	39.35 ± 6.96	35.34 ± 2.98	37.90 ± 9.03	38.57 ± 6.52	T × G$_q$ = 0.07
Group	41.53 ± 2.35	40.03 ± 2.35	35.21 ± 2.35	35.84 ± 2.72		
Time to exhaustion (sec)						
Baseline	1,249 ± 210	1,185 ± 303	963 ± 289	1,093 ± 324	1,125 ± 290	T = 0.30
1 Week	1,294 ± 246	1,196 ± 360	1,020 ± 251	1,032 ± 314	1,142 ± 303	G = 0.24
4 Weeks	1,293 ± 240	1,173 ± 319	1,046 ± 198	1,083 ± 310	1,153 ± 273	T × G$_q$ = 0.13
Group	1,279 ± 97	1,185 ± 97	1,010 ± 97	1,069 ± 112		
METS						
Baseline	11.88 ± 1.60	11.63 ± 2.00	9.79 ± 1.64	10.27 ± 2.77	10.93 ± 2.09	T = 0.56
1 Week	11.88 ± 1.70	11.41 ± 2.19	10.31 ± 1.74	9.63 ± 3.00	10.89 ± 2.21	G = 0.20
4 Weeks	11.85 ± 1.74	11.25 ± 1.98	10.09 ± 0.85	10.83 ± 2.54	11.02 ± 1.86	T × G$_q$ = 0.07
Group	11.87 ± 0.67	11.43 ± 0.67	10.06 ± 0.37	10.24 ± 0.78		
Ventilatory threshold (%VO$_{2peak}$)						
Baseline	86.81 ± 8.73	86.44 ± 10.73	77.01 ± 6.46	85.75 ± 10.64	83.89 ± 9.68	T < 0.001
1 Week	84.06 ± 7.34	85.35 ± 10.47	78.61 ± 10.53	84.78 ± 11.03	83.30 ± 9.79	G = 0.44
4 Weeks	78.59 ± 9.75	78.26 ± 13.02	76.50 ± 11.21	75.30 ± 9.63	77.29 ± 10.58†‡	T × G = 0.19
Group	83.15 ± 2.92	83.35 ± 2.92	77.38 ± 2.92	82.29 ± 3.73		

Individual group and time data are presented as means ± SD while time and group effects are presented as means ± SEM. MANOVA analysis revealed overall Wilks' Lambda time (p < 0.049) and group × time (p = 0.017) effects. Univariate ANOVA p-levels from MANOVA analysis are presented for each variable. BA signifies beta-alanine only group; BAC represents beta-alanine and creatine combined group; CRE represents the creatine only group; PLA represents the placebo group; T represents time p-level; G represents group p-level, and T × G represents interaction. $_q$ represents quadratic p-level. † represents p < 0.05 difference from baseline. ‡ represents p < 0.05 difference from 1 week.

1 and 4 weeks of BA supplementation. There were no significant differences for lactate threshold between groups or over time.

Anaerobic exercise performance

Results from the Wingate anaerobic capacity testing are presented in Table 5 and Figure 3. Peak Power (PP) normalized to body weight demonstrated a significant time × group × Wingate interaction (p = 0.02). Relative mean power, total work, and rate of fatigue significantly decreased from the first to second Wingate anaerobic capacity tests. Significant time × Wingate × group effects were observed among groups in relative peak power (p = 0.02) and rate of fatigue (p = 0.04). Post-hoc analysis demonstrated that placebo relative peak power and rate of fatigue values were lower than other groups at baseline no differences among groups after 1 or 4 weeks of supplementation. Additionally, relative peak power in the second sprint test in the CRE group was significantly greater than PLA values after 4 weeks of supplementation. Rate of fatigue after 4-weeks of supplementation was significant higher in the BA group compared to initial fatigue

values when performing the second Wingate test before supplementation.

Effect size analysis

Results from effect size calculations (Cohen's *d*) are presented in Table 6. Cohen's *d* effect size calculations were performed to compare supplementation group means to placebo after four weeks of supplementation to assess magnitude of effects. In comparison to placebo responses, BA supplementation resulted in large effects sizes for muscle carnosine (–2.00), muscle creatine (1.16), and rate of fatigue after the first (–1.44) and second (–1.25) Wingate test; BAC supplementation resulted in large effect sizes for muscle carnosine (–1.73) and rate of fatigue following the first Wingate test (–0.90); while CRE supplementation resulted in large effect sizes for changes in muscle creatine (–0.83) and moderate effect sizes for changes in muscle carnosine (–0.75), fat free mass (–0.69), and peak power during the first Wingate test (–0.83). These findings indicate that follow-up study with a larger sample size may reveal additional statistically significant findings among groups in these variables.

Table 4 Blood lactate results observed during the maximal exercise test

	BA (n = 8)	BAC (n = 9)	CRE (n = 8)	PLA (n =7)	Time	P value
Resting lactate (mmol/L)						
Baseline	1.44 ± 0.64	1.51 ± 0.44	1.33 ± 0.24	2.03 ± 0.96	1.56 ± 0.63	T = 0.71
1 Week	1.60 ± 0.61	1.43 ± 0.58	1.18 ± 0.28	1.54 ± 0.46	1.43 ± 0.51	G = 0.15
4 Weeks	1.58 ± 0.43	1.36 ± 0.49	1.53 ± 0.47	1.66 ± 0.45	1.52 ± 0.45	T × G = 0.38
Group	1.54 ± 0.12	1.43 ± 0.11	1.34 ± 0.12	1.74 ± 0.13		
Peak lactate (mmol/L)						
Baseline	12.91 ± 4.48[bcd]	8.63 ± 3.34[a]	9.71 ± 1.83[a]	7.54 ± 2.26	9.73 ± 3.64	T = 0.10
1 Week	10.43 ± 2.27	8.93 ± 3.18	9.20 ± 2.15	8.76 ± 1.25	9.33 ± 2.36	G = 0.07
4 Weeks	9.85 ± 1.89†	8.04 ± 2.59	8.99 ± 1.46	8.64 ± 2.28	8.87 ± 2.12	T × G = 0.05
Group	11.06 ± 0.77[bd]	8.54 ± 0.73[a]	9.30 ± 0.77	8.31 ± 0.83[a]		
Lactate threshold (% Peak VO$_2$)						
Baseline	65.18 ± 8.37	67.12 ± 14.08	66.09 ± 7.54	66.40 ± 10.14	66.22 ± 7.45	T = 0.14
1 Week	68.86 ± 5.98	69.92 ± 7.44	67.31 ± 6.64	64.51 ± 6.88	67.82 ± 6/75	G = 0.91
4 Weeks	67.04 ± 7.66	69.04 ± 6.91	69.61 ± 9.42	73.53 ± 5.83	69.67 ± 7.58	T × G = 0.86
Group	67.03 ± 1.73	68.70 ± 1.63	67.67 ± 1.73	68.15 ± 1.85		
Onset of blood lactate (%VO$_{2peak}$)						
Baseline	77.50 ± 9.89	82.94 ± 10.9	81.71 ± 8.82	83.81 ± 8.82	81.47 ± 9.54	T = 0.13
1 Week	78.50 ± 10.1	84.90 ± 9.30	83.48 ± 7.67	75.17 ± 17.43	80.82 ± 11.5	G = 0.58
4 Weeks	84.14 ± 8.35	86.68 ± 8.51	83.76 ± 11.68	84.77 ± 11.93	84.90 ± 9.70	T × G = 0.81
Group	80.05 ± 2.61	84.84 ± 2.46	82.98 ± 2.61	81.25 ± 2.79		
Blood lactate difference from baseline to max (mmol/L)						
Baseline	11.48 ± 4.19[bcd]	7.10 ± 3.52[a]	8.39 ± 1.75[ad]	5.51 ± 2.15[ac]	8.17 ± 3.67	T = 0.08
1 Week	8.83 ± 2.64†	7.43 ± 3.31	8.03 ± 2.03	7.20 ± 1.59	7.88 ± 2.49	G = 0.06
4 Weeks	8.28 ± 1.88†	6.61 ± 2.73	7.46 ± 1.26	6.81 ± 2.24	7.28 ± 2.12	T × G = 0.02
Group	9.53 ± 0.79	7.05 ± 0.74	7.96 ± 0.79	6.51 ± 0.84		

Individual group and time data are presented as means ± SD while time and group effects are presented as means ± SEM. MANOVA analysis revealed overall Wilks' Lambda time (p = 0.33) and group × time (p = 0.34) effects. Univariate ANOVA p-levels from MANOVA analysis are presented for each variable. BA signifies beta-alanine only group; BAC represents beta-alanine and creatine combined group; CRE represents the creatine only group; PLA represents the placebo group; T represents time p-level; G represents group p-level, and T × G represents interaction. † represents p < 0.05 difference from baseline. [a]represents p < 0.05 difference from BA group. [b]represents p < 0.05 difference from BAC group. [c]represents p < 0.05 difference from CRE group. [d]represents p < 0.05 difference from PLA group.

Discussion

The present study sought to determine whether co-supplementation of creatine monohydrate and β-ALA would provide additive ergogenic benefits on body composition, aerobic and/or anaerobic exercise performance in recreationally-active females. We hypothesized that co-supplementation of β-ALA and creatine monohydrate may lead to greater ergogenic and performance adaptations by synergistically enhancing anaerobic threshold, aerobic capacity, time to exhaustion, and/or the ability to perform repeated 30-second sprints. Results revealed that although some benefits were found from β-ALA and creatine supplementation, there appeared to be little additive benefits from co-supplementation in recreationally active women. The following provides additional assessment of results observed.

Muscle carnosine and phosphagens

Harris and colleagues [3] reported that β-ALA supplementation (3.2 g/day) resulted in a 42% increase in muscle carnosine levels after four weeks of supplementation. Results in the present study showed a mean increase in muscle carnosine levels of 35.3 ± 45% following BA supplementation and 42.5 ± 99% following BAC supplementation with average doses of 6.1 ± 0.7 g/day of β-ALA. While these mean changes in muscle carnosine levels following β-ALA supplementation are consistent with values reported in other studies [3,10,37-40] and we found some group effects with large effect sizes, no statistically significant interactions were observed among groups in muscle carnosine levels. The lack of statistical significance was apparently due to the large variability in muscle carnosine levels observed in response to β-ALA supplementation,

Table 5 Anaerobic capacity repeated sprint performance results

	BA (n = 8)	BAC (n = 9)	CRE (n = 8)	PLA (n =7)	Time	P value
Peak power (W/kg)						
Wingate 1						
Baseline	15.24 ± 4.87^d	14.74 ± 5.81^d	15.00 ± 3.95^d	11.09 ± 2.33^{abc}	14.13 ± 4.62	T = 0.67
1 Week	15.68 ± 3.85	13.88 ± 2.95	14.63 ± 2.82	13.43 ± 1.93	14.42 ± 2.97	G = 0.46
4 Weeks	14.77 ± 1.82	13.00 ± 3.40	13.46 ± 2.69	$14.26 \pm 4.73†$	13.83 ± 3.19	T × G = 0.58
Wingate 2	G × W = 0.91					
Baseline	13.51 ± 1.37	13.22 ± 3.15	$12.70 \pm 3.22†$	13.77 ± 3.62	13.28 ± 2.83	W = 0.59
1 Week	14.97 ± 1.95	14.96 ± 3.80	13.30 ± 3.38	12.67 ± 3.04	14.05 ± 3.16	T × W = 0.46
4 Weeks	13.68 ± 1.40	13.60 ± 3.89	15.48 ± 4.47	12.61 ± 2.47	13.87 ± 3.33	T × W × G = 0.02
Mean power (W/kg)						
Wingate 1						
Baseline	6.13 ± 0.97	5.77 ± 0.59	5.87 ± 0.53	5.44 ± 1.21	5.81 ± 0.84	T = 0.46
1 Week	6.25 ± 0.83	5.89 ± 0.65	6.01 ± 0.65	5.39 ± 0.67	5.90 ± 0.74	G = 0.36
4 Weeks	6.07 ± 0.80	5.75 ± 0.61	5.65 ± 0.86	5.69 ± 0.76	5.79 ± 0.74	T × G = 0.48
Wingate 2	G × W = 0.89					
Baseline	5.60 ± 0.87	5.42 ± 0.55	5.20 ± 0.54	5.10 ± 1.01	5.34 ± 0.74	W = 0.006
1 Week	5.48 ± 0.86	5.48 ± 0.62	5.37 ± 0.64	5.21 ± 0.96	5.39 ± 0.74	T × W =0.58
4 Weeks	5.27 ± 0.86	5.34 ± 0.57	5.19 ± 0.71	5.14 ± 1.05	5.24 ± 0.76	T × W × G = 0.70
Total work (J)						
Wingate 1						
Baseline	$11,467 \pm 1,048$	$10,476 \pm 1,499$	$10,764 \pm 1,420$	$9,541 \pm 2,262$	$10,591 \pm 1,653$	T = 0.97
1 Week	$11,793 \pm 1,438$	$10,719 \pm 1,531$	$11,081 \pm 1,726$	$9,566 \pm 1,422$	$10,826 \pm 1,660$	G = 0.07
4 Weeks	$11,494 \pm 1,430$	$10,561 \pm 1,223$	$10,437 \pm 2,071$	$10,152 \pm 1,698$	$10,674 \pm 1,621$	T × G = 0.33
Wingate 2	G × W = 0.92					
Baseline	$10,565 \pm 1,862$	$9,878 \pm 1,678$	$9,545 \pm 1,235$	$8,939 \pm 1,800$	$9,761 \pm 1,678$	W = 0.02
1 Week	$10,363 \pm 1,767$	$9,986 \pm 1,617$	$9,903 \pm 1,605$	$8,220 \pm 1,673$	$9,892 \pm 1,633$	T × W =0.48
4 Weeks	$10,019 \pm 1,785$	$9,835 \pm 1,320$	$9,548 \pm 1,556$	$9,168 \pm 2,041$	$9,663 \pm 1,619$	T × W × G = 0.66
Rate of fatigue (%)						
Wingate 1						
Baseline	107.4 ± 13.9^d	104.1 ± 14.3^d	103.7 ± 21.0	92.4 ± 9.4^{ab}	102.3 ± 15.6	T = 0.40
1 Week	105.8 ± 14.1	102.0 ± 9.9	96.2 ± 16.6	$108.4 \pm 9.4†$	102.9 ± 13.1	G = 0.09
4 Weeks	109.8 ± 10.9^d	103.4 ± 10.3	104.2 ± 15.9	93.1 ± 12.4^a	102.7 ± 13.1	T × G = 0.52
Wingate 2						G × W = 0.96
Baseline	$91.7 \pm 12.0†$	101.9 ± 11.4	96.0 ± 14.8	92.9 ± 13.7	95.9 ± 13.0	W = 0.02
1 Week	102.4 ± 9.5	97.9 ± 13.5	99.6 ± 11.2	90.3 ± 21.0	97.8 ± 14.1	T × W = 0.66
4 Weeks	$108.5 \pm 13.8‡^{bd}$	95.3 ± 16.6^{ad}	99.6 ± 15.9^d	82.8 ± 11.1^{abc}	99.1 ± 15.2	$T × W × G_q = 0.04$

Data are means ± SD. BA signifies beta-alanine only group; BAC represents beta-alanine and creatine combined group; CRE represents the creatine only group; PLA represents the placebo group; T represents time p-level; G represents group p-level, W represents Wingate p-level, T × G represents time by group interaction, T × W × G represents time × group × Wingate interactions, $_q$ represents quadratic p-level. MANOVA analysis revealed overall Wilks' Lambda time (p = 0.004), T × G (0.65), T × W (0.97), and T × G × W effects (p = 0.21). Univariate ANOVA p-levels from MANOVA analysis are presented for each variable. † represents p < 0.05 difference from Wingate 1 baseline while ‡ represents p < 0.05 difference from Wingate 2 baseline. ^{a}represents p < 0.05 difference from BA group. ^{b}represents p < 0.05 difference from BAC group. ^{c}represents p < 0.05 difference from CRE group. ^{d}represents p < 0.05 difference from PLA group. B

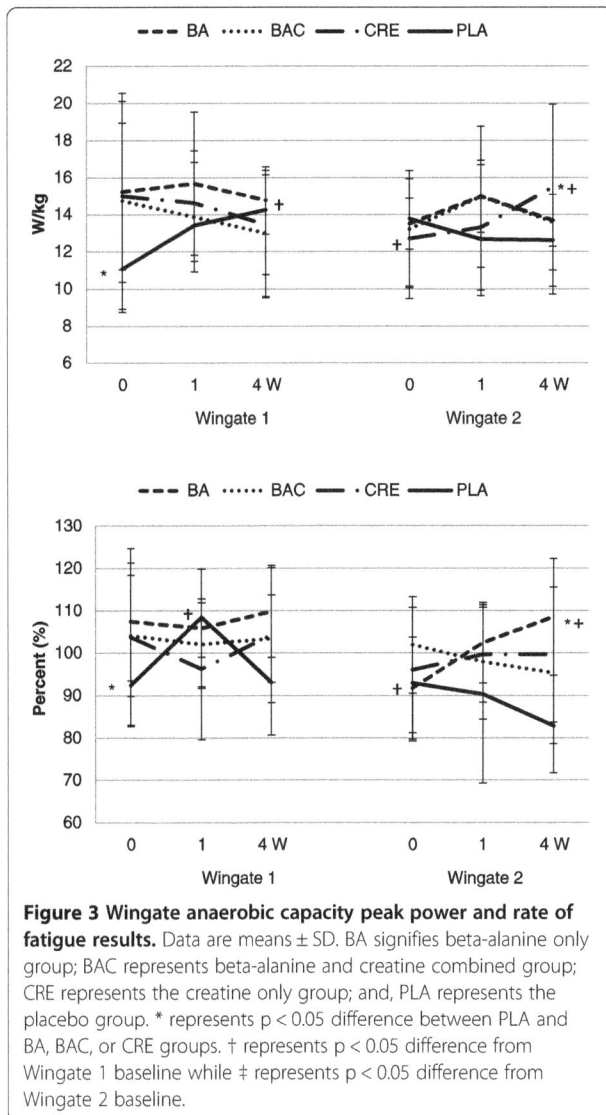

Figure 3 Wingate anaerobic capacity peak power and rate of fatigue results. Data are means ± SD. BA signifies beta-alanine only group; BAC represents beta-alanine and creatine combined group; CRE represents the creatine only group; and, PLA represents the placebo group. * represents p < 0.05 difference between PLA and BA, BAC, or CRE groups. † represents p < 0.05 difference from Wingate 1 baseline while ‡ represents p < 0.05 difference from Wingate 2 baseline.

assay variability, and/or inadequate sample size. More research is needed to determine the effects of β-ALA supplementation on muscle carnosine levels in recreationally-active women.

In terms of muscle phosphagen changes, it is important to note that the sample size for muscle creatine and phosphagen assessment was quite small due to prioritizing muscle carnosine assays as well as some samples not being large enough to run the appropriate assays. Therefore, statistical power is relatively low on these data. The creatine dosages used in the present study (0.3 g/kg/day of creatine for week 1 and 0.1 g/kg/day for weeks 2–4) are similar to those used with previous studies that indicate significant increases in muscle creatine after a loading and maintenance phase [19,21]. Results from the present study found non-significant increases in muscle creatine (+21%, +9.4%) and total creatine content (+6.5%, +14.5%) following creatine and β-ALA plus

creatine supplementation after 1-week of loading and 3-weeks of maintenance doses, respectively. While overall results were not statistically significant, mean changes observed support previous studies that have reported that creatine loading (e.g., 20 g/day or 0.3 g/kg/d for 5 to 7-days) results in an increase in muscle creatine content by 10–40% [16,19-21,31,41] and a large effect size was observed following creatine supplementation. While the lack of significance may have simply been a result of the small sample size, it is also known that there is individual variability in response to creatine supplementation [19-21]. Additionally, measurement of muscle PCr levels can be challenging.

It is also possible that sex may have played a role in response to creatine and/or β-ALA supplementation. In this regard, most studies on creatine and β-ALA supplementation have been conducted on males and there is some evidence that females may respond differently to creatine and/or β-ALA supplementation. For example, Fosberg and colleagues [42] reported that females had greater total creatine amounts relative to tissue weight; however, other studies show there is no difference between males and females [40,43]. There are also some data suggesting that men may have greater muscle carnosine levels than women [4,44]; however, a recent study showed sex did not have an effect on increasing carnosine levels with supplementation [40]. Additionally, Bex and coworkers [45] reported that carnosine loading is more pronounced in trained versus untrained individuals. Thus, it is possible that sex and/or the types and/or amounts of training performed among participants may have influenced response to creatine and/or β-ALA supplementation.

Body composition

As expected, body weight and markers of body composition improved over time during training in all groups. However, no significant differences were observed among groups. These findings support findings that females may experience less changes in body mass and/or fat free mass in response to creatine supplementation during training than is typically observed in men [16]. Present findings also support Kendrick et al. [39] who found that 10-weeks of β-ALA supplementation (6.4 g/day) had no effects on body composition. However, Hoffman and associates [22] reported that supplementation of β-ALA with creatine promoted greater gains in lean body mass compared to creatine alone in male strength/power athletes. Smith and colleagues [12] reported that beta alanine supplementation during high-intensity interval training in men promoted improvements in exercise capacity and lean body mass. Additionally, Kern and Robinson [46] reported that β-ALA supplementation (4 g/day for 8 weeks) in college wrestlers and football players augmented performance and increased lean mass accrual. The reason for the

Table 6 Effect size calculations

	BA	BAC	CRE
Carnosine	−2.00 (large)	−1.73 (large)	−0.75 (moderate)
Creatine	1.16 (large)	−0.30 (low)	−0.83 (large)
Phosphocreatine	−0.39 (low)	0.55 (low)	0.12 (low)
Total Creatine	0.77 (moderate)	−0.22 (low)	0.08 (low)
Body Weight	−0.63 (moderate)	−0.29 (low)	−0.33 (low)
Fat Mass	−0.37 (low)	0.02 (low)	0.15 (low)
Fat Free Mass	−0.36 (low)	−0.46 (low)	−0.69 (moderate)
Percent Body Fat	−0.43 (low)	0.12 (low)	0.34 (low)
VO$_{2peak}$	−0.47 (low)	−0.02 (low)	0.38 (low)
Max Time	−0.76 (moderate)	−0.16 (low)	0.14 (low
Ventilatory Threshold	−0.34 (low	−0.4 (low)	−0.11 (low)
Peak Lactate	−0.58 (moderate)	0.38 (low)	−0.18 (low)
Lactate Threshold	−0.05 (low)	−0.12 (low)	−0.28 (low
Peak Power Wingate 1	−0.36 (low)	0.21 (low)	0.11 (low)
Peak Power Wingate 2	−0.80 (moderate)	−0.39 (low)	−0.83 (moderate)
Total Work Wingate 1	−0.85 (large)	−0.28 (low)	0.15 (low)
Total Work Wingate 2	−0.44 (low)	−0.39 (low)	−0.21 (low)
Rate of Fatigue Wingate 1	−1.44 (large)	−0.90 (large)	−0.78 (low)
Rate of Fatigue Wingate 2	−1.25 (large	−0.17 (low)	−0.49 (low

Cohen's d calculations compared each group mean to PLA.
All calculations used data from week 4.

inconsistency in results observed on body composition in the present study remain unclear but may be due to differences in sex and/or training programs among participants.

Aerobic exercise performance

Creatine supplementation has been purported to provide a mild effect on aerobic exercise capacity possibly through an increase in anaerobic threshold although the literature is mixed on this relationship [16]. Baguet et al. [9], used a similar supplementation protocol for β-ALA as the present study with physically active males and found no effects on VO$_{2peak}$ as a result of supplementation. Stout and colleagues [13] measured the effects of β-ALA supplementation on VT in females. They supplemented for 28 days and found that VT and time to exhaustion were increased in the β-ALA group. The present study was unable to show similar results with β-ALA supplementation groups. There was a slight trend with the creatine only group towards improvement in time to VO$_{2peak}$, but this was not statistically significant. The lack of significance in the present study could be due to differences in training programs among participants and/or low power and effect size of the data. It is unlikely that familiarity was a major factor as all participants underwent familiarization tests on the cycle ergometer prior to starting the study protocol.

Blood lactate and lactate threshold

The increase in muscle carnosine following supplementation would theoretically reduce blood lactate levels during submaximal exercise and/or increase LT since one of the main functions of carnosine is as an intramuscular pH buffer. Although the carnosine results between groups in the present study were not significant, the groups supplemented with β-ALA showed greater percent changes compared to those without. The percent increase also compares closely to previous studies with significant results [3], therefore some inferences can be made based on this trend. The present study found a significant difference in peak lactate achieved during the maximal aerobic capacity test for the group supplementing with β-ALA over the combined supplementation and placebo. However, the study failed to show any differences with LT between the groups, only a trend of β-ALA supplementation improving levels after one week. Previous studies have reported mixed results pertaining to the effect of β-ALA and creatine supplementation on blood lactate accumulation and LT. Van Thienen and colleagues [47] reported no difference between groups in blood lactate levels in healthy males after an incremental maximal cycle ergometer test followed by a 30 second all out sprint after eight weeks of supplementation with β-ALA (2–3 g/d weeks 1–4 and 4 g/d for weeks 4–8) or placebo. Zoeller et al. [15] studied 55 men who supplemented with β-ALA

(3–6 g/d), creatine (5 g/d), a combination or placebo for 28 days and reported a greater VO_{2peak} at LT for the combined supplementation group, suggesting that this supplementation protocol may delay the onset of LT during incremental exercise.

The present study may have failed to show improvements in lactate accumulation and LT with β-ALA alone or the combined β-ALA and creatine supplementation strategy for various reasons. First, the power analysis and effect size calculations were low, which indicates the strength of the data could be improved, possibly with a larger sample size. Also, the present study examined the effects of supplementation in recreationally active females, who did not engage in a standardized training program during the four weeks of the study. Perhaps with a training program, like one seen in other studies, there may have been training effects seen for lactate variables. Finally, since we did not observe statistically significant differences in muscle carnosine or phosphagen levels due to large variation in response to the supplementation protocol, variability in measurement, and/or low statistical power; it is possible that this may have limited the potential ergogenic benefit.

Anaerobic exercise performance

Creatine supplementation has been consistently reported to increase anaerobic sprint and/or exercise capacity [16]. For example, Kreider and colleagues [48] reported that creatine supplementation (15 g/day for 28-days) significantly increased repetitive sprint performance and muscle mass during training in college football players. Wiroth and colleagues [49] reported that creatine supplementation improved maximal power and work during a set of 5×10 second sprints on the cycle ergometer. Green and colleagues [50] reported that creatine supplementation (20 g/day for 6-days) increased PP during the first arm Wingate test and the decline in performance was less after the second leg Wingate test. Ziegenfuss et al. [51] also showed that creatine supplementation in college athletes resulted in increased TW and PP during multiple maximal 10-sec sprints on a cycle ergometer. Results from the present study, however, did not reveal an ergogenic benefit when performing repeated 30-sec anaerobic capacity tests. These findings may be related to the length of the sprint which is generally more dependent on glycolytic capacity rather than phosphagen availability.

A number of studies have also reported that β-ALA supplementation provides ergogenic benefit during high intensity exercise [1,2,5,44,47]. For example, Hill and colleagues [10] reported that 10-weeks of β-ALA supplementation significantly increased total work performed during high-intensity cycling by approximately 13%. Van Thienen et al. [47] reported that β-ALA supplementation (2.4 g/day for 8-weeks) significantly increased sprint

performance at the end of an exhausted endurance cycling exercise bout. Hoffman et al. [52] reported that β-ALA supplementation (4.5 g/day for 3-weeks) in college football players tended to decrease fatigue rate during sprint exercise (p = 0.07). Another study by this group [22] examined the effects of creatine alone, β-ALA and creatine combined and placebo supplementation for 10-weeks in strength power athletes. The researchers reported some beneficial effects on improvements in strength and lean tissue accretion from β-ALA and/or creatine supplementation. Tobias et al. [53] reported that β-ALA supplementation (6.4 g/day for 4-weeks) significantly improved repetitive anaerobic capacity while performing 4×30-sec sprints in judo and jujitsu athletes. Similarly, De Salles Painelli and coworkers [54] reported that β-ALA supplementation (6.4 g/day for 4-weeks) significantly improved anaerobic capacity while performing 4×30-sec sprints in untrained and trained men. In the present study, there was some evidence that β-ALA supplementation may have led to an improvement in rate of fatigue after four weeks of supplementation. However, we did not find that β-ALA with creatine supplementation improved repetitive bouts of 30-sec sprint performance in recreationally active women. It is possible that greater benefits may have been observed from performing more than two 30-sec Wingate sprints as noted above and/or longer sprints. In this regard, Hobson et al. [11] reported that β-ALA supplementation was effective in improving sprint performance in tasks lasting longer than 60-seconds. Saunders et al. [55] tested this theory in a study utilizing the YoYo Intermittent Recovery Test in participants supplementing with β-ALA for 12 weeks. This test is designed to assess the ability to perform and recover from multiple sprints, as seen in many sports. They found supplementation improved performance on this test and suggested it was due to enhanced muscle buffering capabilities between bouts of high intensity exercise resulting from the increased muscle carnosine due to supplementation with β-ALA [55]. However, more research is needed to examine the potential ergogenic value of β-ALA with and without creatine monohydrate supplementation in this population.

Conclusion

This is one of the first studies to use a more individualized dosing strategy for β-ALA supplementation instead of providing a standardized amount β-ALA for all participants irrespective of difference in body mass. Although the mean increases in muscle carnosine levels were similar to those reported in the literature, changes in muscle carnosine levels were not statistically increased in the present study. The lack of significance may have been due to the dosing strategy employed in that the calculated doses may not have been great enough to elicit positive responses.

Additionally, there may be a sex effect with females needing a different amount of β-ALA to consistently increase muscle carnosine levels compared to males. Further, the small sample size of the present study resulting in low power and effect sizes in some instances may have contributed to the lack of significant findings as previous research has demonstrated that four weeks of creatine and β-ALA supplementation was sufficient to increase muscle carnosine and phosphagen levels. Moreover, results of the present study did not show supplementation to have significant effects on body composition, aerobic or anaerobic performance measures. However, perhaps a greater total amount of β-ALA is needed to be ingested over time in women in order for performance adaptations to occur, especially without the addition of a standardized exercise training program. Further studies should be conducted to examine the potential independent and synergistic effects of a combined supplementation of creatine, β-ALA, and other purported nutritional ergogenic aids in untrained and trained male and female populations. Additionally, future studies should examine the effects of combined supplementation on muscle carnosine and phosphagen levels in a larger and/or more active population.

Competing interests

All researchers involved independently collected, analyzed, and interpreted the results from this study and have no financial interests concerning the outcome of the investigation. RBK has received grants as Principal Investigator through institutions with which he has been affiliated to conduct exercise and nutrition related research, has served as a legal and scientific consultant, and currently serves as a scientific consultant for Woodbolt International (Bryan, TX). Remaining co-authors have no competing interests to declare. Data from this study have been presented at the International Society of Sports Nutrition Annual meeting and have not been submitted for publication to any other journals. Publication of these findings should not be viewed as endorsement by the investigators or their institutions of the nutrients investigated.

Authors' contributions

JYK served as the study coordinator, oversaw all testing, and assisted in data analysis and writing of the manuscript. JMO and ARJ assisted in data collection, performed muscle assays, assisted in statistical analysis and manuscript preparation. JF and SR supervised the biopsy procedures. KK supervised muscle assays and CM and ST served as collaborating scientists. CR served as lab coordinator and oversaw data collection and quality control of the study. RBK served as Principal Investigator and contributed to the design of the study, statistical analysis, manuscript preparation, and procurement of external funding. All authors read and approved the final manuscript.

Acknowledgements

We would like to thank the individuals that participated as participants in this study and research assistants who assisted with data collection and/or analysis. We would also like to thank Dr. Roger Harris for providing guidance on muscle carnosine and phosphagen assays.

Funding

This study was supported by a student grant from the Huffines Institute for Sports Medicine and Human Performance and the Exercise & Sport Nutrition Lab at Texas A&M University. Supplements used in this study were provided by AlzChem Trostberg GmbH (Germany) and Natural Alternatives International, Inc. (San Marcos, CA).

Author details

[1]Department of Sports Medicine and Nutrition, School of Health and Rehabilitation Sciences, University of Pittsburgh, Pittsburgh, PA 15260, USA. [2]Kinesiology Department, Texas Christian University, Fort Worth, TX 76129, USA. [3]Department of Exercise & Sport Science, University of Wisconsin – La Crosse, La Crosse, WI 54601, USA. [4]Department of Health and Kinesiology, Muscle Biology Laboratory, Texas A&M University, College Station, TX 77843-4243, USA. [5]Department of Health and Kinesiology, Human Countermeasures Laboratory, Texas A&M University, College Station, TX 77843-4243, USA. [6]Department of Medical Physiology, Texas A&M Health Science Center, College Station, TX 77843-1114, USA. [7]Department of Nutrition and Food Science, Institute for Obesity Research and Program Evaluation, Texas A&M University, College Station, TX 77843-4243, USA. [8]Department of Health and Kinesiology, Exercise and Sport Nutrition Lab, Texas A&M University, College Station, TX 77843-4243, USA.

References

1. Culbertson JY, Kreider RB, Greenwood M, Cooke M: **Effects of beta-alanine on muscle carnosine and exercise performance: a review of the current literature.** *Nutrients* 2010, **2:**75–98.
2. Harris RC, Sale C: **Beta-alanine supplementation in high-intensity exercise.** *Med Sport Sci* 2012, **59:**1–17.
3. Harris RC, Tallon MJ, Dunnett M, Boobis L, Coakley J, Kim HJ, Fallowfield JL, Hill CA, Sale C, Wise JA: **The absorption of orally supplied beta-alanine and its effect on muscle carnosine synthesis in human vastus lateralis.** *Amino Acids* 2006, **30:**279–289.
4. Harris RC, Wise JA, Price KA, Kim HJ, Kim CK, Sale C: **Determinants of muscle carnosine content.** *Amino Acids* 2012, **43:**5–12.
5. Quesnele JJ, Laframboise MA, Wong JJ, Kim P, Wells GD: **The effects of beta-alanine supplementation on performance: a systematic review of the literature.** *Int J Sport Nutr Exerc Metab* 2014, **24:**14–27.
6. Sale C, Artioli GG, Gualano B, Saunders B, Hobson RM, Harris RC: **Carnosine: from exercise performance to health.** *Amino Acids* 2013, **44:**1477–1491.
7. Sale C, Saunders B, Harris RC: **Effect of beta-alanine supplementation on muscle carnosine concentrations and exercise performance.** *Amino Acids* 2010, **39:**321–333.
8. Stellingwerff T, Decombaz J, Harris RC, Boesch C: **Optimizing human in vivo dosing and delivery of beta-alanine supplements for muscle carnosine synthesis.** *Amino Acids* 2012, **43:**57–65.
9. Baguet A, Koppo K, Pottier A, Derave W: **Beta-alanine supplementation reduces acidosis but not oxygen uptake response during high-intensity cycling exercise.** *Eur J Appl Physiol* 2010, **108:**495–503.
10. Hill CA, Harris RC, Kim HJ, Harris BD, Sale C, Boobis LH, Kim CK, Wise JA: **Influence of beta-alanine supplementation on skeletal muscle carnosine concentrations and high intensity cycling capacity.** *Amino Acids* 2007, **32:**225–233.
11. Hobson RM, Saunders B, Ball G, Harris RC, Sale C: **Effects of beta-alanine supplementation on exercise performance: a meta-analysis.** *Amino Acids* 2012, **43:**25–37.
12. Smith AE, Walter AA, Graef JL, Kendall KL, Moon JR, Lockwood CM, Fukuda DH, Beck TW, Cramer JT, Stout JR: **Effects of beta-alanine supplementation and high-intensity interval training on endurance performance and body composition in men; a double-blind trial.** *J Int Soc Sports Nutr* 2009, **6:**5.
13. Stout JR, Cramer JT, Zoeller RF, Torok D, Costa P, Hoffman JR, Harris RC, O'Kroy J: **Effects of beta-alanine supplementation on the onset of neuromuscular fatigue and ventilatory threshold in women.** *Amino Acids* 2007, **32:**381–386.
14. Jordan T, Lukaszuk J, Misic M, Umoren J: **Effect of beta-alanine supplementation on the onset of blood lactate accumulation (OBLA) during treadmill running: Pre/post 2 treatment experimental design.** *J Int Soc Sports Nutr* 2010, **7:**20.
15. Zoeller RF, Stout JR, O'Kroy JA, Torok DJ, Mielke M: **Effects of 28 days of beta-alanine and creatine monohydrate supplementation on aerobic power, ventilatory and lactate thresholds, and time to exhaustion.** *Amino Acids* 2007, **33:**505–510.
16. Kreider RB: **Effects of creatine supplementation on performance and training adaptations.** *Mol Cell Biochem* 2003, **244:**89–94.
17. Gaitanos GC, Williams C, Boobis LH, Brooks S: **Human muscle metabolism during intermittent maximal exercise.** *J Appl Physiol (1985)* 1993, **75:**712–719.
18. Sahlin K: **Metabolic factors in fatigue.** *Sports Med* 1992, **13:**99–107.

19. Greenhaff PL, Bodin K, Soderlund K, Hultman E: Effect of oral creatine supplementation on skeletal muscle phosphocreatine resynthesis. *Am J Physiol* 1994, **266**:E725–730.

20. Harris RC, Soderlund K, Hultman E: Elevation of creatine in resting and exercised muscle of normal subjects by creatine supplementation. *Clin Sci (Lond)* 1992, **83**:367–374.

21. Hultman E, Soderlund K, Timmons JA, Cederblad G, Greenhaff PL: Muscle creatine loading in men. *J Appl Physiol (1985)* 1996, **81**:232–237.

22. Hoffman J, Ratamess N, Kang J, Mangine G, Faigenbaum A, Stout J: Effect of creatine and beta-alanine supplementation on performance and endocrine responses in strength/power athletes. *Int J Sport Nutr Exerc Metab* 2006, **16**:430–446.

23. Kendrick IP, Kim HJ, Harris RC, Kim CK, Dang VH, Lam TQ, Bui TT, Wise JA: The effect of 4 weeks beta-alanine supplementation and isokinetic training on carnosine concentrations in type I and II human skeletal muscle fibres. *Eur J Appl Physiol* 2009, **106**:131–138.

24. Smith AE, Moon JR, Kendall KL, Graef JL, Lockwood CM, Walter AA, Beck TW, Cramer JT, Stout JR: The effects of beta-alanine supplementation and high-intensity interval training on neuromuscular fatigue and muscle function. *Eur J Appl Physiol* 2009, **105**:357–363.

25. Smith AE, Stout JR, Kendall KL, Fukuda DH, Cramer JT: Exercise-induced oxidative stress: the effects of beta-alanine supplementation in women. *Amino Acids* 2012, **43**:77–90.

26. Walter AA, Smith AE, Kendall KL, Stout JR, Cramer JT: Six weeks of high-intensity interval training with and without beta-alanine supplementation for improving cardiovascular fitness in women. *J Strength Cond Res* 2010, **24**:1199–1207.

27. Bergstrom J: Percutaneous needle biopsy of skeletal muscle in physiological and clinical research. *Scand J Clin Lab Invest* 1975, **35**:609–616.

28. Almada AL, Kreider RB, Ransom J, Rasmussen C, Tutko R, Milnor P: Comparison of the reliability of repeated whole body DEXA scans to repeated spine and hip scans. *J Bone Miner Res* 1999, **14**:243.

29. Crouter SE, Antczak A, Hudak JR, DellaValle DM, Haas JD: Accuracy and reliability of the ParvoMedics TrueOne 2400 and MedGraphics VO2000 metabolic systems. *Eur J Appl Physiol* 2006, **98**:139–151.

30. Tanner RK, Fuller KL, Ross ML: Evaluation of three portable blood lactate analysers: Lactate Pro, Lactate Scout and Lactate Plus. *Eur J Appl Physiol* 2010, **109**:551–559.

31. Jagim AR, Oliver JM, Sanchez A, Galvan E, Fluckey J, Riechman S, Greenwood M, Kelly K, Meininger C, Rasmussen C, Kreider RB: A buffered form of creatine does not promote greater changes in muscle creatine content, body composition, or training adaptations than creatine monohydrate. *J Int Soc Sports Nutr* 2012, **9**:43.

32. Harris RC, Hultman E, Nordesjo LO: Glycogen, glycolytic intermediates and high-energy phosphates determined in biopsy samples of musculus quadriceps femoris of man at rest. Methods and variance of values. *Scand J Clin Lab Invest* 1974, **33**:109–120.

33. Soderlund K, Hultman E: Effects of delayed freezing on content of phosphagens in human skeletal muscle biopsy samples. *J Appl Physiol (1985)* 1986, **61**:832–835.

34. Tarnopolsky MA, Parise G: Direct measurement of high-energy phosphate compounds in patients with neuromuscular disease. *Muscle Nerve* 1999, **22**:1228–1233.

35. Dunnett M, Harris RC: High-performance liquid chromatographic determination of imidazole dipeptides, histidine, 1-methylhistidine and 3-methylhistidine in equine and camel muscle and individual muscle fibres. *J Chromatogr B Biomed Sci Appl* 1997, **688**:47–55.

36. Twisk J, de Vente W: Attrition in longitudinal studies. How to deal with missing data. *J Clin Epidemiol* 2002, **55**:329–337.

37. Baguet A, Bourgois J, Vanhee L, Achten E, Derave W: Important role of muscle carnosine in rowing performance. *J Appl Physiol (1985)* 2010, **109**:1096–1101.

38. Derave W, Ozdemir MS, Harris RC, Pottier A, Reyngoudt H, Koppo K, Wise JA, Achten E: beta-Alanine supplementation augments muscle carnosine content and attenuates fatigue during repeated isokinetic contraction bouts in trained sprinters. *J Appl Physiol (1985)* 2007, **103**:1736–1743.

39. Kendrick IP, Harris RC, Kim HJ, Kim CK, Dang VH, Lam TQ, Bui TT, Smith M, Wise JA: The effects of 10 weeks of resistance training combined with beta-alanine supplementation on whole body strength, force production, muscular endurance and body composition. *Amino Acids* 2008, **34**:547–554.

40. Stegen S, Bex T, Vervaet C, Vanhee L, Achten E: Derave W: beta-Alanine dose for maintaining moderately elevated muscle carnosine levels. *Med Sci Sports Exerc* 2014, **46**:1426–1432.

41. Buford TW, Kreider RB, Stout JR, Greenwood M, Campbell B, Spano M, Ziegenfuss T, Lopez H, Landis J, Antonio J: International Society of Sports Nutrition position stand: creatine supplementation and exercise. *J Int Soc Sports Nutr* 2007, **4**:6.

42. Forsberg AM, Nilsson E, Werneman J, Bergstrom J, Hultman E: Muscle composition in relation to age and sex. *Clin Sci (Lond)* 1991, **81**:249–256.

43. Balsom PD, Soderlund K, Sjodin B, Ekblom B: Skeletal muscle metabolism during short duration high-intensity exercise: influence of creatine supplementation. *Acta Physiol Scand* 1995, **154**:303–310.

44. Derave W, Everaert I, Beeckman S, Baguet A: Muscle carnosine metabolism and beta-alanine supplementation in relation to exercise and training. *Sports Med* 2010, **40**:247–263.

45. Bex T, Chung W, Baguet A, Stegen S, Stautemas J, Achten E, Derave W: Muscle carnosine loading by beta-alanine supplementation is more pronounced in trained vs. untrained muscles. *J Appl Physiol (1985)* 2014, **116**:204–209.

46. Kern BD, Robinson TL: Effects of beta-alanine supplementation on performance and body composition in collegiate wrestlers and football players. *J Strength Cond Res* 2011, **25**:1804–1815.

47. Van Thienen R, Van Proeyen K, Vanden Eynde B, Puype J, Lefere T, Hespel P: Beta-alanine improves sprint performance in endurance cycling. *Med Sci Sports Exerc* 2009, **41**:898–903.

48. Kreider RB: Creatine supplementation: analysis of ergogenic value, medical safety, and concerns. *J Exerc Physiol Online* 1998, **1**:7–18.

49. Wiroth JB, Bermon S, Andrei S, Dalloz E, Hebuterne X, Dolisi C: Effects of oral creatine supplementation on maximal pedalling performance in older adults. *Eur J Appl Physiol* 2001, **84**:533–539.

50. Green JM, McLester JR, Smith JE, Mansfield ER: The effects of creatine supplementation on repeated upper- and lower-body Wingate performance. *J Strength Cond Res* 2001, **15**:36–41.

51. Ziegenfuss TN, Rogers M, Lowery L, Mullins N, Mendel R, Antonio J, Lemon P: Effect of creatine loading on anaerobic performance and skeletal muscle volume in NCAA Division I athletes. *Nutrition* 2002, **18**:397–402.

52. Hoffman JR, Ratamess NA, Faigenbaum AD, Ross R, Kang J, Stout JR, Wise JA: Short-duration beta-alanine supplementation increases training volume and reduces subjective feelings of fatigue in college football players. *Nutr Res* 2008, **28**:31–35.

53. Tobias G, Benatti FB, de Salles PV, Roschel H, Gualano B, Sale C, Harris RC, Lancha AH Jr, Artioli GG: Additive effects of beta-alanine and sodium bicarbonate on upper-body intermittent performance. *Amino Acids* 2013, **45**:309–317.

54. de Salles PV, Saunders B, Sale C, Harris RC, Solis MY, Roschel H, Gualano B, Artioli GG, Lancha AH Jr: Influence of training status on high-intensity intermittent performance in response to beta-alanine supplementation. *Amino Acids* 2014, **46**:1207–1215.

55. Saunders B, Sunderland C, Harris RC, Sale C: beta-alanine supplementation improves YoYo intermittent recovery test performance. *J Int Soc Sports Nutr* 2012, **9**:39.

6

Performance during a 20-km cycling time-trial after caffeine ingestion

Henrique Bortolotti[1,2,4], Leandro Ricardo Altimari[1,2,3], Marcelo Vitor-Costa[1,2] and Edilson Serpeloni Cyrino[1,2,3*]

Abstract

Background: The objective of this study was to analyze the effect of caffeine ingestion on the performance and physiological variables associated with fatigue in 20-km cycling time trials.

Methods: In a double-blind placebo-controlled crossover study, 13 male cyclists (26 ± 10 y, 71 ± 9 kg, 176 ± 6 cm) were randomized into 2 groups and received caffeine (CAF) capsules (6 mg.kg^{-1}) or placebo (PLA) 60 min before performing 20-km time trials. Distance, speed, power, rpm, rating of perceived exertion (RPE), electromyography (EMG) of the quadriceps muscles and heart rate (HR) were continuously measured during the tests. In addition, BRUMS questionnaire was applied before and after the tests.

Results: Significant interactions were found in power and speed ($P = 0.001$), which were significantly higher at the end of the test (final 2 km) after CAF condition. A main effect of time ($P = 0.001$) was observed for RPE and HR, which increased linearly until the end of exercise in both conditions. The time taken to complete the test was similar in both conditions (PLA = 2191 ± 158 s vs. CAF = 2181 ± 194 s, $P = 0.61$). No significant differences between CAF and PLA conditions were identified for speed, power, rpm, RPE, EMG, HR, and BRUMS ($P > 0.05$).

Conclusion: The results suggest that caffeine intake 60 min before 20-km time trials has no effect on the performance or physiological responses of cyclists.

Keywords: Ergogenic aid, Sports performance, Perceived exertion, Electromyography, Exercise testing

Background

Recent studies have shown that caffeine (CAF) can act as an ergogenic aid, both in short and long-term exercise [1-4] at both central and peripheral level [4-6]. Conversely to what was initially thought, CAF intake does not seem to be able to accelerate fat metabolism and to spare muscle glycogen during exercise, which would explain the increased performance observed in endurance tasks [4,7]. Currently, this potential effect of CAF is credited to its affinity to adenosine receptors (A_1 and A_{2a}). When CAF molecules bind with these pre and post synaptic receptors, it inhibits adenosine action, promoting the release of excitatory neurotransmitters, increasing corticomotor excitability [8,9]. This stimulatory effect of CAF on the central nervous system may be responsible for modifying the motivation parameters that cause sustain discomfort during physical exercise, reducing the rating of perceived exertion (RPE) during exercise [10].

Although the ergogenic effect of CAF on the neuromuscular system has been discussed in detail in a previous review study [11], it is noteworthy that the majority of studies have so far adopted open-loop protocols. Despite being a sensitive test that quantifies changes in performance [12], it does not represent the reality of sports competitions. Although closed-loop protocols have been less frequently used in investigations on the effect of CAF on physical performance [13-16], they have greater ecological validity than open-loop protocols due to its similarity with actual competitive situations, as well as having the ability to evaluate athletes' pacing strategy [17]. Moreover, few studies have investigated the effect of CAF on RPE on time trials, where the subject can choose and plan his pacing strategy during the effort. As

* Correspondence: emcyrino@uel.br

[1]Metabolism, Nutrition, and Exercise Research Group, Londrina State University, Londrina, Paraná, Brazil

[2]Neuromuscular System and Exercise Research Group, Londrina State University, Londrina, Paraná, Brazil

Full list of author information is available at the end of the article

a result, it has been difficult to extrapolate information on the use of CAF to competitive situations.

Therefore, the objective of the present study was to analyze the effect of CAF ingestion on the performance and physiological variables associated with fatigue in 20-km cycling time trials using a closed-loop protocol.

Methods

Experimental design

A double-blind, randomized, placebo-controlled cross-over study with previous familiarization was approved by the Londrina State University Ethics Committee. Thirteen male cyclists (71 ± 9 kg; 176 ± 5 cm; 253 ± 142 km.week^{-1}) with at least two years of competitive experience were recruited for the study. All participants had been free of injuries for at least six months before the tests. Prior to tests, the subjects visited the laboratory to become aware of the purpose of the study and sign an informed consent. Schedules were set, and subjects returned to the laboratory to perform anthropometric measurements and a pre-experimental trial to become familiarized with the equipment and the experimental protocol.

Participants were randomized into 2 groups and received caffeine (CAF) capsules (6 mg.kg^{-1}) or placebo (PLA) 60 min before performing 20-km time trials in two different occasions separated by a minimum interval of 72 h. Therefore, the amount of CAF or PLA (malto-dextrin) that the volunteers should ingest was determined from the body weight (i.e. a subject weighing 70 kg would ingest 420 mg of caffeine or placebo). Subjects were instructed to abstain from any CAF in the 48 h before the test. Furthermore, instructions were also given to abstain from alcohol intake and strenuous exercise in the 24 h prior to visiting the laboratory. For inclusion in the study, volunteers should not use other nutritional supplements. Ambient temperature and relative humidity in the laboratory were maintained between 21-24°C and 55-60%, respectively, in all tests. The subjects performed the tests always in the same period of the day to avoid the potential influence of circadian cycle.

During the time between ingesting the capsules and starting the test (60 min), the participants answered the Brunel mood scale (BRUMS) questionnaire, electrodes were placed, specific tests for EMG signal normalization were performed, and a 10-min warm-up was carried out.

Pre-experimental test

Prior to the experimental tests, a maximal incremental test for determination of maximum parameters (power and HR) and physiological thresholds was performed, using specific software (Velotron CS 2008™ - Racer-Mate®, Seattle, WA, USA). After warming-up for 2 min at 100 W, the load was increased in 50 W at every

2 min until exhaustion or the inability to maintain the stipulated minimum cadence (70 rpm) for more than 5 s, despite verbal encouragement. The power reached in the last complete stage added to the product of the percentage of the time spent in the exhaustion stage by the standardized increment (50 W) was considered the maximum power (345.0 ± 41.6 W). The highest HR value at the last minute of test was recorded as the maximum HR (192 ± 11.6 bpm).

Experimental protocol

Time trials were performed in a cyclosimulator (Velotron™ - RacerMate®, Seattle, WA, USA), which was calibrated prior to each test, according to manufacturer's recommendations. The 20-km time trial was built in a straight line and 0° tilt using the same software used in the pre-experimental tests.

The subjects came to the laboratory on scheduled days and underwent a closed-loop test, in which they had to complete the 20-km time trial, in the shortest possible time with free choice of cadence and gear ratio, simulating an actual race. All participants received feedback on the time, power, RPM and distance traveled during the test on a monitor. Before, during and after the tests the following variables were analyzed: electromyographic activity of the muscles rectus femoris (RF), vastus medialis (VM) and vastus lateralis (VL), RPE, mood, and HR.

Surface electromyography (EMG)

The torque-velocity test (T-V test) was performed to normalize the electromyographic activity [18]. After a 10-min warm-up at 100 W, each subject performed two maximum bouts with duration of 8 s each, with an interval of 5 min between bouts. The load during the test was 7.5% of the volunteer's body mass. Participants were instructed to remain seated throughout the test. The electromyographic activity of each muscle was examined between the second and eighth seconds of each maximum bout, and the highest peak amplitude found, expressed in root mean square (RMS), was used as the normalization factor.

Electromyographic activity was monitored continuously during the tests in both experimental conditions (CAF or PLA) using an eight-channel electromyograph (TeleMyo 2400 T G2 - Noraxon Inc., USA). The sampling frequency for EMG records was 2000 Hz and the factor of common-mode rejection ratio was greater than 95 dB. The muscles examined were the superficial quadriceps femoris (QF), RF, VM and VL. The signal was recorded following the recommendations by ISEK. After site preparation by shaving, cleansing with alcohol and curettage to reduce skin impedance, active electrodes (TeleMyo 2400 - Noraxon Inc., USA) were fixed to the skin, with inter-electrode distance (center to center) of two centimeters. The reference electrode was positioned over the iliac crest. The location of the anatomical landmarks for electrode placement followed the standardization proposed by SENIAM [19].

Analysis and processing of the EMG signal

RMS (μV) values were averaged for each 30-s period and were used for the analysis of electromyographic signals from RF, VM, and VL muscles and the integrated QF [(RF + VM + VL) / 3]. Data were processed using a mathematical simulation environment (Matlab 7.0 - MathWorks ®, South Natick, MA, USA). To obtain the values expressed in RMS, raw EMG signals were digitally filtered, using a band-pass filter of 20Hz and 500Hz, according to the procedures proposed by Dantas et al. [20].

Measurement of perceived exertion

All subjects were instructed to report their perceived exertion according to the 6–20 point Borg scale [21] at each 2 km of exercise. From these data, we determined the intercept on the y axis (y-intercept), the coefficient of determination (R^2) and the slope between the time and the individual perceived exertion values attributed during each test obtained by linear regression analysis.

Psychological-motivational changes

On test days, subjects responded to the Brunel Mood Scale (BRUMS) when they arrived and after the experimental trial. This questionnaire was used for the detection of mood based on 24 questions, stratified into six areas, namely: confusion, anger, depression, fatigue, tension and vigor. Each domain score was normalized by the score obtained prior to the exercise by subtracting the scores at the end of the trial from the scores before the trial.

Heart rate

During all testing protocols HR was monitored and recorded in RR intervals (ms) and beats per minute (bpm), using a heart rate monitor (Polar RS800CX - Polar®, Kempele, Finland). Data were recorded and stored for later beat-by-beat analysis of the heart's R-wave signals through a coded Polar WearLink transmitter, positioned on the subject's chest, allowing the transmission of data by telemetry.

Statistical analyses

The normality of data was assessed by Shapiro-Wilk's test. Levene's test was used to analyze the homogeneity of variances. Two-way analysis of variance (ANOVA) for repeated measures was used for comparisons between conditions (CAF and PLA) and over time. The Bonferroni post hoc test was used when a significant F ratio was found for the main or interaction effect. A significance level of 5% was used for all analyzes.

Additionally, the practical inference based on magnitudes was also applied [22]. The chance of a given value to be beneficial (positive) or detrimental (negative) effect [e.g., higher or lower than the smallest worthwhile changes (0.20 multiplied by the initial standard deviation based on the effect size)] was calculated [23]. Thus, the change was assessed qualitatively as follows: <1% almost certainly not; 1-5% very unlikely, 5-25% unlikely, 25-75% possible, 75-95% likely, 95-99% very likely and > 99% almost certainly yes. When the negative and positive values showed results greater than 10%, the inference was considered inconclusive. The effect size (Cohen's d) was also calculated for the time trial performance and interpreted using the recommendations suggested by Hopkins et al. [22] as follows: 0 = Trivial; 0.2 = Small; 0.6 = Moderate; 1.2 = Large; 2.0 = Very large; 4.0 = Nearly perfect.

Results

Information on power, speed, pedaling cadence, HR and 20-km time trial test duration for PLA and CAF conditions are presented in Table 1. No significant differences were observed between CAF and PLA concerning HR and all the performance variables ($P > 0.05$). The results of the qualitative analysis proved inconclusive (unclear). The effect size was 0.06, being considered trivial. Power output and speed at every two kilometers in the 20-km time-trial, for CAF and PLA, are illustrated in Figure 1. Although a similar response was observed among groups ($P > 0.05$), a significant distance main effect in the last two kilometers of the test was observed with increased power and speed ($P < 0.001$). However, no significant group main effect or group by moment interaction was identified ($P > 0.05$).

The EMG pattern during the tests is presented in Figure 2. No difference was found between the two experimental conditions (PLA and CAF) for the VL, RF, VM and QF muscles. Thus, no significant group main effect or group by moment interaction was identified ($P > 0.05$). There was a progressive increase in the RPE during the test in both groups, without any statistically significant differences between them ($P > 0.05$). Only a significant distance main effect was identified for HR and RPE ($P < 0.001$). No statistically significant difference ($P > 0.05$) was detected in the RPE increase rate between groups (PLA = 0.88 points.km^{-1} vs. CAF = 0.95 points. km^{-1}). Mood changes before and after the 20-km time trials are illustrated in Figure 3.

Discussion

The main result obtained in this study was that the oral administration of 6 mg.kg^{-1} of body mass of CAF

Table 1 Cycling performance indicators during the 20-km time trials, after acute ingestion of CAF (n = 13) or PLA (n = 13). Values are expressed as mean ± standard deviation

Variables	Condition		
	PLA	CAF	P
Power (watts)	206.9 ± 28.5	204.6 ± 43.9	0.79
Speed (km.h^{-1})	33.5 ± 1.8	33.3 ± 2.8	0.72
Cadence (rpm)	105.3 ± 8.4	103.4 ± 4.1	0.96
HR (beats.min^{-1})	171 ± 9.9	171 ± 8.0	0.94
Duration (s)	2191 ± 157.6	2181 ± 193.9	0.61
% difference (IC 90%)	−10.1 (−45 to 24.9)		
% difference positive/trivial/negative	2/85/12		
Qualitative Inference	Unclear		

CAF = caffeine; PLA = placebo.

60 min before the effort had no effect on the performance of cyclists in the 20-km time trial. The results also indicated that the use of CAF did not promote any changes in pacing strategy during the test or attenuation of RPE.

Although our results are interesting, comparisons with previous studies are really very difficult due to differences in the protocols. In a time trial study performed by McNaughton et al. [16], although the distance was similar to that used here, the authors included some uphill stretches, which made the test harder, naturally forcing their athletes to assume different pacing strategies.

Additionally, their subjects ingested CAF in the form of a low-kilojoule flavored drink, and the authors did not mention whether the subjects were able to distinguish between the drink containing CAF or PLA. In another study conducted by Ivy et al. [15], CAF was used in combination with other substances (labeled as an "energy drink") to compete a fixed amount of work on a cycle ergometer in significantly less time than after consuming a placebo. Thus, the results of these studies cannot be compared with our results.

The stimulatory effect of CAF on the central nervous system appears not only to modify the parameters of motivation, but also to attenuate RPE, enabling cyclists to sustain the discomfort caused by exercise. The magnitude of this effect has been reported to be close to 6% during constant load exercise, increasing time to exhaustion [10]. However, this effect was not observed in this study. Our results showed that RPE showed no differences when the two trial conditions were compared. The RPE increase rate verified by the slope on the regression plot for RPE values throughout the test, showed no significant differences between conditions (0.88 points.km^{-1} vs. 0.95 points.km^{-1}, for PLA and CAF, respectively).

In open protocols, individuals usually must maintain a fixed work rate to exhaustion. Thus, the fact that there is no defined end prevents pacing strategy planning [14]. However, when the subject does not necessarily need to keep a fixed intensity, this allows the development of strategies during the race aiming at finishing in the

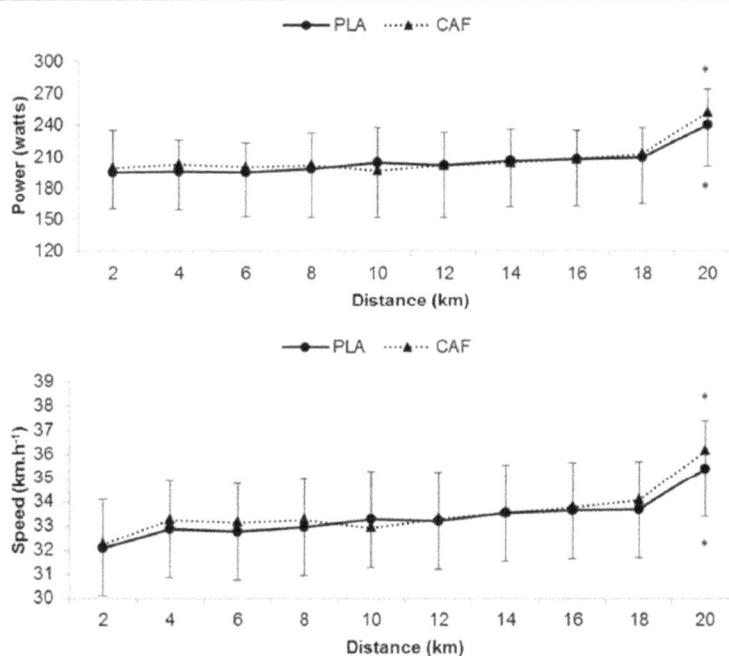

Figure 1 Responses of power and speed on 20-km time-trial test under the conditions CAF (n = 13) and PLA (n = 13). *$P < 0.05$ vs. 20 km. Significant main effect of time ($P < 0.001$).

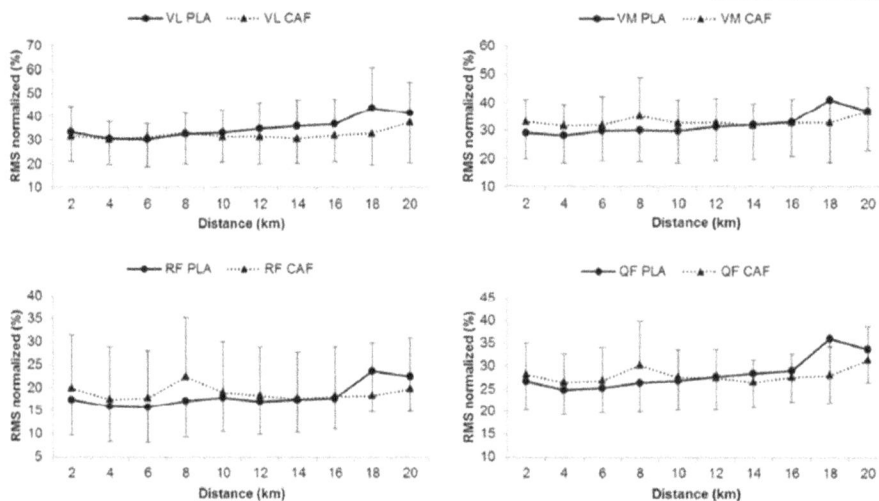

Figure 2 Pattern of EMG activity of the VL, RF, VM and QF muscles during the 20-km time-trial test under the conditions CAF (n = 12) and PLA (n = 12). No main effect or group vs. time interaction was identified (P > 0.05).

shortest possible time. Therefore, investigations on CAF effect on performance in tests that mimic the actual conditions found in competitions could be more relevant and strengthen the importance of the results found.

Pacing strategy planning is centrally mediated. Due to its direct action on the nervous system, CAF should, therefore, influence and change pacing strategy during 20-km time trials. These changes should be observed by different power, speed and/or rpm behaviors during the tests. However, our results failed to show any influence of his level of CAF intake on pacing planning. This confirms

the results of Hunter et al. [14], who demonstrated that CAF not only had no effect on EMG, RPE, HR and performance (time) parameters during 100-km time trials, but it also had no influence on pacing strategy. Only in the final part of the test were significant differences in pacing strategy observed when compared to the remainder of the exercise. This has already been shown in a previous study where pacing strategy varied only minimally in the last 30 s of a 30-min time trial [24].

Few studies have investigated the effect of CAF without combination with carbohydrates on medium and

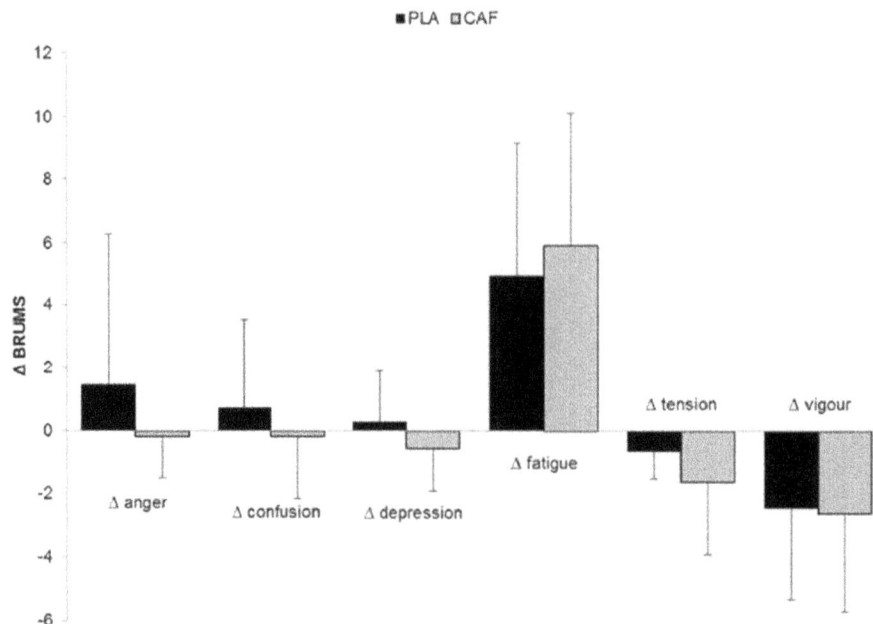

Figure 3 Variation delta of mood (BRUMSpost − BRUMSpre) in their various domains in the 20-km time-trial (n = 13).

long time trial distances (>5 km) Bruce et al. [13] demonstrated that CAF ingestion significantly improved the performance of rowers in the first 500 of 2000 m trials. The authors suggested that CAF may act directly on subconscious brain centers responsible for pacing strategy planning during exercise [13]. On the other hand, Cohen et al. [25] showed a decrease in performance of 0.7% in a 21-km race protocol, after the subjects had ingested capsules of CAF (9 mg.kg^{-1}) 60 min prior to the beginning of the exercise. In a 20-km race protocol, 60 min after the ingestion of CAF capsules (6 mg.kg^{-1}), individuals improved performance in 1.7%, but this increase was not significant [26]. In this study, we found an improvement of only 0.46% (~10 s) in the performance, again not significant.

Throughout the test, EMG showed no differences between the experimental conditions and along the 20 km. Muscle activation during the tests was ~25% of the values obtained in the TV-test, with no significant changes at any time. This suggests the absence of peripheral fatigue during testing. Similarly, Hunter et al. [14] also failed to identify changes in EMG at any point along the 100 km time trial. During exercise, there is a decrease in muscular strength, and the amplitude of the EMG signal should increase to sustain the same intensity of exercise and/or stay on the task, increasing the firing rate. As a result, the amplitude of the EMG signal should be higher for the same power. But we could not confirm the absence of neuromuscular fatigue during the test as RPE gradually increased. These could be better discussed with the use of different techniques for the assessment of central and/or peripheral fatigue, such as the level of maximal voluntary activation measured by the twitch interpolation technique [27].

In the present study, the BRUMS's scale, which is intended to allow a quick measure of mood [28], was applied immediately before and after the tests in order to verify possible changes promoted by the administration of CAF (Figure 3). We expected that CAF would modify mood variation, relieving fatigue, and/or strength symptoms, which would explain possible improvements in performance. However, no significant differences were found between the experimental conditions.

In the present study we aimed at controlling key variables previously mentioned in the literature, to generate reliable and reproducible information. Thus, some methodological precautions were taken. It is known that several factors appear to influence CAF's potential and magnitude ergogenic effects, such as the way the substance is administered (capsules, drink, or gum), the moment the substance administered (prior and/or during exercise), whether CAF is associated with some other substances (carbohydrate) or not, fasting status, and habituation, among others [3]. In the present study,

subjects were asked to avoid eating foods containing CAF 48 hours before the test to minimize the possible influence of the level of habituation on the results. However, the level of habituation to CAF and the subjects' eating habits were not directly controlled. It has been shown that after a period of 2 to 4 days of CAF withdrawal, a tendency to potentiate the effects of CAF on the protocol until exhaustion does exist, when compared to 0 days, but without any differences between those times [29]. However, in an animal model, an increase in the number and affinity of adenosine receptors after 7 days of CAF abstinence was observed [30]. Hence, studies seeking to demonstrate the effect of a prolonged period (>7 days) of CAF abstinence on performance in humans could be of interest. In sports, it might be speculated that when habituation to CAF exists, a restriction in the consumption of this substance for a period of approximately seven days may provide gains and/or potentiate the effect of CAF. But this hypothesis has yet to be verified.

Another limitation of this study was that athletes in the present sample only participate in local competitions making it difficult to extrapolate our findings to well-trained athletes, who compete internationally. This probably explains the low power values found here compared to studies that used well-trained athletes [31]. Unfortunately, studies with tests of similar duration that demonstrated an ergogenic effect of CAF alone [16] or in combination with other substances [15] have reported no data on the average power observed during the time trial, or the maximum power in the incremental test, again making comparison difficult.

In conclusion, our results do not encourage the supplementation with CAF in a cycling time trial setting. Studies involving shorter protocols, similar to cycling events, should be tested for better understanding the use of CAF in closed-loop protocols. Furthermore, future studies should also seek to demonstrate whether CAF abstinence for longer periods could enhance performance on closed protocols and the mechanisms involved in fatigue during exercise.

Competing interests
The authors declare that they have no competing of interests.

Authors' contributions
HB, LRA, MVC and ESC were significant manuscript writers; HB, LRA and ESC participated in the concept and design; HB and MVC were responsible for data acquisition; HB, LRA, MVC and ESC participated in data analysis and interpretation. All authors read and approved the final manuscript.

Acknowledgments
We would like to express thanks to all the participants for their engagement in this study and also the Coordination of Improvement of Higher Education Personnel (CAPES/Brazil) for the master scholarship conferred to H.B. and M.V.C. and the National Council of Technological and Scientific Development (CNPq/Brazil) for the grants conceded to E.S.C. and L.R.A.

Author details

[1]Metabolism, Nutrition, and Exercise Research Group, Londrina State University, Londrina, Paraná, Brazil. [2]Neuromuscular System and Exercise Research Group, Londrina State University, Londrina, Paraná, Brazil. [3]Department of Physical Education, Centre for Physical Education and Sport, Londrina State University, Londrina, Paraná, Brazil. [4]School of Physical Education and Sport, University of São Paulo, São Paulo, Brazil.

References

1. Burke LM: **Caffeine and sports performance.** *Appl Physiol Nutr Metab* 2008, **33:**1319–1334.
2. Bentley DJ, McNaughton LR, Thompson D, Vleck VE, Batterham AM: **Peak power output, the lactate threshold, and time trial performance in cyclists.** *Med Sci Sports Exerc* 2001, **33:**2077–2081.
3. Doherty M, Smith PM: **Effects of caffeine ingestion on exercise testing: a meta-analysis.** *Int J Sport Nutr Exerc Metab* 2004, **14:**626–646.
4. Ganio MS, Klau JF, Casa DJ, Armstrong LE, Maresh CM: **Effect of caffeine on sport-specific endurance performance: a systematic review.** *J Strength Cond Res* 2009, **23:**315–324.
5. Graham TE: **Caffeine and exercise: metabolism, endurance and performance.** *Sports Med* 2001, **31:**785–807.
6. Gandevia S, Taylor J: **Supraspinal fatigue: the effects of caffeine on human muscle performance.** *J Appl Physiol* 2006, **100:**1749–1750.
7. Kalmar J, Cafarelli E: **Effects of caffeine on neuromuscular function.** *J Appl Physiol* 1999, **87:**801–808.
8. Graham TE, Helge JW, MacLean DA, Kiens B, Richter EA: **Caffeine ingestion does not alter carbohydrate or fat metabolism in human skeletal muscle during exercise.** *J Physiol* 2000, **529:**837–847.
9. Cerqueira V, De Mendonça A, Minez A, Dias AR, De Carvalho M: **Does caffeine modify corticomotor excitability?** *Neurophysiol Clin* 2006, **36:**219–226.
10. Kalmar JM, Cafarelli E: **Caffeine: a valuable tool to study central fatigue in humans?** *Exerc Sport Sci Rev* 2004, **32:**143–147.
11. Doherty M, Smith P: **Effects of caffeine ingestion on rating of perceived exertion during and after exercise: a meta-analysis.** *Scand J Med Sci Sports* 2005, **15:**69–78.
12. Tarnopolsky MA: **Effect of caffeine on the neuromuscular system-potential as an ergogenic aid.** *Appl Physiol Nutr Metab* 2008, **33:**1284–1289.
13. Amann M, Hopkins WG, Marcora SM: **Similar sensitivity of time to exhaustion and time-trial time to changes in endurance.** *Med Sci Sports Exerc* 2008, **40:**574–578.
14. Bruce CR, Anderson ME, Fraser SF, Stepto NK, Klein R, Hopkins WG, Hawley JA: **Enhancement of 2000-m rowing performance after caffeine ingestion.** *Med Sci Sports Exerc* 2000, **32:**1958–1963.
15. Hunter AM, St Clair GA, Collins M, Lambert M, Noakes TD: **Caffeine ingestion does not alter performance during a 100-km cycling time-trial performance.** *Int J Sport Nutr Exerc Metab* 2002, **12:**438–452.
16. Ivy JL, Kammer L, Ding Z, Wang B, Bernard JR, Liao YH, Hwang J: **Improved cycling time-trial performance after ingestion of a caffeine energy drink.** *Int J Sport Nutr Exerc Metab* 2009, **19:**61–78.
17. McNaughton LR, Lovell RJ, Siegler J, Midgley AW, Moore L, Bentley DJ: **The effects of caffeine ingestion on time trial cycling performance.** *Int J Sports Physiol Perform* 2008, **3:**157–163.
18. Laursen PB, Francis GT, Abbiss CR, Newton MJ, Nosaka K: **Reliability of time-to-exhaustion versus time-trial running tests in runners.** *Med Sci Sports Exerc* 2007, **39:**1374–1379.
19. Rouffet DM, Hautier CA: **EMG normalization to study muscle activation in cycling.** *J Electromyogr Kinesiol* 2008, **18:**866–878.
20. Hermens HJ, Freriks B, Disselhorst-Klug C, Rau G: **Development of recommendations for SEMG sensors and sensor placement procedures.** *J Electromyogr Kinesiol* 2000, **10:**361–374.
21. Dantas JL, Camata TV, Brunetto MAOC, Moraes AC, Abrão T, Altimari LR: **Fourier and Wavelet spectral analysis of EMG signals in isometric and dynamic maximal effort exercise.** *Conf Proc IEEE Eng Med Biol Soc* 2010, **2010:**5979–5982.
22. Borg GA: **Psychophysical bases of perceived exertion.** *Med Sci Sports Exerc* 1982, **14:**377–381.
23. Hopkins WG, Marshall SW, Batterham AM, Hanin J: **Progressive statistics for studies in sports medicine and exercise science.** *Med Sci Sports Exerc* 2009, **41:**3–13.
24. Buchheit M, Chivot A, Parouty J, Mercier D, Al Haddad H, Laursen PB, Ahmaidi S: **Monitoring endurance running performance using cardiac parasympathetic function.** *Eur J Appl Physiol* 2010, **108:**1153–1167.
25. Chaffin ME, Berg K, Zuniga J, Hanumanthu VS: **Pacing pattern in a 30-minute maximal cycling test.** *J Strength Cond Res* 2008, **22:**2011–2017.
26. Cohen BS, Nelson AG, Prevost MC, Thompson GD, Marx BD, Morris GS: **Effects of caffeine ingestion on endurance racing in heat and humidity.** *Eur J Appl Physiol* 1996, **73:**358–363.
27. Berglund B, Hemmingsson P: **Effects of caffeine ingestion on exercise performance at low and high altitudes in cross-country skiers.** *Int J Sports Med* 1982, **3:**234–236.
28. Hales J, Gandevia S: **Assessment of maximal voluntary contraction with twitch interpolation: an instrument to measure twitch responses.** *J Neurosci Methods* 1988, **25:**97–102.
29. Rohlfs ICPM: *Validation of Brums test for mood evaluation in Brazilian athletes and non-athletes [dissertation].* Florianópolis: State University of Santa Catarina; 2006:110.
30. Van Soeren M, Graham T: **Effect of caffeine on metabolism, exercise endurance, and catecholamine responses after withdrawal.** *J Appl Physiol* 1998, **85:**1493–1501.
31. Kaplan GB, Greenblatt DJ, Kent MA, Cotreau-Bibbo MM: **Caffeine treatment and withdrawal in mice: relationships between dosage, concentrations, locomotor activity and A1 adenosine receptor binding.** *J Pharmacol Exp Ther* 1993, **266:**1563–1572.

7

Validity of the Rapid Eating Assessment for Patients for assessing dietary patterns in NCAA athletes

Jonathan M Kurka, Matthew P Buman and Barbara E Ainsworth[*]

Abstract

Background: Athletes may be at risk for developing adverse health outcomes due to poor eating behaviors during college. Due to the complex nature of the diet, it is difficult to include or exclude individual food items and specific food groups from the diet. Eating behaviors may better characterize the complex interactions between individual food items and specific food groups. The purpose was to examine the Rapid Eating Assessment for Patients survey (REAP) as a valid tool for analyzing eating behaviors of NCAA Division-I male and female athletes using pattern identification. Also, to investigate the relationships between derived eating behavior patterns and body mass index (BMI) and waist circumference (WC) while stratifying by sex and aesthetic nature of the sport.

Methods: Two independent samples of male (n = 86; n = 139) and female (n = 64; n = 102) collegiate athletes completed the REAP in June-August 2011 (n = 150) and June-August 2012 (n = 241). Principal component analysis (PCA) determined possible factors using wave-1 athletes. Exploratory (EFA) and confirmatory factor analyses (CFA) determined factors accounting for error and confirmed model fit in wave-2 athletes. Wave-2 athletes' BMI and WC were recorded during a physical exam and sport participation determined classification in aesthetic and non-aesthetic sport. Mean differences in eating behavior pattern score were explored. Regression models examined interactions between pattern scores, participation in aesthetic or non-aesthetic sport, and BMI and waist circumference controlling for age and race.

Results: A 5-factor PCA solution accounting for 60.3% of sample variance determined fourteen questions for EFA and CFA. A confirmed solution revealed patterns of Desserts, Healthy food, Meats, High-fat food, and Dairy. Pattern score (mean ± SE) differences were found, as non-aesthetic sport males had a higher (better) Dessert score than aesthetic sport males (2.16 ± 0.07 vs. 1.93 ± 0.11). Female aesthetic athletes had a higher score compared to non-aesthetic female athletes for the Dessert (2.11 ± 0.11 vs. 1.88 ± 0.08), Meat (1.95 ± 0.10 vs. 1.72 ± 0.07), High-fat food (1.70 ± 0.08 vs. 1.46 ± 0.06), and Dairy (1.70 ± 0.11 vs. 1.43 ± 0.07) patterns.

Conclusions: REAP is a construct valid tool to assess dietary patterns in college athletes. In light of varying dietary patterns, college athletes should be evaluated for healthful and unhealthful eating behaviors.

Keywords: Athlete, Nutrition, Factor analysis

* Correspondence: Barbara.Ainsworth@asu.edu
Exercise and Wellness Program, School of Nutrition and Health Promotion, Arizona State University, 500 N Third Street, Mail Code 3020, Phoenix, AZ 85004, USA

Background

Young adults with unhealthful eating behaviors are at risk for poor health outcomes [1]. Those involved in team sports requiring strength and power (i.e., football) may be at risk for being overweight and for developing chronic conditions [2]. Approximately 50% of amateur football linemen may be obese (body mass index ≥ 30) [2] and more likely to have insulin resistance compared to their non-obese counterparts [3]. Healthful eating behaviors should be encouraged in young adulthood [4]. The college lifestyle includes barriers to healthful eating behaviors such as limited cooking skills and limited finances leading to meal skipping or frequent snacking on readily accessible unhealthful food [5,6]. College athletes are particularly vulnerable to poor eating habits due to the added demands of competitive sport and the need for nutritional services and education on healthful dietary habits in members of athletic teams and sports is evident [6].

Disease risk factors associated with diet are often attributed to increased intake or lack of consumption of singular nutrients (e.g., saturated fat, dietary fiber) or food groups (e.g., fruits and vegetables) [7]. However, including or excluding individual food items or food groups to or from the diet is difficult due to its complex nature. Because of these complex interactions, dietary habits are becoming increasingly characterized as latent variables or constructs. Latent variable analysis is the emerging standard of measuring dietary habits or "dietary patterns" using pattern identification protocols (i.e. cluster and factor analysis) [8]. Latent variable analysis has contributed to the understanding of dietary composition related to health outcomes [9], as healthful dietary patterns reduce risks for CVD markers [10].

Our purpose was to determine construct validity of the nutrition component of the Rapid Eating and Activity Assessment for Patients (REAP) to describe dietary patterns of NCAA Division-I athletes using pattern identification protocol. Secondly, dietary pattern scores were examined in males and females between sport types, with the hypothesis that athletes in sports where success is partially dependent on an amenable physique (e.g., gymnastics) exhibit different scores than athletes in sports where an appealing physique has no impact on success (e.g., baseball/softball). Lastly, we explored whether dietary pattern score was a predictor of CVD markers of body mass index (BMI) and waist circumference.

Methods

Data were obtained during two separate waves of collection, June-August 2011 (n = 150) and June-August 2012 (n = 241). In each wave, convenience samples of male and female NCAA Division-I athletes were asked to complete an informed consent and the REAP either immediately before or after a pre-participation physical examination. The protocol was approved by the University Office of Research Integrity and Assurance. Demographic information was approved for extraction from the athlete's electronic medical record (EMR) by the lead researcher and included sex, age, race/ethnicity, and sport.

Data from the first wave (n = 150) of completed REAP surveys identified possible dietary patterns using principal components analysis (PCA). Data from the second wave (n = 241) confirmed dietary patterns using exploratory (EFA) and confirmatory (CFA) factor analysis. Mean differences in dietary pattern scores of athletes after stratifying by gender and the aesthetic nature of the sport were compared. The interactive role of dietary pattern score x aesthetic nature of the sport on markers of CVD (BMI and waist circumference) was examined within these subpopulations.

Measurements

The REAP was originally developed to evaluate the dietary behaviors with the goal to identify a comprehensive nutritional profile [11]. The original survey includes 27 questions assessing the eating frequency of breakfast and meals not prepared in the home, intake of whole grains, fruits and vegetables, calcium-rich foods, saturated fat and cholesterol, sugar-rich food and beverages, sodium, alcohol beverages, and physical activity level. The survey takes approximately 10 minutes to complete and is written at the sixth-grade reading level. Practicing physicians consider the survey a feasible tool to assess patients' dietary habits and it is valid against the Healthy Eating Index in medical students and against food frequency questionnaires in the general population [12]. Good test-retest reliability ($r = 0.86$) was reported in ethnically and educationally diverse groups [12]. In the current study, only nutrition questions were examined. Answers were coded according to previous studies with usually/often = 1, sometimes = 2, rarely/never = 3, and blank answers = 3 [13]. Questions are phrased so higher scores indicate healthier eating behaviors. The alcohol use answers were categorized by frequency of alcohol consumption over the past month. Frequency of consuming >1-2 drinks were categorized as 0–1 times = rarely/never(3), 1–6 times = sometimes(2), and >6 times = usually/often(1).

Body weight (to the nearest 0.5 lbs.) and height (to the nearest 0.5 inch) were collected during the athlete's pre-participation physical examination. Waist circumference was obtained by using a standard tailor's tape measuring the narrowest portion of the waist between the xyphoid process and naval, recorded to the nearest quarter inch and expressed in centimeters. Weight was measured on a laboratory scale.

Data analysis

PCA was conducted with the first wave of data using the scree plot to determine the number of components to retain. EFA was conducted on the second wave of data to represent the realistic nature of the study measurement. Proportion of common variance >0.75 and chi-square significance test of retained factors against the inclusion of an additional factor were criteria used to determine the number of factors to retain. The second wave of athletes was surveyed to avoid dependency among the data. Last, a CFA, designed to test the fit of the exploratory factor model was performed. Factor score coefficients were obtained from the confirmed model output and scores were computed for each participant on each dietary pattern.

After progressing through the model identification steps to establish the construct validity of the REAP, male and female athletes were stratified by participation in aesthetic, or appearance-oriented sport; or non-aesthetic sport, in which success is not related to appearance. Aesthetic sports included gymnastics, swimming, diving, and wrestling. Non-aesthetic sports included golf, basketball, baseball, softball, soccer, football, volleyball, cross-country/track and field, water polo, and tennis. Mean differences between pattern scores were explored between aesthetic classification (aesthetic sport vs. non-aesthetic sport) for males and females using a two-way ANOVA. Regression prediction models to examine if an interaction between pattern scores and participation in aesthetic or non-aesthetic sport impact BMI and waist circumference were conducted. All data were analyzed using SAS 9.3 (Cary, NC) with significance set at $p < 0.05$.

Results

Comparison of wave-1 (n = 150) and wave-2 (n = 241) (Table 1) showed that participants were similar across waves for age, gender, race, and aesthetic vs. non-aesthetic sport status.

Principal components analysis (PCA)

A PCA oblique rotation (promax) was conducted on the 25 nutrition items of the wave-1 REAP. The initial analysis indicated seven components be retained based on eigenvalues >1 that explained 62.01% of the variance in the sample. The scree plot showed an inflection point suggesting five components be retained [14] that explained 53.2% of the data variance. Small communalities (<0.4) suggested that questions two ($h^2 = 0.31$) and 28 ($h^2 = 0.34$) be eliminated. Due to small loadings (<0.4) questions 22 (loading = 0.29) and 24 (loading = 0.22) were eliminated and cross loading (>0.35 on more than one factor) indicated questions 12 (loadings = 0.36, 0.35) and 13 (loadings = 0.38, 0.35) be eliminated. The final PCA resulted in 19 questions loading on five factors explaining 60.3% of the sample variance. Based on item

factor loadings, factor one represented a dessert pattern (DES; sweets, dessert consumption), factor two represented a high-fat food pattern (FAT; fried foods, high-fat snack consumption), factor three represented a healthful eating pattern (HP; whole grain, fruit, vegetable consumption), factor four represented a meat choice pattern (MEAT; frequency, amount, and fat content of meats), and factor five represented a dairy pattern (DARY; whole milk, regular cheese, salad dressing consumption).

Exploratory factor analysis (EFA)

Additional file 1: Table S2 displays the final rotated 5-factor pattern solution using 14 REAP items. The initial EFA on wave-2 data determined four factors should be retained based on proportion criterion (>0.75) although the chi-square was significant ($\chi^2 = 165.2$, $p < 0.0001$) indicating a rejection of the null-hypothesis ($H_0 = 4$-factor model) and the testing of a 5-factor model. Low communalities on questions one ($h^2 = 0.13$), three ($h^2 = 0.13$), six ($h^2 = 0.12$), seven ($h^2 = 0.24$), 18 ($h^2 = 0.32$), and 23 ($h^2 = 0.33$) suggested they be eliminated from further analyses; but in keeping with the goal of achieving a simple solution (high loading on only factor with low loadings on all others), questions three (loading = 0.36) and seven (loading = 0.54) were retained. Questions 17, 18, and 23 were removed due to non-loading (<0.40). The EFA was rerun revealing model fit statistics (chi-square $p > 0.05$, Tucker-Lewis = 0.99) and the scree plot inflection point conducive to a 5-factor model with the 14 remaining variables. DES explained most of the shared variance and DARY, MEAT, HP, and FAT explained the remaining shared variance.

Confirmatory factor analysis (CFA)

The wave-2 data was a good fit (RMSEA = 0.055, CFI = 0.934) to the 5-factor model with the 14 REAP items. The initial CFA conducted on the second wave of data showed the model to be good fit based on common fit indices (GFI = 0.936, CFI = 0.929, RMSEA = 0.058), however warning messages indicated fit statistics might not be accurate. A second-order CFA was conducted to examine the existence of a hierarchical model, but resulted in unclear factor score coefficients and worse model fit (GFI = 0.925, CFI = 0.906, RMSEA = 0.064). A multigroup CFA was conducted to determine if model fit improved with gender stratification. Fit indices indicated the gender-stratified model to be a slightly better fit overall (RMSEA = 0.055, CFI = 0.934), for males (GFI = 0.904), and females (GFI = 0.918). This gender-differentiated group structure was used based on improved fit indices (reported above). Pattern scores were computed by summing the product of each survey item score coefficient by the item's numerical response.

Table 1 Descriptives of male, female, and total sample of 2 waves of data

WAVE 1

		Males (n=86)	Females (n-64)	Total (n=150)
		Mean SD	Mean SD	Mean SD
Age		19.6 (1.4)	19.5 (1.2)	19.5 (1.3)
Height (cm)		183.4 (8.6)	169.9 (7.9)	177.6 (10.6)
Weight (kg)		87.3 (20.9)	67.4 (46.4)	78.8 (20.5)
BMI		25.8 (5.2)	23.2 (3.5)	24.7 (4.7)
		N %	N %	N %
Race				
	Caucasian	50 (33.3)	51 (34.0)	101 (67.3)
	African American	23 (15.3)	6 (4.0)	29 (19.3)
	Other	13 (8.7)	7 (4.7)	20 (13.3)
Sport				
	Aesthetic	28 (32.6)	13 (20.3)	41 (27.3)
	Non-aesthetic	58 (67.4)	51 (79.7)	109 (72.7)

WAVE 2

		Men (n=139)	Women (n=102)	Total (n=241)
		Mean SD	Mean SD	Mean SD
	Age	20.0 (1.6)	19.1 (1.3)	19.6 (1.5)
	Height (cm)	186.3 (26.6)	170.1 (8.5)	179.4 (22.4)
	Weight (kg)	90.9 (20.8)	66.5 (10.3)	80.6 (21.0)
	Waist Circumference (cm)*	84.8 (9.1)	74.8 (7.5)	31.9 (3.9)
	BMI (kg/m2)	26.6 (5.1)	22.9 (2.5)	25.0 (4.5)
		N %	N %	N %
Race				
	Caucasian	82 66.13	73 80.22	155 72.09
	African-American	34 27.42	13 14.29	47 21.86
	Other	8 6.45	5 5.49	13 6.05
	Not Reported	15	11	26
Sport				
	Aesthetic	26 18.98	28 27.45	54 22.59
	Nonaesthetic	111 81.02	74 72.55	185 77.41
	Not Reported	2	0	2

*N=81 Men, N=48 Women, N=129 Total.

Pattern score differences, BMI and waist circumference

For males (Figure 1), a significant mean difference ($p < .05$) in DES pattern scores (mean ± SE) were observed between aesthetic (1.93 ± 0.11) and non-aesthetic sport (2.16 ± 0.07) athletes while controlling for age and race. No other significant differences were found in males. Figure 2 shows female aesthetic athletes had higher (better) scores compared to non-aesthetic female athletes for the DES (2.11 ± 0.11; 1.88 ± 0.08), MEAT (1.95 ± 0.10; 1.72 ± 0.07), FAT (1.70 ± 0.08, 1.46 ± 0.06), and DARY (1.70 ± 0.11, 1.43 ± 0.07) patterns while controlling for age and race. HP was not significantly different between female aesthetic and non-aesthetic athletes. Interactions between the pattern score and aesthetic/non-aesthetic sport in predicting BMI or waist circumference were not observed ($p > .05$).

Discussion

Using pattern identification protocols, the REAP had construct validity for dietary pattern assessment in a population of NCAA athletes and distinguished different dietary habits between aesthetic and non-aesthetic athletes, particularly in females. Five factors were observed to reflect dietary intake: consumption of desserts, healthy foods, high-fat foods, dairy, and meat choices. Dietary patterns between aesthetic and non-aesthetic athletes were different

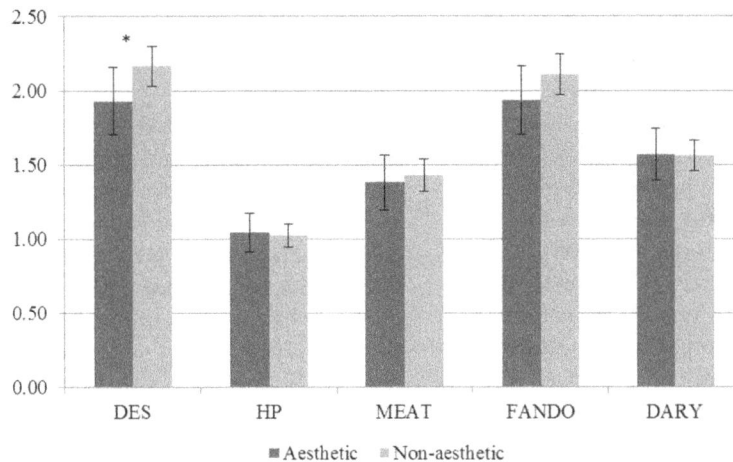

Figure 1 Means and standard errors for dietary pattern scores of aesthetic and non-aesthetic sport male athletes. All models adjust for age and race. *$p < .05$.

in males and females. Aesthetic-sport males reported lower dessert pattern scores than non-aesthetic-sport males, while aesthetic-sport females reported higher pattern scores for the dessert, meat, high fat food, and dairy patterns. No interaction between dietary patterns and waist circumference and BMI were observed, indicating that the relationship between health metrics and pattern scores do not differ by sport type.

Several approaches can be used to measure individuals' dietary patterns and multiple analyses should be used on multiple samples to verify the findings [15]. PCA is a useful screening procedure to reduce the initial pool of questions and trim those that do not contribute to eating patterns [15] while representing as much of the variation

within the data as possible. EFA seeks to explore the number of factors underlying the data that best reproduce the correlations while accounting for error variance. PCA and factor analysis have been used previously to assess food intake patterns in relation to waist circumference and triglycerides [16], hence they are useful when examining associations between dietary patterns and health metrics. One approach to assessing diet is to examine intake compared to guidelines. However, our analysis took a data-driven approach, a method that has become acceptable over the past decade [10]. Using a series of multivariate analysis techniques, the underlying structure of this survey was determined in an under-studied yet high risk population of NCAA athletes [6].

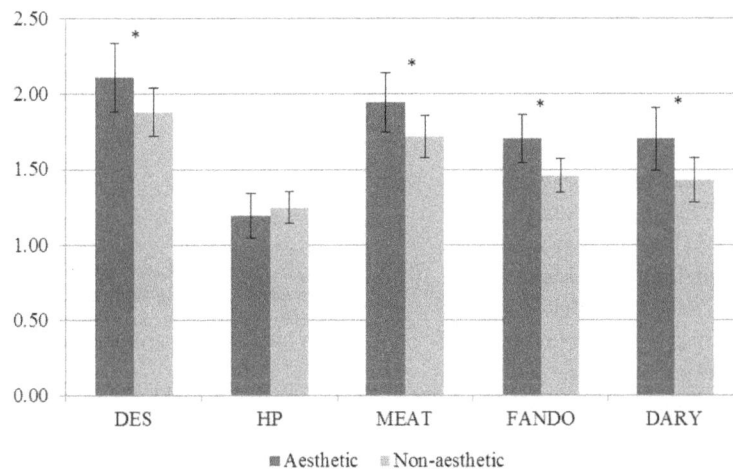

Figure 2 Means and standard errors for dietary pattern scores of aesthetic and non-aesthetic sport female athletes. All models adjust for age and race. *$p < .05$.

The 5-factor solution is a unique finding among factor-analyzed dietary studies, possibly because college athletes' eating behaviors are seldom examined using these methods. Most studies using the PCA/factor analysis approach involve middle-aged men and women and often find a limited amount of sample variance represented by components [8]. Our 5-factor PCA represented 60% of the sample variance. While variance accounted for is important in deriving dietary patterns, the interpretability of the solution is just as important [17]. Our solution is comparable to other studies in regards to pattern characteristics. Red meat consumption and vegetable/fruit intake patterns have been identified previously [18] as has a dairy pattern [19], but the dessert pattern has yet to be identified to our knowledge. Our results agree with previous studies concluding females have better diet scores than males [8], although this was evident in non-aesthetic sport females. Male non-aesthetic sport athletes had higher dessert, high-fat food, and dairy consumption scores than non-aesthetic sport females, indicating better eating choices for these three dietary patterns in this sub-group of male athletes.

In comparison to their recreational athlete and non-athletic counter parts, college athletes are at increased risk for poor dietary patterns. Lack of discipline, social obligations, time constraints, perception of the impact of a healthful diet, and ready access to healthful food are cited as barriers to healthful eating among college athletes [5]. Sports discipline is an important moderator when evaluating athlete nutrition, as unhealthful eating behaviors may be modeled from teammates [20]. Athletes often transition out of sport without adequate nutrition knowledge that may follow them for the rest of their lives [21], increasing risk of poor health outcomes.

There are some limitations to the data-driven approach to dietary pattern examination. Most studies use PCA, EFA, or CFA to derive latent factors. This study employed all three methods, a strength of the study. However, the patterns derived from these methods are not often predictive of a tangible outcome variable, such as BMI or waist circumference. This is likely due to the fact that while dietary patterns explain variation in eating behaviors, they are not specific to nor explain variation in nutrients consumed. The lack of variability in BMI (wave-1 SD = 4.7; wave-2 SD = 4.5) may have suppressed differences between dietary patterns as well. Specific to this population of college athletes, energy needs may not be the same across different types of sport. Therefore, a diet consisting of more higher-fat foods may be more appropriate in the more physically demanding sports. Other methods of analyses and specific diet composition measurement methods should be considered as a valuable alternative [22]. Also, bias may exist in the self-reporting of dietary habits, possibly

contributing to under-reporting of unhealthful eating behaviors and over-reporting of healthier behaviors.

Conclusions

The REAP demonstrated construct validity when measuring dietary patterns in a population of NCAA Division-I athletes. College athletes are a group that requires guidance in light of the increasing demands and expectations given dual roles as athlete and student. It is recommended that all athletes, regardless of sport, be screened for dietary intake behaviors. Education regarding healthful eating should be provided by a sport dietician to prevent unhealthful eating behaviors from being adopted. Young adults should continue to be monitored and advised on healthful dietary choices to encourage the development of healthful dietary habits that may persist into middle and late adulthood.

Consent

Written informed consent was obtained from the patient for the publication of this report and any accompanying images.

Additional file

Additional file 1: Table S2. Exploratory factor analysis: rotated factor pattern of item loadings and communalities.

Competing interests

The authors declare no financial support for the work supported in the manuscript, sources of substantial technical assistance, or sources from which some or all of the data were taken.

Authors' contributions

JMK contributed to the acquisition of data, analysis and interpretation of data, drafting of the manuscript, and revising the manuscript for intellectual content. MPB contributed to the analysis and interpretation of the data and revising the manuscript for intellectual content. BEA contributed to the conception and design of the study and revising the manuscript for intellectual content. All authors read and approved the final manuscript.

Acknowledgements

The authors wish to thank the University athletics department for their cooperation with this project.

References

1. Julia C, Vernay M, Salanave B, Deschamps V, Malon A, Oleko A, Hercberg S, Castetbon K: Nutrition patterns and metabolic syndrome: a need for action in young adults (French Nutrition and Health Survey - ENNS, 2006-2007). Prev Med 2010, 51:488–493.
2. Bovard RS: Risk behaviors in high school and college sport. Curr Sports Med Rep 2008, 7:359–366.
3. Borchers JR, Clem KL, Habash DL, Nagaraja HN, Stokley LM, Best TM: Metabolic syndrome and insulin resistance in Division 1 collegiate football players. Med Sci Sports Exerc 2009, 41:2105–2110.
4. Harvey JS Jr: Nutritional management of the adolescent athlete. Clin Sports Med 1984, 3:671–678.
5. Greaney ML, Less FD, White AA, Dayton SF, Riebe D, Blissmer B, Shoff S, Walsh JR, Greene GW: College students' barriers and enablers for

healthful weight management: a qualitative study. *J Nutr Educ Behav* 2009, **41**:281–286.

6. Quatromoni PA: Clinical observations from nutrition services in college athletics. *J Am Diet Assoc* 2008, **108**:689–694.

7. Amini M, Esmaillzadeh A, Shafaeizadeh S, Behrooz J, Zare M: Relationship between major dietary patterns and metabolic syndrome among individuals with impaired glucose tolerance. *Nutrition* 2010, **26**:986–992.

8. Kant AK: Dietary patterns and health outcomes. *J Am Diet Assoc* 2004, **104**:615–635.

9. Berg CM, Lappas G, Strandhagen E, Wolk A, Torén K, Rosengren A, Aires N, Thelle DS, Lissner L: Food patterns and cardiovascular disease risk factors: the Swedish INTERGENE research program. *Am J Clin Nutr* 2008, **88**:289–297.

10. Kant AK: Dietary patterns: biomarkers and chronic disease risk. *Appl Physiol Nutr Metab* 2010, **35**:199–206.

11. Gans KM, Ross E, Barner CW, Wylie-Rosett J, McMurray J, Eaton C: REAP and WAVE: new tools to rapidly assess/discuss nutrition with patients. *J Nutr* 2003, **133**:556S–562S.

12. Gans KM, Risica PM, Wylie-Rosett J, Ross EM, Strolla LO, McMurray J, Eaton CB: Development and evaluation of the nutrition component of the Rapid Eating and Activity Assessment for Patients (REAP): a new tool for primary care providers. *J Nutr Educ Behav* 2006, **38**:286–292.

13. Segal-Isaacson CJ, Wylie-Rosett J, Gans KM: Validation of a short dietary assessment questionnaire: the Rapid Eating and Activity Assessment for Participants short version (REAP-S). *Diabetes Educ* 2004, **30**:774. 776, 778 passim.

14. Cattell RB: The scree test for the number of factors. *Multivariate Behav Res* 1966, **1**:245–276.

15. Matsunaga M: How to factor-analyze your data right: do's, don'ts, and how-to's. *Int J Psychol Res* 2010, **3**:97–110.

16. Panagiotakos DB, Pitsavos C, Skoumas Y, Stefanadis C: The association between food patterns and the metabolic syndrome using principal components analysis: The ATTICA Study. *J Am Diet Assoc* 2007, **107**:979–987. quiz 997.

17. McCann SE, Marshall JR, Brasure JR, Graham S, Freudenheim JL: Analysis of patterns of food intake in nutritional epidemiology: food classification in principal components analysis and the subsequent impact on estimates for endometrial cancer. *Public Health Nutr* 2001, **4**:989–997.

18. Tseng M, DeVellis RF: Fundamental dietary patterns and their correlates among US whites. *J Am Diet Assoc* 2001, **101**:929–932.

19. Schulze MB, Hoffmann K, Kroke A, Boeing H: Dietary patterns and their association with food and nutrient intake in the European Prospective Investigation into Cancer and Nutrition (EPIC)-Potsdam study. *Br J Nutr* 2001, **85**:363–373.

20. Nazni P, Vimala S: Nutrition knowledge, attitude and practice of college sportsmen. *Asian J Sports Med* 2010, **1**:93–100.

21. Shoaf LR, McClellan PD, Birskovich KA: Nutrition knowledge, interests, and information sources of male athletes. *J Nutr Educ* 1986, **18**:243–245.

22. Moeller SM, Reedy J, Millen AE, Dixon LB, Newby PK, Tucker KL, Krebs-Smith SM, Guenther PM: Dietary patterns: challenges and opportunities in dietary patterns research an Experimental Biology workshop, April 1, 2006. *J Am Diet Assoc* 2007, **107**:1233–1239.

8

Dietary supplement usage and motivation in Brazilian road runners

José Vítor Vieira Salgado[1,3*], Pablo Christiano Barboza Lollo[2], Jaime Amaya-Farfan[2] and Mara PatríciaTraina Chacon-Mikahil[1]

Abstract

Background: The consumption of dietary supplements is highest among athletes and it can represent potential a health risk for consumers.

Objective: The aim of this study was to determine the prevalence of consumption of dietary supplements by road runners.

Methods: We interviewed 817 volunteers from four road races in the Brazilian running calendar. The sample consisted of 671 male and 146 female runners with a mean age of 37.9 ± 12.4 years.

Results: Of the sample, 28.33% reported having used some type of dietary supplement. The main motivation for this consumption is to increase in stamina and improve performance. The probability of consuming dietary supplements increased 4.67 times when the runners were guided by coaches. The consumption of supplements was strongly correlated ($r = 0.97$) with weekly running distance, and also highly correlated ($r = 0.86$) with the number of years the sport had been practiced. The longer the runner had practiced the sport, the higher the training volume and the greater the intake of supplements. The five most frequently cited reasons for consumption were: energy enhancement (29.5%), performance improvement (17.1%), increased level of endurance (10.3%), nutrient replacement (11.1%), and avoidance of fatigue (10.3%). About 30% of the consumers declared more than one reason for taking dietary supplements. The most consumed supplements were: carbohydrates (52.17%), vitamins (28.70%), and proteins (13.48%).

Conclusions: Supplement consumption by road runners in Brazil appeared to be guided by the energy boosting properties of the supplement, the influence of coaches, and the experience of the user. The amount of supplement intake seemed to be lower among road runners than for athletes of other sports. We recommend that coaches and nutritionists emphasise that a balanced diet can meet the needs of physically active people.

Keywords: Road race, Road runners, Dietary supplements, Performance, Running

Background

The consumption of dietary supplements is highest among athletes [1,2]. The practice has become increasingly popular in Brazil, and is prevalent not only among athletes but among those who practice physical activity for recreational purposes and non-professional athletes [3] such as road runners [4]. The abusive consumption

of food supplements can represent a health risk for consumers in general and also for road runners. The analysis of dietary supplements conducted by the International Olympic Committee's anti-doping lab found that of 634 supplements tested, 14.8% contained precursors of hormones such as testosterone and nandrolone, substances not declared on the product labels. Similar findings have been reported by other authors [5].

Both the supply of dietary supplements and road racing are growing trends, as can be seen from the number of competitions and the steady increase in the number of participants [6,7] since the "jogging boom" of the early 1970s, as inspired by the theory of Kenneth

* Correspondence: josevitorvs@gmail.com
[1]Exercise Physiology Laboratory - FISEX, FEF-UNICAMP Cidade Universitária, Physical Education Faculty, State University of Campinas, Cep:13083-851, Campinas SP 6134, Brazil
[3]Sport's Sciences Department, University of Campinas, Physical Education Faculty, Erico Veríssimo Av., 701., Campinas, Brazil
Full list of author information is available at the end of the article

Cooper [8]. According to the Marathons and Distance Races International Association [9], both marathons and road races are increasingly being seen as participative recreations. This is evident in Brazil, especially in São Paulo City where road races have grown exponentially; in 2012 there were 311 competitions compared with 11 in 2001 [5,6]. Thus, the objective of this study was to verify the prevalence of the use of commercial dietary supplements among Brazilian road runners.

Methods

A previously structured interview was conducted with 817 registered runners who agreed to participate voluntarily in the study and signed a consent term. The research project was previously approved by the UNICAMP university's Ethics Research Committee (n° 5372005). The targeted group of runners took part in the following races in the national official calendar of competitions (Table 1): "Integração" race (10 km), Campinas-SP; "Maratona Pão de Açúcar de Revezamento" race (10 km), São Paulo-SP; "Volta Internacional da Pampulha" race (17,8 km), Belo Horizonte-MG; and "São Silvestre" race (15 km), São Paulo-SP. The average age (±SD) of the sample was 37.9 ± 12.4 years. The oldest subject interviewed was 92 and the youngest was 15 years old. Of all the subjects interviewed, 82.1% (n = 671) were men and 17.9% (n = 146) were women.

Sample selection

The sample design used was defined according to the calculation of the sample size to a proportion, considering a value of 50% for the proportion (p = 50%) for the athletes to submit to nutritional supplementation, with a variation of 7% (v = 7%) and confidence level of 5% (alpha = 5%), also considering 10% of loss and rejection. Thus a total of 840 interviews was determined as necessary, distributed throughout the four races (210 interviews/race). The sampling was random for each race, and only amateur athletes were considered for filling in the questionnaire.

Questionnaire

The questionnaire used for the interviews was structured according to a pre-competition scenario, following the recommendations of Foddy, 1994 [10]. The questionnaire

Table 1 Road races where the data were collected

City	State	Road race	Distance
Campinas	SP	Integração	10 km
São Paulo	SP	Maratona Pão de Açúcar de Revezamento	42,195 km
Belo Horizonte	MG	Volta da Pampulha	17,8 km
São Paulo	SP	São Silvestre	15 km

comprised 10 questions, including both closed questions such as, "Do you use any type of food supplement?" (with reply options of "yes" or "no"), and open questions such as, "Which supplement(s) do you use?" The questionnaire was tested and validated before its application, and the validation (pre-test) and training of the evaluation team took place at the "Corrida da Independência" in Campinas - SP, Brazil.

Data analysis

A descriptive analysis, inferential statistics and hypothesis test: Pearson's Correlation test and the Odds Ratio (OR) test were carried out using the software SPSS 13.0 for Windows, Release 13.0, and adopting a value of $p < 0.05$.

Results

The average age (±SD) of the sample was 37.9 ± 12.4 years. The oldest interviewed subject was 92 and the youngest 15 years old. Of all the interviewed subjects, 82.1% (n = 671) were men and 17.9% (n = 146) were women.

Those who reported to be dietary supplement consumers (n = 230) represented 28.3% of the entire sample, of which 81.7% were men (n = 188) and 18.3% women (n = 42). Of the total sample, 71.7% (n = 687) were non-consumers of supplements, constituted by men 82.3% (n = 483) and 17.7% (n = 104) women. We did not find any significant differences between genders among dietary supplement consumers and non-consumers.

When asked whether they received some guidance from managers or coaches in their physical activities, 27.3% of the subjects stated that they did not receive guidance from either source. Among those with professional guidance for race training, the dietary supplement consumers represented almost twice the number of those with no guidance (42.60 to 22.39%), as seen in Figure 1.

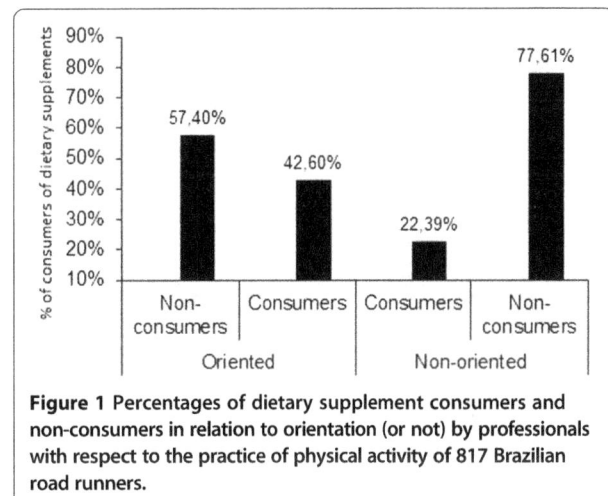

Figure 1 Percentages of dietary supplement consumers and non-consumers in relation to orientation (or not) by professionals with respect to the practice of physical activity of 817 Brazilian road runners.

The fact that a runner had been trained by a coach increased the chances of the runner being a dietary supplements consumer (OR = 4.67, p < 0.0001) by more than 4.5 times. When correlating the dietary supplements consumption with the volume of weekly training (km/week), the coefficient found was r = 0.97, indicating that the higher the training volume, the higher the frequency of dietary supplement consumption (Figure 2).

A similar tendency can be found in Figure 3, where the frequency of consumers was plotted against the number of years of road-racing practice. The correlation in this case was r = 0.86. Therefore, consumers of supplements were more frequently found among subjects that had been regularly training for a longer period of time, to the detriment of beginners.

As noticed in Figure 3, only about 20% of the runners with no specific training for road races, though frequently participating in competitions, did consume supplements. Comparing the prevalence of dietary supplement consumption separately in each race, significant differences were observed only among competitors of the São Silvestre and the Integração competitions (p = 0.003), as seen in Table 2.

Of the subjects using supplements (28.3% of the sample), the five reasons mentioned as causes for supplement consumption were: to obtain energy (29.5%; n = 69), to increase performance (17.1%; n = 40), to replace nutrients (11.1%; n = 26), to increase stamina (10.3%; n = 24), and to avoid fatigue (10.3%; n = 24). Of the consumers, 29.5% (n = 69) used more than one supplement and declared more than one reason for consuming them.

We have noticed that behind the reasons quoted to induce consumption (obtaining energy, increasing stamina, and avoiding fatigue), there were allusions to boosting performance. Grouping the reasons, the athletic performance was the most quoted one; i.e., 17.1% and 54.7% of the consumers, respectively, quoted it either

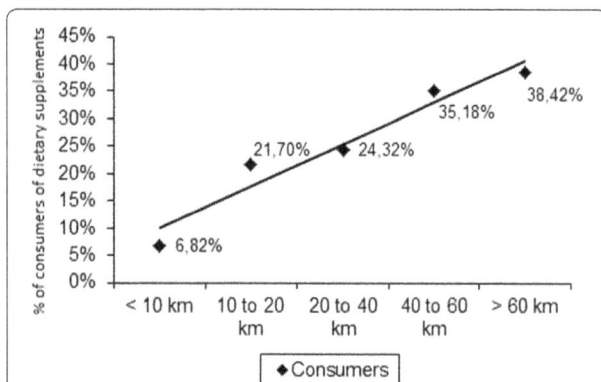

straightforwardly or indirectly. The dietary supplements that the road runners admitted using the most were carbohydrates (52.17%).

From the reasons quoted (obtaining energy, increasing stamina, and avoiding fatigue), it was thought that the enhancement of performance was the main factor in taking supplements. Grouping the reasons, athletic performance was the most quoted, with 17.1% and 54.7% of consumers respectively quoting it either straightforwardly or indirectly. We found only five subjects who mentioned the consumption of isotonic drinks, but this low number may result from the non-association of isotonic drinks with dietary supplements.

Discussion

The aim of the present study was to verify the prevalence of use of commercial dietary supplements amongst Brazilian road runners and 28.3% of the road runners questioned were found to be dietary supplement consumers. No studies of a similar population (Brazilian road runners) were found, but the percentage of road runners (amateurs) consuming dietary supplements in this study was similar to the prevalence found in the Los Angeles Marathon of 1987, which was 29% [11]. This

Figure 3 Pearson's Correlation between dietary supplement consumption as a function of the road racer's history of practice in 817 Brazilian road runners.

Figure 2 Pearson's Correlation between dietary supplement consumption and training volume (km/week) in 817 Brazilian road runners.

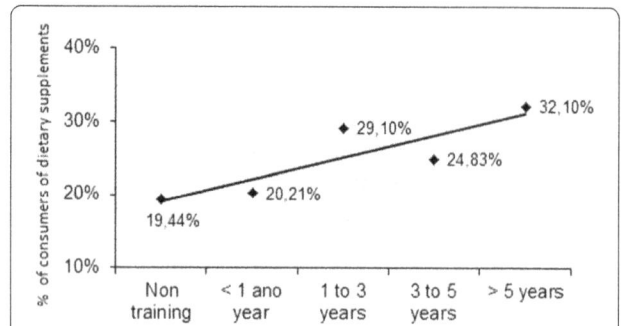

Table 2 Supplements used by the athletes in 4 road races in Brazil

	Integração	PA	Pampulha	SS	TOTAL
Non consumers	79.6%	69.0%	73.0%	66.0%	81.7%
Consumers	20.4%	31.0%	27.0%	34.0%	28.3%
Vitamins and Minerals	16.7%	25.8%	29.8%	42.5%	28.7%
Carbohydrate	26.7%	16.1%	17.0%	10.0%	17.5%
Protein	20.0%	12.9%	17.0%	15.0%	16.2%
BCAA*	33.3%	29.0%	21.3%	20.0%	25.9%
Creatine	3.3%	12.9%	10.6%	10.0%	9.2%
Others	0.0%	3.2%	4.3%	2.5%	2.5%

*Branched chain amino acids.

prevalence is significantly low as compared to elite athletes, the use of nutritional supplements in professional long and middle distance track and field athletes being 82% [12]. The general use of nutritional supplements by athletics has been reported to be about 60% in adults and junior athletes [13]. This suggests that supplement consumption in Brazil is a relatively recent phenomenon, and lower than in developed countries. The data show there is a substantial consumption of dietary supplements amongst road runners, although lower than amongst gym goers (36.8%) [14–16] and basketball players (58%) [17]. Studies carried out with samples that were equally significant to those used in the present study [14,15] reported consumption rates in gyms that varied between 36.8 and 61.2%. The greater consumption amongst runners with professional coaching was obvious, suggesting that physical education teachers or managers may be stimulating this consumption in some way. The authors would like to clarify that in this study the interviewees were not asked to reveal who recommended this practice. However, data from gyms clearly identified these professionals as strong inducers of supplement consumption [14–18]. For an adequate consumption, road racers should ask for professional advice in the use of supplements, since some supplements have been shown to contain doping substances [5], and it is unclear whether the coaches or athletes know about this.

We detected only five subjects who mentioned the consumption of isotonic drinks, but this low number may result from the non-association of isotonic drinks with dietary supplements. During races, these products are frequently handed out for free. To the contrary of the present data, the consumption of isotonic drinks was 32% amongst gymnasium users [14], 27.5% amongst university students [19] and 90.1% amongst university athletes from Singapore [20]. The present study showed that the frequency of consumption increased with either the distance of weekly training or the training time. This outcome may be related to the perception that this type of training is associated with high energy requirements.

Considering that the races analyzed covered a minimum distance of 10 km, hydration and electrolyte loss may be considered as relevant factors, since about 2% dehydration already causes an important loss of performance, dehydration between 4 and 6% may cause thermal fatigue, and dehydration above 6% causes a risk of thermal shock, coma and even death [21]. Nevertheless, amongst those interviewed, only 2.1% (n=5) reported straightforwardly having consumed some kind of supplement with this intention. The authors believe that in addition to the above, the higher exposure of newcomers to environments where supplement consumption is commonplace could place the more experienced athlete in a truly influential position to promote new

dietary techniques, in order for beginners to achieve their desired performances. Supplement consumption by road runners in Brazil appears to have been guided by the energy boosting properties of the supplement (38.6%), the influence of physical educators, the training volume and by the experience of the user in road races. The volumes intakes seemed to be lower than those practiced by athletes of other sports.

Conclusion

The authors believe that the higher exposure of newcomers to environments where supplement consumption is commonplace could place the more experienced athlete in an influential position to promote new dietary techniques, in order for beginners to achieve their desired performance. Supplement consumption by road runners in Brazil appears to have been guided by the energy boosting properties of the supplement, the influence of coaches, the training volume, and the experience of the user in road races. The amount of supplement intake seemed to be lower than for athletes of other sports. Coaches and nutritionists should emphasise that a balanced diet can meet the needs of physically active people to avoid inadequate use of dietary supplements by road racers.

Competing interests
The authors declare that they have no competing of interest.

Authors' contributions
Conception and design of the study by JWS and MPTCM. Generation, collection, assembly, analysis and interpretation of data by JSW and PCBL. Revision of the manuscript by JAF. Approval of the final version of the manuscript by MPTCM. All authors read and approved the final manuscript.

Acknowledgments
The authors are thankful to CNPq/SAE-UNICAMP and Physical Education Faculty of University of Campinas for the support, and all the runners that participated in this study, as well as the team involved in the data collection.

Author details
[1]Exercise Physiology Laboratory - FISEX, FEF-UNICAMP Cidade Universitária, Physical Education Faculty, State University of Campinas, Cep:13083-851, Campinas SP 6134, Brazil. [2]Food's Engineering Faculty, Department of Food and Nutrition, State University of Campinas - UNICAMP, Campinas, SP, Brazil. [3]Sport's Sciences Department, University of Campinas, Physical Education Faculty, Erico Veríssimo Av., 701., Campinas, Brazil.

References
1. Braun H, Koehler K, Geyer H, Kleiner J, Mester J, Schanzer W: **Dietary supplement use among elite young German athletes.** *Int J Sport Nutr Exerc Metab* 2009, **19**:97–109.
2. Wiens K, Erdman KA, Stadnyk M, Parnell JA: **Dietary supplement usage, motivation, and education in young, Canadian athletes.** *Int J Sport Nutr Exerc Metab* 2014, http://www.ncbi.nlm.nih.gov/pubmed/24667342.
3. Guidelines of the Brazilian Society of Sports Medicine: **Dietary changes, fluid replacement, dietary supplements and drugs: demonstration of ergogenic action and potential health risks.** *Rev Bras Med Esporte* 2003, **9**:52–58.
4. Salgado JVV, Lollo PC, Miyasaka CK, Chacon-Mikahil MPT: **Prevalence of the Dietary Supplements Intake in Brazilian Road Runners.** In *13th annual*

congress of the European College Sport Science. 1st edition. Portugal: Taylor & Francis in Estoril; 2008:718.

5. Kohler M, Thomas A, Geyer H, Petrou M, Schanzer W, Thevis M: **Confiscated black market products and nutritional supplements with non-approved ingredients analyzed in the Cologne Doping Control Laboratory 2009.** *Drug Test Anal* 2010, **2**:533–537.

6. Hespanhol Junior LC, Costa LOP, Carvalho ACA, e Lopes AD: **A description of training characteristics and its association with previous musculoskeletal injuries in recreational runners: a cross-sectional study.** *Rev Bras Fisioter [online]* 2012, **16**:46–53.

7. Salgado JVV: **Comparison of functional and biochemical indicators in middle aged men undergoing aerobic training and long distance runners.** *Ms thesis. University of Campinas, Physical Education Faculty* 2009, http://libdigi.unicamp.br/document/?code=000467613.

8. Salgado JVV, Chacon-Mikahil MPT: **Street race: analyses of the growth of the number of competitions and pratictioners.** *Conexões* 2006, **4**:100–109.

9. AIMS 1982 – 2007: *Association of International Marathons and Distance Race: 25 Years of Running History.* 2007.

10. Foddy L, Mantle J: *Constructing questions for interviews and questionnaires: theory and practice in social research.* Cambridge: Cambridge University Press; 1993.

11. Nieman DC, Gates JR, Butler JV, Pollett LM, Dietrich SJ, Lutz RD: **Supplementation patterns in marathon runners.** *J Am Diet Assoc* 1989, **89**:1615–1619.

12. Tscholl P, Alonso J, Dolle G, Junge A, Dvorak J: **The use of drugs and nutritional supplements in top-level track and field athletes.** *Am J Sports Med* 2010, **38**:133–140.

13. Corrigan B, Kazlauskas R: **Medication use in athletes selected for doping control at the Sydney Olympics (2000).** *Clin J Sport Med* 2003, **13**:33–40.

14. Goston JL, Correia MI: **Intake of nutritional supplements among people exercising in gyms and influencing factors.** *Nutrition* 2010, **26**:604–611.

15. Maughan RJ, Depiesse F, Geyer H: **The use of dietary supplements by athletes.** *J Sports Sci* 2007, **25**(Suppl 1):S103–S113.

16. Lollo PCB, Tavares MCGCF: **Profile of the consumers of dietary supplements in the fitness centers of Campinas.** *Rev Dig* 2004, **5**:105–111.

17. Schroder H, Navarro E, Mora J, Seco J, Torregrosa JM, Tramullas A: **The type, amount, frequency and timing of dietary supplement use by elite players in the First Spanish Basketball League.** *J Sports Sci* 2002, **20**:353–358.

18. Smith-Rockwell M, Nickols-Richardson SM, Thye FW: **Nutrition knowledge, opinions, and practices of coaches and athletic trainers at a division university.** *Int J Sport Nutr Exerc Metab* 2001, **11**:174–185.

19. Malinauskas BM, Overton RF, Carraway VG, Cash BC: **Supplements of interest for sport-related injury and sources of supplement information among college athletes.** *Adv Med Sci* 2007, **52**:50–54.

20. Tian HH, Ong WS, Tan CL: **Nutritional supplement use among university athletes in Singapore.** *Singapore Med J* 2009, **50**:165–172.

21. Shirreffs SM: **The importance of good hydration for work and exercise performance.** *Nutr Rev* 2005, **63**:S14–S21.

9

Effects of 28-days ingestion of a slow-release energy supplement versus placebo on hematological and cardiovascular measures of health

Adam J Wells, Jay R Hoffman*, Adam M Gonzalez, Kyle S Beyer, Adam R Jajtner, Jeremy R Townsend, Leonardo P Oliveira, David H Fukuda, Maren S Fragala and Jeffrey R Stout

Abstract

Background: Recently, slow release tablets have been developed to prolong energy release throughout the day. The efficacy of the delivery of slow-release caffeine alone is fairly well documented; however, an assessment of safety and tolerability of prolonged use of slow-release energy supplements is lacking. Therefore the objective of this study was to investigate the effect of daily ingestion of a slow-release energy supplement for 28 days on blood chemistry and resting cardiovascular measures in healthy men and women.

Methods: Forty healthy individuals (20 males, 20 females; age: 22.73 ± 3.06 years; height: 171.68 ± 10.45 cm; mass: 74.49 ± 15.51 kg; BMI: 25.08 ± 3.66 $(kg \cdot m^2)^{-1}$) participated in this randomized, double-blind, placebo controlled study. Following a 12-hour fast, participants reported for pre-testing. Testing consisted of resting heart rate (RHR) and blood pressure (BP) measures, followed by assessment of metabolic blood chemistry, blood lipids and complete cell counts. Participants then supplemented with either Energize™ (SUPP) or placebo (PL) for 28 days. Post-testing occurred 24-hours after ingestion of the final dose and consisted of the same protocol at the same time of day as pre-testing.

Results: No significant changes in outcome measures were observed. A significant difference between groups was observed for plasma glucose concentrations; however, follow-up testing revealed that pre- to post-supplementation changes were not significant for either SUPP or PL. All variables remained within normal adult reference ranges. No adverse events were reported.

Conclusions: These findings indicate that 28 consecutive days ingestion of a slow release energy supplement containing caffeine in caffeine users is both safe and tolerable.

Keywords: Energy supplement, Slow-release, Caffeine, Health, Safety, Comprehensive blood chemistry, Lipid profile, Complete blood counts, Resting heart rate, Blood pressure

Background

Caffeine is the most frequently consumed pharmacologically active substance in the world [1,2], where approximately 80 percent of the adult population consumes between 200–250 mg of caffeine on a daily basis [3]. Moderate doses of caffeine can lead to an increase in both physical and mental task performance [4-10], making caffeine an ideal compound for combating both fatigue and sub-optimal arousal. Caffeine's effect is likely attributable to its function as a mild central nervous system (CNS) stimulant [11], whereby it competitively binds to adenosine receptors, leading to a suppression of its inhibitory effect on CNS activity [12]. Accordingly, caffeine is the main physiologically active ingredient in many commercially available energy supplements [13]. Nevertheless, caffeine and caffeine-containing energy supplements alike, typically induce only 90–120 minutes of increased alertness

* Correspondence: jay.hoffman@ucf.edu
Institute of Exercise Physiology and Wellness, University of Central Florida, 4000 Central Florida Blvd., Orlando, FL 32816, USA

[14,15], and are often associated with an acute "crash" state following their metabolism [16,17]. Additionally, the amounts of these ingredients are often undisclosed and unregulated [18]. As a consequence, repeat administration of such energy supplements may lead to more aversive effects and dysphoric reactions over time [3]. Of particular concern are the effects of prolonged use on resting cardiovascular parameters, as well as on hepatic and renal function.

Recently, slow release tablets have been developed to prolong energy release throughout the day [14,19]. Pharmacokinetic studies have demonstrated that these tablets are able to provide a steady release of caffeine and other compounds over a longer period of time [20], likely eliminating the need for repeat administration and possibly reducing any potential adverse effects associated with repeated use [21]. Therefore, the use of these tablets to deliver an energy supplement may be beneficial for workers involved in sustained operations that demand peak cognitive and physical performance, and provide a safer alternative to repeated dosing.

The efficacy of the delivery of slow-release caffeine alone is fairly well documented [3,21-23]. However, an assessment of safety and tolerability of prolonged use of slow-release energy supplements is lacking. Therefore, the purpose of this study was to investigate the effects of 28-days ingestion of a commercially available slow-release energy supplement on blood lipid profiles, comprehensive blood chemistry, and complete blood counts in young, healthy men and women.

Methods

Participants

Forty healthy individuals (20 men, 20 women; age: 22.73 ± 3.06 years; height: 171.68 ± 10.45 cm; mass: 74.49 ± 15.51 kg; BMI: 25.08 ± 3.66 (kg $\cdot$ m^2) $^{-1}$) who were regular consumers of caffeine volunteered to participate in this randomized, double-blind, placebo controlled study. Anthropometric data by group is presented in Table 1. The research protocol was approved by the New England Institutional Review Board. Following an explanation of all risks and benefits associated with the experimental protocol, each participant gave his or her informed consent to participate in this study. For inclusion in the

study, participants had to be regular caffeine consumers (between 60–180 mg per day). Participants were excluded if they had any history of cardiovascular disease, metabolic, renal, hepatic, or musculoskeletal disorders or were taking any other medication (other than oral contraceptives) as determined by a confidential medical history questionnaire. Participants were also excluded as a result of any intolerance or known allergy to the supplement ingredients. While enrolled in the study, participants were permitted to maintain their normal caffeine intake.

Experimental design

The experimental design is depicted in Figure 1. Following the initial screening visit, participants reported to the Human Performance Laboratory (HPL) on 22 separate occasions. Testing was conducted at pre- (visit 1) and post- (visit 22) supplementation only. Testing sessions were separated by 28 days. For each testing session, participants were required to report to the HPL following a 12-hour fast. Resting heart rate (RHR) and blood pressure (BP) were recorded, followed by a venous blood draw. Upon completion of pre-testing during visit 1, participants were required to consume the first dosage of Energize™ (iSatori, Golden, CO, USA) (SUPP) or placebo (PL) witnessed by one of the research personnel. Participants then continued supplementation for an additional 27 days. Supplement and placebo were provided by the sponsor in coded bottles. Each bottle contained 28-days' worth of supplement or placebo. Subject numbers were assigned to each code chronologically following obtainment of consent. Subject numbers were permanently marked on their respective bottles, and each daily serving for each participant was taken from the same bottle until completion of the study. Participants were required to report to the HPL on all weekdays (20 total visits) to receive either SUPP or PL. On weekends, participants were provided 2 dosages of SUPP or PL to consume on each weekend day. Weekend supplementation was provided in zip lock bags with clear instructions on how to take the supplement. All participants were required to consume the supplement before 4 pm each day to avoid disturbance of sleep cycles and return the bags the following Monday to demonstrate adherence. Post-testing (visit 22) occurred the day following ingestion of the last dosage. Following a 12-hour fast, participants completed the same testing protocol as at pretesting, at the same time of day. Recent reviews suggest that a daily caffeine dosage of 400 mg $\cdot$ d^{-1} is not associated with risk of toxicity, changes in behavior or adverse cardiovascular effects [2,24]. Since participants in the present study reported an average daily consumption of 60–180 mg of caffeine, the addition of the supplement placed average daily consumption below this threshold. As a result, changes in hematological and/or cardiovascular variables are likely related to the time-release nature of

Table 1 Participant anthropometric characteristics

Variable	SUPP (n = 20)	PL (n = 20)
	(10 men, 10 women)	(10 men, 10 women)
Age (years)	22.95 ± 3.05	22.5 ± 3.13
Height (cm)	172.83 ± 8.84	170.54 ± 11.97
Mass (kg)	73.77 ± 12.65	75.21 ± 18.23
BMI (kg $\cdot$ m^2)$^{-1}$	24.62 ± 3.35	25.53 ± 3.97

Data presented as mean ± SD.

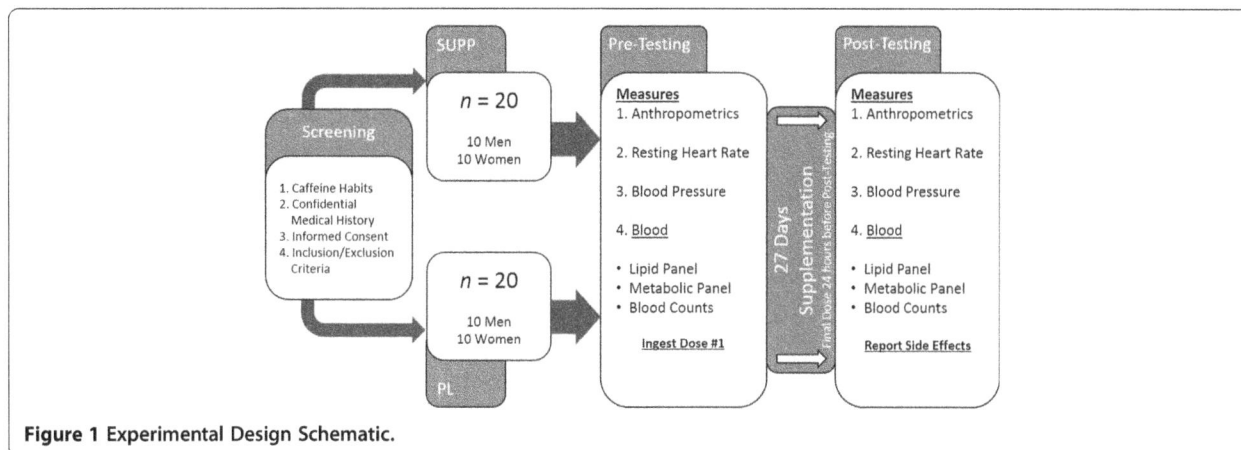

Figure 1 Experimental Design Schematic.

the supplement. All participants were asked to report any adverse effects they felt were directly attributable to ingestion of the supplement at post-testing.

Testing sessions

During visits 1 and 22, anthropometrics, RHR and BP were assessed. Upon arrival to the HPL, body mass ($\pm$ 0.1 kg) and height ($\pm$ 0.1 cm) were measured using a Health-O-Meter professional scale (Patient Weighing Scale, Model 500 KL; Pelstar, Alsip, IL, USA). Following 15-minutes of rest in a supine position, RHR and BP were assessed using a digital blood pressure monitor (Omron Healthcare, Inc, HEM-712C, Vernon Hills, Illinois, USA). A resting blood sample was then obtained from an antecubital vein in the superficial forearm using a 21-gauge disposable needle stick by an experienced lab technician. Blood was drawn into serum separator tubes (SST), serum tubes, and EDTA tubes. SST and serum tubes were allowed to clot for 30 minutes prior to centrifugation and then separated at $3000 \times g$ for 15 minutes at room temperature. The resulting serum from the serum tube was then transferred to a 5 mL transport tube. Samples were then packaged along with a requisition form for analysis at a commercial laboratory (Quest Diagnostics, Tampa, FL, USA) for blood lipids, metabolic blood chemistry, and complete blood counts.

Supplement

The SUPP and PL were ingested in tablet form, and two tablets were consumed per dose. Tablets were identical in appearance and taste. The ingredients in SUPP are presented in Table 2, while the placebo consisted of only rice powder. Participants were provided one dose per day according to manufacturer recommendations. Supplementation began immediately following the blood draw at pre- and ceased the day before post-testing. Participants did not ingest supplement or placebo on the day of post-testing. Supplement administration was witnessed by

research personnel during all weekdays. Additional work in our laboratory showed elevated plasma caffeine and theobromine concentrations for 8 hours following ingestion of Energize™ versus placebo, as determined via high performance liquid chromatography (HPLC) [25].

Statistical analyses

Statistical analysis of the data was accomplished using a 2 by 2 repeated measures analysis of variance (ANOVA) to determine between groups differences (SUPP vs. PL). In the event of significant differences between groups at baseline, data from the corresponding pre-values were used as a covariate in subsequent analysis. In the event of a significant F-ratio, dependent t-tests were used for pairwise comparisons. A criterion α-level of $p \leq 0.05$ was used to determine statistical significance. Pre- and post- mean values for all blood variables were compared against

Table 2 Supplement Ingredients (per serving size)

Ingredients	Amount	
Thiamine (vitamin B1) (as thiamine hydrochloride)	5.2	mg
Vitamin B6 (as pyridoxine hydrochloride)	25	mg
Folate (as folic acid)	200	µg
Vitamin B12 (as cyanocobalamin)	3	µg
Magnesium (as magnesium oxide)	150	mg
Proprietary Energizer Formula:	**1600**	**mg**
L-Tyrosine		
Glucuronolactone		
Natural Caffeine (coffee arabica) (seed)-sustained release	194	mg
Theobromine (theobroma cacao) (seed)		
Rhodiola Rosea Extract (root) (standardized to contain 3% rosavins & 1% salidroside)		
Korean Ginseng Powder (root)		
Octacosonal (from sugar cane polycosanol)		

mg = milligrams; µg = micrograms.

clinically accepted normative data. Data are presented as mean ± SD.

Results

Compliance among all participants was 98.3%. No significant between-group differences were observed at baseline for blood lipid variables, metabolic blood chemistry or complete blood counts. Study participants reported no adverse events during supplementation with either SUPP or PL.

Heart rate and blood pressure measures

Pre- to post-supplementation changes for RHR and BP are presented in Table 3. No significant differences between the groups were observed for RHR, SBP or DBP ($p = 0.945$, $p = 0.327$, and $p = 0.678$, respectively) from pre- to post-supplementation.

Lipid panel

Pre- to post-supplementation changes in blood lipids are presented in Table 4. No significant differences between the groups were observed for total cholesterol ($p = 0.523$), HDL cholesterol ($p = 0.235$), triglycerides ($p = 0.752$), LDL cholesterol ($p = 0.850$), non-HDL cholesterol ($p = 0.977$) or the cholesterol to HDL ratio ($p = 0.861$) from pre-to post-supplementation. All values for all blood lipid measures remained within reference norms.

Metabolic blood chemistry

Pre- to post-supplementation changes in metabolic blood chemistry are presented in Table 5. A significant difference between groups was observed for plasma glucose concentrations ($p = 0.028$); however, follow-up testing revealed that pre- to post-supplementation changes were not significant for either SUPP ($p = 0.077$) or PL ($p = 0.116$). No other changes in any blood chemistry variables were noted. All values for the metabolic blood chemistry measures remained within reference norms.

Complete blood counts

Pre- to post-supplementation changes in complete blood counts are presented in Table 6. No significant differences between the groups were observed for any of the cell count variables. Values for all blood count variables remained within reference norms.

Discussion

This is the first study to examine health and safety markers following prolonged daily ingestion of a slow-release energy supplement. The results of this study indicate that daily ingestion of a slow-release energy supplement containing approximately 200 $mg \cdot day^{-1}$ caffeine in combination with other ingredients for 28 days does not significantly affect blood lipids, metabolic blood chemistry profiles or blood counts. In addition, no changes in resting cardiovascular measures were noted, suggesting that prolonged use of the commercially available slow-release energy supplement Energize™, is apparently safe in young healthy adults.

Previous investigations have primarily focused on the efficacy of ingesting a single, moderate dose of slow release caffeine (SRC) in sleep-deprived subjects [3,10,23]. Although a number of these studies have reported SRC tolerability [21] and some have reported adverse events [21,26], studies have been limited to the acute response following a single 150–600 mg dose of SRC [3,20]. Lagarde and colleagues [20] examined a number of cardiovascular parameters including heart-rate, blood pressure and blood chemistry prior to and following the acute ingestion of 150, 300 and 600 mg of SRC in healthy male and female participants. Participants were subjected to 32-hours of sleep-deprivation in a cross-over design with a 1-week wash out period. During this time, participants underwent regular clinical evaluations, while tolerance was evaluated by complaints reported by the participants. Adverse events were reported by 8 of the 24 participants (7 female, 1 male), which included numbness, shaking, muscular pains, heart palpitations, and headaches. Two adverse events were reported in the placebo group. No significant changes in blood chemistry were observed; however, the authors did not delineate the blood tests performed. Reports of shivering and tachycardia were recorded in the 600 mg group; however, a clear break-down of adverse events by dosage was not presented. Additionally, it is not clear whether the adverse effects were related to the SRC (at any dosage), or due to the effects of sleep-deprivation.

Patat and colleagues [3] compared the effects of 600 mg SRC to placebo in a number of psychomotor and cognitive tasks in sleep-deprived subjects. Similar to our study, they utilized routine laboratory tests including complete blood counts and general blood chemistry in order to assess any

Table 3 Changes in resting heart rate and blood pressure

Variable	SUPP (n = 20)		PL (n = 20)	
	Pre	Post	Pre	Post
Resting Heart Rate (bpm)	67.45 ± 16.70	64.40 ± 11.67	68.10 ± 9.40	64.85 ± 9.09
Systolic Blood Pressure (mmHg)	123.25 ± 10.96	120.10 ± 11.06	122.25 ± 13.01	113.15 ± 26.95
Diastolic Blood Pressure (mmHg)	70.10 ± 8.33	68.65 ± 7.47	71.25 ± 7.85	68.95 ± 5.83

Pre = pre-supplementation; Post = post-supplementation; Data presented as mean ± SD.

Table 4 Changes in blood lipids

Variable	SUPP (n = 20)		PL (n = 20)		Reference Range
	Pre	Post	Pre	Post	
Total Cholesterol (mg/dL)	163.5 ± 22.8	163.8 ± 24.1	155.5 ± 25.6	152.2 ± 25.2	125-170 mg/dL
HDL Cholesterol (mg/dL)	57.9 ± 12.3	60.4 ± 16.5	56.9 ± 16.0	55.9 ± 10.7	≥ 40^M, ≥ 46^F mg/dL
Triglycerides (mg/dL)	71.0 ± 25.8	74.7 ± 30.6	70.5 ± 27.9	77.0 ± 37.6	38-152^M, 40-136^F mg/dL
LDL Cholesterol (mg/dL)	91.3 ± 25.0	88.5 ± 22.4	84.7 ± 21.1	81.0 ± 23.4	<130 mg/dL (calc)
Risk Ratio (CHOL/HDL)	3.0 ± 0.8	2.9 ± 0.7	2.9 ± 0.8	2.8 ± 0.8	≤ 5.0 (calc)
Non-HDL cholesterol	105.6 ± 25.6	103.5 ± 23.5	98.7 ± 24.6	96.4 ± 28.2	n/a mg/dL (calc)

Pre = pre-supplementation; Post = post-supplementation; ^{M} = Male; ^{F} = Female; Data presented as mean ± SD.

potential negative effects of supplementation on resting cardiovascular parameters. In line with our findings, they observed no clinically relevant changes in routine laboratory tests and reported no safety related drop-out issues. However, in contrast to our findings, three adverse events were reported for the SRC group, including an episode of anxiety in one subject, and one episode of trembling and diarrhea in another. The observed differences between the results of the present study, and those of Lagarde et al. [20] and Petat et al. [3], is likely related to the differences in the dosage used. By comparison, we used a relatively moderate dose (approx. 200 mg SRC) compared to the larger 600 mg dose utilized by others. Lagarde et al. [20] suggest that the optimal dose, defined as the maximum effect without any side effects, is 300 mg of SRC.

Considering that no adverse events were reported in the present study, our results appear to support the conclusions from Lagarde and colleagues [20]. Tolerability issues reported in previous studies appear to be transient in nature, with spontaneous remission occurring soon after the symptoms present [3,20]. This did not appear to be a concern in our study suggesting that tolerability in caffeine users is not an issue at moderate doses of SRC.

Comparable results have been observed in other studies investigating the safety aspects of similar multi-ingredient energy/thermogenic supplements [27,28]. Following 28-days ingestion of a popular multi-ingredient thermogenic drink, Roberts and colleagues [28] reported no significant group by time interactions for lipid profiles, complete blood counts or general blood chemistry in a group of

Table 5 Changes in blood chemistry

Variable	SUPP (n = 20)		PL (n = 20)		Reference Range
	Pre	Post	Pre	Post	
Glucose	88.3 ± 5.2	85.8 ± 6.1	83.2 ± 10.2	88.1 ± 6.24 ‡	65-99 mg/dL
Urea Nitrogen (BUN)	15.1 ± 4.2	15.4 ± 4.3	16.4 ± 4.1	16.4 ± 4.39	7-20 mg/dL
Creatinine	0.9 ± 0.2	1.0 ± 0.2	0.9 ± 0.2	1.0 ± 0.21	0.60-1.35^M, 0.50-1.10^F mg/dL
eGFR Non-Afr. American	107.3 ± 15.6	94.5 ± 15.8	103.6 ± 18.2	95.8 ± 14.82	≥ 60 mL/min/1.73 m^2
eGFR Afr. American	124.4 ± 18.2	109.5 ± 18.2	119.9 ± 21.0	110.9 ± 17.19	≥ 60 mL/min/1.73 m^2
Sodium	142.3 ± 2.9	143.2 ± 3.1	141.8 ± 3.2	143.1 ± 2.79	135-146 mmol/L
Potassium	4.6 ± 0.5	5.1 ± 0.5	4.7 ± 0.4	4.9 ± 0.57	3.8-5.1 mmol/L
Chloride	104.9 ± 2.6	105.7 ± 2.7	104.5 ± 2.2	104.9 ± 3.79	98-110 mmol/L
Carbon Dioxide	24.4 ± 2.7	25.4 ± 2.5	24.8 ± 2.0	26.1 ± 1.86	19-30 mmol/L
Calcium	9.6 ± 0.4	9.8 ± 0.3	9.7 ± 0.4	9.7 ± 0.33	8.6-10.3^M, 8.6-10.2^F mg/dL
Protein (TOTAL)	7.0 ± 0.4	7.1 ± 0.4	7.2 ± 0.5	7.0 ± 0.41	6.1-8.1 g/dL
Albumin	4.5 ± 0.3	4.4 ± 0.3	4.5 ± 0.3	4.4 ± 0.28	3.6-5.1 g/dL
Globulin	2.5 ± 0.4	2.6 ± 0.3	2.7 ± 0.3	2.6 ± 0.27	1.9-3.7 g/dL (calc)
Albumin/Globulin Ratio	1.8 ± 0.4	1.7 ± 0.3	1.7 ± 0.2	1.7 ± 0.19	1.0-2.5 (calc)
Bilirubin (TOTAL)	0.8 ± 0.5	0.7 ± 0.3	0.7 ± 0.4	0.7 ± 0.41	0.2-1.1 mg/dL
Alkaline Phosphatase	67.6 ± 17.2	65.4 ± 18.8	59.4 ± 21.4	57.0 ± 21.58	40-115^M, 33-115^F U/L
AST	25.9 ± 15.7	24.5 ± 12.0	20.1 ± 8.8	20.0 ± 10.2	12-32 U/L
ALT	21.4 ± 11.2	22.2 ± 13.3	17.8 ± 7.9	18.8 ± 12.63	9-46^M, 6-29^F U/L

‡ = Between groups interaction, p ≤ 0.05; Pre = pre-supplementation; Post = post-supplementation; eGFR = epidermal growth factor receptor; AST = aspartate aminotransferase; ALT = alanine aminotransferase; ^{M} = Male; ^{F} = Female; Data presented as mean ± SD.

Table 6 Changes in complete blood counts

Variable	SUPP (n = 20)		PL (n = 20)		Reference Range
	Pre	Post	Pre	Post	
WBC Count	6.0 ± 1.4	6.4 ± 1.7	6.1 ± 1.3	6.0 ± 1.5	4.5-13.0 Thousand/uL
RBC Count	4.6 ± 0.5	4.6 ± 0.6	4.7 ± 0.6	4.7 ± 0.6	4.10-5.70^M, 3.80-5.10^F Million/uL
Hemoglobin	13.7 ± 2.0	13.5 ± 2.1	13.8 ± 1.0	13.6 ± 1.5	12.0-16.9^M, 11.5-15.3^F g/dL
Hematocrit	39.7 ± 7.5	41.2 ± 5.7	41.6 ± 2.6	41.1 ± 4.1	36.0-49.0^M, 34.0-46.0^F%
MCV	89.0 ± 5.5	89.0 ± 5.8	88.8 ± 6.8	89.1 ± 6.9	78.0-98.0 fL
MCH	29.5 ± 2.6	29.3 ± 2.4	29.5 ± 2.7	29.5 ± 2.7	25.0-35.0 pg
MCHC	33.1 ± 1.3	32.8 ± 0.9	33.2 ± 1.0	33.1 ± 0.9	31.0-36.0 g/dL
RDW	14.1 ± 1.5	14.1 ± 1.3	13.7 ± 1.0	13.9 ± 0.9	11.0-16.0%
Platelet Count	215.5 ± 47.3	222.8 ± 54.6	207.3 ± 45.9	207.6 ± 47.1	150-400 Thousand/uL
Abs Neutrophils	3403.9 ± 1131.6	3790.1 ± 1660.3	3289.9 ± 1194.9	3482.3 ± 1198.5	1800-8000 cells/uL
Abs Lymphocytes	1947.6 ± 471.3	1934.3 ± 570.4	2006.3 ± 640.6	1954.7 ± 533.1	1200-5200 cells/uL
Abs Monocytes	428.9 ± 122.0	419.2 ± 124.2	414.3 ± 109.0	388.0 ± 118.4	200-900 cells/uL
Abs Eosinophils	179.6 ± 122.2	213.0 ± 268.7	124.4 ± 98.6	131.5 ± 105.4	15-600 cells/uL
Abs Basophils	30.2 ± 19.9	28.7 ± 15.1	25.4 ± 12.5	23.8 ± 7.9	0-250 cells/uL
Neutrophils	56.0 ± 7.4	57.8 ± 11.5	57.6 ± 6.7	57.4 ± 7.4	%
Lymphocytes	33.0 ± 6.5	31.6 ± 9.8	33.1 ± 6.9	33.3 ± 7.4	%
Monocytes	7.2 ± 1.5	6.7 ± 1.5	6.9 ± 1.6	6.7 ± 1.9	%
Eosinophils	3.2 ± 2.4	3.4 ± 4.4	2.0 ± 1.4	2.2 ± 1.8	%
Basophils	0.5 ± 0.4	0.5 ± 0.4	0.4 ± 0.2	0.4 ± 0.2	%

Pre = pre-supplementation; Post = post-supplementation; WBC = white blood cell; RBC = red blood cell; MCV = mean corpuscular volume; MCH = mean corpuscular hemoglobin; MCHC = mean corpuscular hemoglobin concentration; RDW = red blood cell distribution width; Abs = absolute; ^{M} = Male; ^{F} = Female; Data presented as mean ± SD.

sixty college aged males. Further, no significant effects were reported in resting cardiovascular measures (RHR, SBP and DBP). Similarly, Lockwood and colleagues [27] observed no significant changes in clinical safety markers following 10-weeks of daily supplementation with a low-calorie multi-ingredient energy drink. Both of these studies utilized supplements that contained similar amounts of caffeine (approx. 200 mg) along with other ingredients. The safety data in the present study appears to be consistent with that of similar energy blend supplements delivered in a non-time-released manner.

Conclusions

In summary, this appears to be the first investigation on the health and safety aspects of prolonged ingestion of a commercially available slow-release energy supplement. A 28-day ingestion protocol resulted in no changes in lipid profile, blood chemistry, blood counts and resting cardiovascular measures, and all measures remained within normal, established reference ranges for adults. These findings indicate that 28 consecutive days ingestion of a moderate amount of caffeine, as part of a multi-ingredient time-release supplement, in caffeine users is both safe and tolerable. This may have important relevance in

professions, where continuous operations demand peak cognitive and physical performance for sustained periods of time.

Abbreviations
SRC: Slow-release caffeine; CNS: Central nervous system; SUPP: Supplement (Energize™); PL: Placebo; HPL: Human performance laboratory; BP: Blood pressure; RHR: Resting heart rate; SBP: Systolic blood pressure; DBP: Diastolic blood pressure; EDTA: Ethylenediaminetetraacetic acid.

Competing interests
The authors declare that they have no competing interests

Authors' contributions
AJW, JRH, AMG, DHF, MSF and JRS were involved in study design, data analysis, manuscript preparation and gave final approval to the manuscript. AJW, KSB, ARJ and JRT were involved in data collection and gave final approval to the manuscript. LPO was involved in study design and served as medical monitor. All authors read and approved the final manuscript.

Acknowledgements
Financial support and supplements for this study were provided by iSatori, Golden, CO, USA. The authors would like to thank Mattan Hoffman, Michael La Monica and Amelia Miramonti for their efforts in assuring participant adherence to the supplement protocol.

References

1. Osei KA, Ovenseri-Ogbomo G, Kyei S, Ntodie M: **The effect of caffeine on tear secretion.** *Optom Vis Sci* 2014, **91**(2):171–177.

2. Nawrot P, Jordan S, Eastwood J, Rotstein J, Hugenholtz A, Feeley M: **Effects of caffeine on human health.** *Food Addit Contam* 2003, **20**(1):1–30.

3. Patat A, Rosenzweig P, Enslen M, Trocherie S, Miget N, Bozon MC, Allain H, Gandon JM: **Effects of a new slow release formulation of caffeine on EEG, psychomotor and cognitive functions in sleep-deprived subjects.** *Hum Psychopharmacol* 2000, **15**(3):153–170.

4. McLellan TM, Bell DG, Kamimori GH: **Caffeine improves physical performance during 24 h of active wakefulness.** *Aviat Space Environ Med* 2004, **75**(8):666–672.

5. Lieberman HR: **The effects of ginseng, ephedrine, and caffeine on cognitive performance, mood and energy.** *Nutr Rev* 2001, **59**(4):91–102.

6. Wells AJ, Hoffman JR, Gonzalez AM, Stout JR, Fragala MS, Mangine GT, McCormack WP, Jajtner AR, Townsend JR, Robinson EH IV: **Phosphatidylserine and caffeine attenuate postexercise mood disturbance and perception of fatigue in humans.** *Nutr Res* 2013, **33**:464–472.

7. Warburton DM, Bersellini E, Sweeney E: **An evaluation of a caffeinated taurine drink on mood, memory and information processing in healthy volunteers without caffeine abstinence.** *Psychopharmacology (Berl)* 2001, **158**(3):322–328.

8. Maridakis V, O'Connor PJ, Tomporowski PD: **Sensitivity to change in cognitive performance and mood measures of energy and fatigue in response to morning caffeine alone or in combination with carbohydrate.** *Int J Neurosci* 2009, **119**(8):1239–1258.

9. Maridakis V, Herring MP, O'Connor PJ: **Sensitivity to change in cognitive performance and mood measures of energy and fatigue in response to differing doses of caffeine or breakfast.** *Int J Neurosci* 2009, **119**(7):975–994.

10. McLellan TM, Kamimori GH, Voss DM, Bell DG, Cole KG, Johnson D: **Caffeine maintains vigilance and improves run times during night operations for Special Forces.** *Aviat Space Environ Med* 2005, **76**(7):647–654.

11. Avois L, Robinson N, Saudan C, Baume N, Mangin P, Saugy M: **Central nervous system stimulants and sport practice.** *Br J Sports Med* 2006, **40**(Suppl 1):i16–i20.

12. Fisone G, Borgkvist A, Usiello A: **Caffeine as a psychomotor stimulant: mechanism of action.** *Cell Mol Life Sci* 2004, **61**(7–8):857–872.

13. Reissig CJ, Strain EC, Griffiths RR: **Caffeinated energy drinks–a growing problem.** *Drug Alcohol Depend* 2009, **99**(1–3):1–10.

14. Tan D, Zhao B, Moochhala S, Yang Y: **Sustained-release of caffeine from a polymeric tablet matrix: an in vitro and pharmacokinetic study.** *Mater Sci Eng B* 2006, **132**:143–146.

15. Penetar D, McCann U, Thorne D, Kamimori G, Galinski C, Sing H, Thomas M, Belenky G: **Caffeine reversal of sleep deprivation effects on alertness and mood.** *Psychopharmacology (Berl)* 1993, **112**(2–3):359–365.

16. Herrick J, Shecterle LM, St Cyr JA: **D-ribose–an additive with caffeine.** *Med Hypotheses* 2009, **72**(5):499–500.

17. Malinauskas BM, Aeby VG, Overton RF, Carpenter-Aeby T, Barber-Heidal K: **A survey of energy drink consumption patterns among college students.** *Nutr J* 2007, **6**:35.

18. Seifert SM, Schaechter JL, Hershorin ER, Lipshultz SE: **Health effects of energy drinks on children, adolescents, and young adults.** *Pediatrics* 2011, **127**(3):511–528.

19. Chauffard F, Enslen MYA, Tachon P: *Sustained Release Microparticulate Caffeine Formulation.* Washington, DC: US Patent No. 5,700,484. U.S. Patent and Trademark Office; 1997:1–17.

20. Lagarde D, Batejat D, Sicard B, Trocherie S, Chassard D, Enslen M, Chauffard F: **Slow-release caffeine: a new response to the effects of a limited sleep deprivation.** *Sleep* 2000, **23**(5):651–661.

21. Beaumont M, Batejat D, Coste O, Doireau P, Chauffard F, Enslen M, Lagarde D, Pierard C: **Recovery after prolonged sleep deprivation: residual effects of slow-release caffeine on recovery sleep, sleepiness and cognitive functions.** *Neuropsychobiology* 2005, **51**(1):16–27.

22. De Valck E, Cluydts R: **Slow-release caffeine as a countermeasure to driver sleepiness induced by partial sleep deprivation.** *J Sleep Res* 2001, **10**(3):203–209.

23. Beaumont M, Batejat D, Pierard C, Coste O, Doireau P, Van Beers P, Chauffard F, Chassard D, Enslen M, Denis JB, Lagarde D: **Slow release caffeine and prolonged (64-h) continuous wakefulness: effects on vigilance and cognitive performance.** *J Sleep Res* 2001, **10**(4):265–276.

24. Heckman MA, Weil J, Gonzalez de Mejia E: **Caffeine (1, 3, 7-trimethylxanthine) in foods: a comprehensive review on consumption, functionality, safety, and regulatory matters.** *J Food Sci* 2010, **75**(3):R77–R87.

25. Gonzalez AM, Hoffman JR, Wells AJ, Mangine GT, Townsend JR, Jajtner AR, Wang R, Miramonti AA, Pruna GJ, LaMonica MB, Bohner JD, Hoffman MW, Oliviera LP, Fukuda DH, Fragala MS, Stout JR: **Pharmacokinetics of caffeine administered in a time-release versus regular tablet form [abstract].** *J Int Soc Sports Nutr* 2014, **11**(Suppl 1):P23.

26. De Valck E, De Groot E, Cluydts R: **Effects of slow-release caffeine and a nap on driving simulator performance after partial sleep deprivation.** *Percept Mot Skills* 2003, **96**(1):67–78.

27. Lockwood CM, Moon JR, Smith AE, Tobkin SE, Kendall KL, Graef JL, Cramer JT, Stout JR: **Low-calorie energy drink improves physiological response to exercise in previously sedentary men: a placebo-controlled efficacy and safety study.** *J Strength Cond Res* 2010, **24**(8):2227–2238.

28. Roberts MD, Dalbo VJ, Hassell SE, Stout JR, Kerksick CM: **Efficacy and safety of a popular thermogenic drink after 28 days of ingestion.** *J Int Soc Sports Nutr* 2008, **5**(19):1–11.

10

Knowledge and attitudes to vitamin D and sun exposure in elite New Zealand athletes: a cross-sectional study

Nicole Walker[1], Thomas D Love[2], Dane Francis Baker[3], Phillip Brian Healey[3], Jillian Haszard[1], Antony S Edwards[4] and Katherine Elizabeth Black[1*]

Abstract

Background: Sun safety and vitamin D status are important for prolonged health. They are of particular interest to those working with athletes for whom for whom safe sun practices maybe limited.
The aim of this cross-sectional study was to describe the attitudes of elite New Zealand athletes to both vitamin D and sun exposure.

Methods: 110 elite New Zealand outdoor athletes volunteered to participate in an interview with a trained interviewer. The interviewer asked the athletes questions on their Vitamin D knowledge, attitudes and practices regarding sun exposure as well as their concerns about skin cancer.

Results: Athletes were more concerned about their risk of skin cancer (66%) than their vitamin D status (6%). Although the majority (97%) were aware of Vitamin D and could identify the sun as a source (76%) only 17% could name another source of Vitamin D.
Only 10 (9%) reported always applying sunscreen before going out in the sun. No athlete reported reapplying sunscreen every hour and 25 suggesting that they never reapply sunscreen.

Conclusions: Athletes are concerned about skin cancer however, their use of sunscreen is not optimal suggesting reapplication of sunscreen could be targeted in order to reduce the risk of sun cancer. Awareness of sources of Vitamin D other than the sun may also need to be improved potentially through educational interventions and possibly in conjunction with sun smart messages.

Keywords: Sun exposure, Cancer, Vitamin D, Athletes

Background

The Vitamin D status of athletes has been described for various athletic populations [1]. History shows that Vitamin D deficiency or insufficiency may be detrimental to performance [2-4] and more recent evidence suggests health implications for those with inadequate compared to those with an adequate serum vitamin D concentration [5]. Insufficient serum Vitamin D concentration has been associated with lower muscle strength and endurance capacity, further it is known that Vitamin D plays an important role in bone health [1,2,6]. However, the awareness of athletes to Vitamin D and their knowledge of its potential implications for health and performance is currently unknown. An understanding of an athlete's awareness, knowledge and attitudes towards Vitamin D could help guide interventions aimed at ensuring adequate Vitamin D status in elite athletes.

Vitamin D is produced in the skin when ultraviolet B (UVB) radiation from sunlight converts cutaneous 7-dehydrocholesterol to previtamin D [7]. Given the importance of sun exposure for vitamin D synthesis and skin cancer risk, an athletes attitudes towards skin cancer risk may influence their vitamin D status. At present no study has investigated elite athletes' attitudes to sun exposure and skin cancer. Sun safety messages are commonplace in New Zealand and Australia due to the

* Correspondence: katherine.black@otago.ac.nz
[1]Department of Human Nutrition, University of Otago, PO Box 56, Dunedin 9054, New Zealand
Full list of author information is available at the end of the article

high rates of skin cancer in these countries from sun exposure [8-10]. Outdoor athletes may have a increased risk of skin cancer as they spend many hours training in the sun [11-13], are limited in the sun protective clothing they are able to wear [13,14], and often cannot seek shade during training or games, with the effectiveness of sunscreen reduced by sweating [13,15] all factors which increase the risk of skin cancer. Therefore these athletes are likely to be at higher risk of skin cancer than the general population. On the contrary, information about Vitamin D is not as strongly promoted and is much less understood by the public [8,9]. It is therefore important to understand an athletes knowledge and concerns for Vitamin D and sun exposure prior to initiating educational programs.

Methods

110 elite outdoor athletes volunteered and provided written, informed consent to participate. Elite was defined as competing internationally. Ethical approval was obtained from the University of Otago Ethics Committee before athletes were approached to participate in the study. Athletes were recruited from rugby, field hockey and rowing and all provided written consent prior to any data collection. Data was collected at the team training bases located around 37° latitude (Hamiliton, Auckland and Lake Karapioro) during a New Zealand summer.

Participants were interviewed in private on topics including Vitamin D and sun exposure. In total there were 57 multiple-choice or short answer questions based on previous questionnaires [16-19]. The interview sessions were peer reviewed by a registered sports dietitian and pilot tested for clarity via a focus group prior to the main study.

Participants were asked to identify their ethnicity (self-selected based on the New Zealand census) [20]. Athletes were also asked to describe the colour of their natural, untanned skin using the Fitzgerald scale [21].

Knowledge of vitamin D was initiated by first asking the participants if they "had ever heard of vitamin D?", followed by questions "are you able to name any health benefits of vitamin D?", and "do you know any personal characteristics that could affect an individual's vitamin D levels?". A knowledge score was created by summing the number of correct responses for both these questions. Participants were not informed if their responses were correct and no help or prompts were provided by the interviewer.

Participants were also asked "are you concerned about your Vitamin D status?"

A section of the questionnaire was designed to assess athletes attitudes towards sun exposure. This section included questions on the participant's concern about their risk of skin cancer from sun exposure, concern about their vitamin D status and whether they intentionally spend time in the sun to improve their vitamin D status or to tan; sunscreen use and, if appropriate, reasons for not using sunscreen or the sunscreen protection factor and reapplication were asked; clothing during training sessions including questions on sunglasses and hat use was collected.

Statistical analyses were undertaken using Stata 12.0 (StataCorp, USA). Chi-squared tests were used to determine if answers to questions on knowledge of vitamin D, attitudes to vitamin D and sun exposure differed between sports, ethnicity and gender. Where significant differences (p < 0.05) within groups were found, post-hoc binomial probability tests were used to determine whether there were proportional differences in the answers given between each of the three sports and four ethnic groups. Bonferroni adjustment was used to account for multiple comparisons. The Kruskal-Wallis test was used to determine differences between sport, ethnicity and gender for the questions related to sun exposure and sunscreen use which had five possible answers "Never", "Rarely", "Sometime", "Often", "Always". The data are presented as the number of participants (percentage of that category of participants) unless otherwise stated.

Results

The characteristics of athletes are shown in Table 1. Ethnic groups were; New Zealand (NZ) European, Maori, Pacific Island and "Other" which included all other ethnicities.

The majority 107 of the 110 (97%) athletes reported that they had heard of vitamin D and there were no significant differences between these groups.

Table 1 Number (%) of participants in each gender, ethnicity, skin colour and sport category and mean (±SD) age (years)

Characteristic	Category	All n = 110
Gender*	Male	76 (69%)
	Female	34 (31%)
Age (years)†		23.53 ± 3.11
Ethnicity*	NZ European	76 (69%)
	Māori	19 (17%)
	Pacific Island	11 (10%)
	Other	4 (4%)
Skin Colour*	Fair	35 (32%)
	Medium	42 (38%)
	Olive	18 (16%)
	Dark	15 (14%)
Sport*	Rugby	35 (32%)
	Hockey	22 (20%)
	Rowing	53 (48%)

*number (%), † mean ± SD.

84 (76%) of athletes were able to identify the sun as source of vitamin D as shown in Table 2. There were differences in ethnicity (p < 0.001) as more NZ European and Māori athletes knew the sun was a source of vitamin D compared to Pacific Island athletes (p < 0.008). However, only 18 (17%) of the total sample was able to name another source of vitamin D such as food sources (6%) or supplements (10%). Examples of the correct food sources the participants identified included: milk, meat, fish and eggs. Incorrect answers included a variety of fruits and vegetables. One athlete correctly mentioned sunbeds as a source. There were no differences between males and females or the four ethnicities in athletes' knowledge of sources of vitamin D, other than the sun. However, there was a difference between sports (p = 0.038) with rowers more likely to know another source than hockey players (p = 0.017).

Almost half (n = 45) (45%) of the sample who had heard of vitamin D were able to correctly name at least one personal characteristic that affects vitamin D status such as: skin colour (n = 30, 27%), sun exposure (n = 22, 20%), diet (n = 9, 8%), body fat (n = 2, 2%) and age (n = 2, 2%). Fourteen percent of athletes could name two or more characteristics and although three quarters of these athletes were rowers this was not a significantly different between sports. There were no differences in athletes' knowledge of personal characteristics affecting vitamin D status according to gender, sport or ethnicity.

Of those athletes who had heard of vitamin D, one quarter (n = 27, 25%) were able to name at least one health benefit of having an adequate vitamin D status. The health benefits named included: bone health (n = 18, 16%), immunity (n = 7, 6% of athletes), mood (n = 6, 5%), and muscle strength (n = 2, 2%).

Many of those who named bone health as a benefit were rowers (94%). There was a significant difference in knowledge of the health benefits of having an adequate vitamin D status between sports (p = 0.031) with rowing having greater knowledge than hockey.

One third of athletes (n = 36, 33%) reported intentionally spending time in the sun in order to get a tan and two thirds (n = 74, 66%) were concerned about the risk of skin cancer when exposing their skin to the sun as shown in Table 3. This compared to only 6% (7 athletes) who were concerned with their Vitamin D status. There were gender differences (p < 0.01), sport differences (p < 0.01) and ethnic differences (p = 0.031) for the athletes that spent time in the sun to tan. Over half of female athletes (n = 22) spend time in the sun to tan in comparison to 18% (n = 14) of males (p < 0.01). No Pacific Island athletes reported spending time in the sun to tan compared to 65% (n = 31) of NZ Europeans (p < 0.01). Hockey players (n = 16, 73%) were significantly more likely to spend time in the sun to tan than rowers (n = 14, 26%) or rugby players (n = 6, 17%) (p < 0.01). Male hockey players reported spending more time in the sun than male rowers and rugby players (p < 0.001). In addition, female hockey players spent more time in sun to tan than female rowers (p = 0.018).

As displayed in Table 3, there was a difference between sports in those that were concerned about their risk of skin cancer with sun exposure (p = 0.047). Half (n = 18) of rugby players were concerned about the risk of skin cancer when exposed to the sun which was significantly less than the proportion of concerned hockey players (n = 18, 82%) or rowers (n = 37, 70%) (p < 0.01). There was no difference between gender or ethnicity.

Ninety-nine of 110 athletes reported using some sunscreen, however only 10 (9%) athletes reported that they always apply sunscreen before going out in the sun. There was a significant difference between ethnicity for sunscreen use with those of Pacific Island ethnicity reporting less sunscreen use compared to the NZ European (p < 0.001) and tending to less regularly use sunscreen compared to NZ Maori (P = 0.076). No participant reported reapplying sunscreen every hour, 5 reported reapplying it at breaks in training and the same number only if they were reminded to do so. A further 8 (7%) reported reapplying sunscreen if they felt their skin burning and another 15 saying they only

Table 2 Proportion of athletes able to name a source of Vitamin D

	Able to name the sun as a source of vitamin D		Able to name another source of vitamin D	
	n (%)	p-value^	n (%)	p-value^
All	84 (76%)		19 (17%)	
Gender		0.323		0.634
Male	56 (74%)		14 (18%)	
Female	28 (82%)		5 (15%)	
Ethnicity		<0.001		0.119
NZ European	64 (84%)		13 (17%)	
Māori	16 (84%)		6 (31%)	
Pacific Island	2 (18%)*[1,2]		0	
Other	2 (50%)		0	
Sport		0.058		0.038
Rugby	22 (63%)		6 (17%)	
Hockey	17 (77%)		0	
Rowing	45 (85%)		13 (25%)*[3]	

n = 110.
*p < 0.05 with Bonferroni adjustment.
^Chi-squared test.
[1]Significant difference between NZ European and Pacific Island ethnicity (p < 0.05).
[2]Significant difference between Māori and Pacific Island ethnicity (p < 0.05).
[3]Significant difference between Rowing and Hockey (p < 0.05).

Table 3 Elite athletes' attitudes towards sun exposure and differences between gender, ethnicity and sport n = 110

	Spend time in the sun to tan		Concerned about risk of skin cancer with sun exposure	
	Yes n(%)	p-value^	Yes n(%)	p-value^
Total	36 (33%)		73 (66%)	
Gender		<0.01		0.806
Male	14 (18%)		51 (67%)	
Female	22 (65%)		22 (65%)	
Ethnicity		0.031		0.430
NZ European	31 (41%)[1]		53 (70%)	
Māori	4 (21%)		12 (63%)	
Pacific Island	0		5 (45%)	
Other	1 (25%)		3 (75%)	
Sport		<0.01		0.047
Rugby	6 (17%)		18 (51%)[4,5]	
Hockey	16 (73%)[2,3]		18 (82%)	
Rowing	14 (26%)		37 (70%)	

^Chi-squared test.
[1]Significant difference between NZ European and Pacific Island ethnicity (p < 0.05).
[2]Significant difference between Hockey and Rugby (p < 0.05).
[3]Significant difference between Hockey and Rowing (p < 0.05).
[4]Significant difference between Rugby and Hockey (p < 0.05).
[5]Significant difference between Rugby and Rowing (p < 0.05).

did it randomly when they remembered. However, 48 (44%) reported that they never reapply sunscreen and 25 (23%) did not know how regularly they reapplied sunscreen. Of those that were concerned about skin cancer (n = 73), only 45% (n = 33) reported using sunscreen always or most of the time, which was not significantly different (p = 0.312) to those that were not concerned about skin cancer (n = 37), with 13 athletes (35%) reporting that they used sunscreen most or all of the time. There was no difference in sunscreen use by gender (p = 0.094) nor by sport when controlling for ethnicity (p = 0.471). The majority of athletes stated that they used an SPF30 for protection (range SPF15-100). Time and availability were the two main reasons provided for not applying sunscreen with 75 (68%) and 67 (61%) athletes respectively providing these as a barrier to sunscreen use. Despite lack of availability being cited as a reason for not using sunscreen 65 athletes did state that it was available at training. Sunglasses were always worn by 40 athletes but 36 responded that they never wear sunglasses. Only two athletes stated that they always seek the shade and 68 never actively seeking the shade for protection. NZ European sought shade more frequently than Maori (p = 0.028) and Pacific Island (p = 0.001). There was also a gender difference with females less frequently seeking shade

than males (p < 0.001). In terms of sun protection for the head only one athlete always wore a hat and 56 never wore one. The most common type of hat was a baseball type cap.

Discussion

This study showed that more elite New Zealand athletes were concerned about their future skin cancer risk than concerned about their vitamin D status. Yet despite their skin cancer concerns, the athletes' practices in the sun, especially around sunscreen re-application could be elevating their risk of skin cancer.

It seems that they are more aware of Vitamin D than the general population. Almost all (97%) athletes in this study had heard of vitamin D, in comparison, published literature from the general population reports only 69-84% have heard of vitamin D [16,19,22]. The differences between the general population and this athletic population may reflect the dietetic and medical support available to these elite athletes, which is less available to the general population. Future studies should investigate the source of information. Further, athletes generally had good knowledge of the sun as a source of vitamin D (76%) which was similar to previous findings in the general population [16,22,23]. However in contrast to the published research in the general population, a smaller proportion of participants could name a correct food source or supplements as a source of vitamin D in the present study [16,22,24]. Although vitamin D intake from food sources alone would not provide sufficient vitamin D for optimal serum concentrations, intake from food could assist when sun exposure is limited. Elite New Zealand athletes have greater access to nutritional support and education than the general population and given the potential role for Vitamin D in health and performance it is interesting that their knowledge of food sources of Vitamin D was not higher than the general population. However, these results must be interpreted with caution as the type of questionnaire used to assess knowledge may influence the scores. The present study utilised an open ended question style whereas others have used a multi-choice type questionnaire [16,22], which generally overestimated the participants knowledge. When groups are asked prompted questions they seem to have a greater knowledge of vitamin D [16,19,22] than when asked open-ended questions [19,22], indicating the ability to express vitamin D knowledge might be highly dependent on the question format. This is highlighted by Kung and Lee [19] who asked older (>50 years) Chinese women either open-ended questions or prompted responses about Vitamin D, the proportion of correct responses varied depending on the type of questioning [16,22]. Only one-quarter named the sun as a source of vitamin D, less than 10% named correct food sources and less than 1% were aware vitamin D could be obtained from supplements. Interestingly, when they were then prompted, responses were inconsistent as over half of the group claimed to know the sun is a source of vitamin D. Furthermore, caution must be taken when comparing studies as the results may reflect the sun smart messages individual to each country [9,23]. Regardless of previous studies, athletes' vitamin D knowledge was poor especially when considering the potential risk of low vitamin D status to health and sporting performance [25].

Despite the role vitamin D plays in health, only a small percentage of athletes were concerned about vitamin D status (6%) which is similar to studies in the general population in which 9% [16] and 12% [22] were concerned with their vitamin D status. In the current study, those who had a greater knowledge score were concerned about vitamin D. Therefore they may have understood their risk of deficiency and educated themselves on potential solutions. Another study [24] found those who knew more about the sources of vitamin D tended to consume more vitamin D-containing foods and supplements. Therefore educating athletes about the importance of vitamin D for helath and importance may increase concern for their vitamin D status and subsequently, behaviours that have the potential to improve vitamin D status, either through food, supplementation, safe sun exposure or a combination of factors, will be undertaken. There have been no studies to date investigating the effectiveness of educational interventions on behaviour change and vitamin D status.

The proportion of athletes who intentionally spend time in the sun to improve their vitamin D status (12%) was similar to the general population (9%) of New Zealand [26]. One Australian study [22] found 16% of participants intended to increase their sun exposure due to concerns about their vitamin D status and 21% had already changed their behaviour. This practice could increase the risk for skin cancer; which is well-known to be associated with sun exposure [27]. Advice to athletes regarding Vitamin D should be provided alongside messages about sunscreen use to ensure athletes are not further increasing their risk of skin cancer in attempt to improve vitamin D status [9,28].

In contrast to the number of athletes concerned with their vitamin D status, a greater number were concerned about skin cancer as the result of sun exposure (66%), this possibly reflects the strongly promoted sun safety messages and the high prevalence of skin cancer in New Zealand [29,30]. The high rate of concern for skin cancer may be the reason for the high proportion of athletes who report sunscreen use. This suggests an awareness of sunscreen use to attenuate the risk of skin cancer. However, the lower proportion who use sunscreen all the time and the even smaller amount who regularly reapply sunscreen is of concern especially given the higher risk

of skin cancer in New Zealand [29,30]. The data suggest that even those who are concerned about skin cancer risk are not fully aware of the optimal application of sunscreen. In order to promote a more effective use of sunscreen ie frequent reapplication, the reasons for not using sunscreen need to be addressed. Factors such as ensuring sunscreen is available at the training location and that the athletes are provided with training breaks in order to reapply sunscreen along with towels to wipe excess cream off their hands therefore minimizing the impact on training could help promote sunscreen use and attenuate the risk of skin cancer. Factors such as seeking shade and the wearing of sunglasses maybe more difficult to address in some sports due to the training venue or sporting regulations, however, in such cases education about attenuating the risk of skin cancer whilst away from training may be beneficial.

Conclusion

The current guidelines in New Zealand and the United Kingdom suggest casual summer sun exposure is enough to maintain vitamin D in a healthy population [9,12,28], therefore there is no reason that sun safety messages and vitamin D cannot be promoted in unison.

Abbreviations
UVB: UltraViolet B; NZ: New Zealand; SPF: Sun protection factor.

Competing interests
The authors declare that they have no competing interests.

Authors' contributions
KEB was invloved with the study design, data collection and analysis, manuscript preparation and gave final approval to the manuscript. TDL was invloved with the study design, data analysis, manuscript preparation and gave final approval to the manuscript. DFB was invloved with the study design, data collection, manuscript preparation and gave final approval to the manuscript. PBH was invloved with the study design, data collection, manuscript preparation and gave final approval to the manuscript. ASE was invloved with the study design, manuscript preparation and gave final approval to the manuscript. NW was invloved with data collection and analysis, manuscript preparation and gave final approval to the manuscript. JH was invloved with statisical analysis, manuscript preparation and gave final approval to the manuscript.

Acknowledgements
This study was funded by the Department of Human Nutrition, University of Otago, New Zealand. The authors have no competing interests.

Author details
[1]Department of Human Nutrition, University of Otago, PO Box 56, Dunedin 9054, New Zealand. [2]College of Engineering, Swansea University, Swansea, UK. [3]Chiefs Super Rugby Franchise, Hamilton, New Zealand. [4]High Performance Sport New Zealand, Auckland, New Zealand.

References
1. Larson-Meyer DE, Willis KS: **Vitamin D and athletes.** *Curr Sports Med Rep* 2010, 9(4):220–226.
2. Foo LH, Zhang Q, Zhu K, Ma G, Hu X, Greenfield H, Fraser DR: **Low vitamin D status has an adverse influence on bone mass, bone**

turnover, and muscle strength in Chinese adolescent girls. *J Nutr* 2009, **139**(5):1002–1007.

3. Glerup H, Mikkelsen K, Poulsen L, Hass E, Overbeck S, Andersen H, Charles P, Eriksen E: **Hypovitaminosis D myopathy without biochemical signs of osteomalacic bone involvement.** *Calcif Tissue Int* 2000, **66**(6):419–424.

4. Hamilton B: **Vitamin D and human skeletal muscle.** *Scand J Med Sci Sports* 2010, **20**(2):182–190.

5. Cannell JJ, Hollis BW, Sorenson MB, Taft TN, Anderson JJB: **Athletic performance and vitamin D.** *Med Sci Sports Exerc* 2009, **41**(5):1102–1110.

6. Ruohola JP, Laaksi I, Ylikomi T, Haataja R, Mattila VM, Sahi T, Tuohimaa P, Pihlajamäki H: **Association between serum 25(OH)D concentrations and bone stress fractures in Finnish young men.** *J Bone Miner Res* 2006, **21**(9):1483–1488.

7. Engelsen O: **The relationship between ultraviolet radiation exposure and vitamin D status.** *Nutrients* 2010, **2**(5):482–495.

8. Bonevski B, Bryant J, Lambert S, Brozek I, Rock V: **The ABC of Vitamin D: a qualitative study of the knowledge and attitudes regarding vitamin D deficiency amongst selected population groups.** *Nutrients* 2013, **5**(3):915–927.

9. New Zealand Ministry of Health: **Consensus Statement vitamin D and Sun Exposure in NZ.** In *MoHaCSoN*. Edited by Zealand. Wellington: Ministry of Health; 2012.

10. O'Dea D: *The costs of skin cancer to New Zealand [Internet].* 2009. [updated 2009 Oct; cited 2012 Sept 25]. Available from: http://www.cancernz.org.nz/reducing-your-cancer-risk/sunsmart/about-skin-cancer/costs-of-skin-cancer/.

11. Moehrle M: **Ultraviolet exposure in the Ironman triathlon.** *Med Sci Sports Exerc* 2001, **33**(8):1385–1386.

12. Herlihy E, Gies PH, Roy CR, Jones M: **Personal dosimetry of solar UV radiation for different outdoor activities.** *Photochem Photobiol* 1994, **60**(3):288–294.

13. Moehrle M: **Outdoor sports and skin cancer.** *Clin Dermatol* 2008, **26**(1):12–15.

14. Lawler S, Spathonis K, Eakin E, Gallois C, Leslie E, Owen N: **Sun exposure and sun protection behaviours among young adult sport competitors.** *Aust N Z J Public Health* 2007, **31**(3):230–234.

15. Moehrle M, Koehle W, Dietz K, Lischka G: **Reduction of minimal erythema dose by sweating.** *Photodermatol Photo* 2000, **16**(6):260–262.

16. Vu LH, van der Pols JC, Whiteman DC, Kimlin MG, Neale RE: **Knowledge and attitudes about vitamin D and impact on sun protection practices among urban office workers in Brisbane, Australia.** *Cancer Epidemiol Biomark Prev* 2010, **19**(7):1784–1789.

17. Froiland K, Koszewski W, Hingst J, Kopecky L: **Nutritional supplement use among college athletes and their sources of information.** *Int J Sport Nutr Exerc Metab* 2004, **14**:104–120.

18. Glanz K, Yaroch EL, Dancel M, Saraiya M, Crane LA, Buller DB, Manne S, O'Riordan DL, Heckman CJ, Hay J, Robinson JK: **Measures of sun exposure and sun protection practices for behavioral and epidemiologic research.** *Arch Dermatol* 2008, **144**(2):217.

19. Kung AWC, Lee KK: **Knowledge of vitamin D and perceptions and attitudes toward sunlight among Chinese middle-aged and elderly women: a population survey in Hong Kong.** *BioMed Central Public Health* 2006, **6**:226–232.

20. Statistics New Zealand: **New Zealand 2013 Census.** Edited by Statistics. Auckland: New Zealand Governement; Statistics New Zealand.

21. Fitzpatrick TB: **The validity and practicality of sun-reactive skin types I through VI.** *Arch Dermatol (1960)* 1988, **124**(6):869.

22. Youl PH, Janda M, Kimlin M: **Vitamin D and sun protection: the impact of mixed public health messages in Australia.** *Int J Cancer* 2009, **124**(8):1963–1970.

23. Dixon H, Warne C, Scully M, Dobbinson S, Wakefield M: **Agenda-setting effects of sun-related news coverage on public attitudes and beliefs about tanning and skin cancer.** *Health Commun* 2013, **27**(3):261–269.

24. Toher C, Lindsay K, McKenna M, Kilbane M, Curran S, Harrington L, Uduma O, McAuliffe FM: **Relationship between vitamin D knowledge and 25-hydroxyvitamin D levels amongst pregnant women.** *J Hum Nutr Diet* 2013, **29**(2):173–181.

25. Angeline ME, Gee AO, Shindle M, Warren RF, Rodeo SA: **The effects of vitamin D deficiency in athletes.** *Am J Sports Med* 2013, **41**(2):461–464.

26. Gray R: *Does Concern about Vitamin D Affect People's Sun Protection Behaviour? [In Fact].* Wellington: Health Sponsorship Council; 2010.

27. Moehrle M: **Extreme UV exposure of professional cyclists.** *Dermatology (Basel)* 2000, **201**(1):44.

28. British Association of Dermatoligists, Cancer Research UK, Diabetes UK, Multiple Sclerosis Society, National Heart Forum, National Osteoporosis Society, Society. PCD: **Consensus vitamin D position statement.** In *NHS livewell.* Edited by UK CR. United Kingdom: Cancer Research UK; 2010.

29. Diffey BL: **When should sunscreen be reapplied?** *J Am Acad Dermatol* 2001, **45**(6):882–885.

30. Pruim B, Green A: **Photobiological aspects of sunscreen re-application.** *Australas J Dermatol* 1999, **40**(1):14–18.

11

Effects of soluble milk protein or casein supplementation on muscle fatigue following resistance training program: a randomized, double-blind, and placebo-controlled study

Nicolas Babault[1,2,6*], Gaëlle Deley[1,2], Pascale Le Ruyet[3], François Morgan[3] and François André Allaert[4,5]

Abstract

Background: The effects of protein supplementation on muscle thickness, strength and fatigue seem largely dependent on its composition. The current study compared the effects of soluble milk protein, micellar casein, and a placebo on strength and fatigue during and after a resistance training program.

Methods: Sixty-eight physically active men participated in this randomized controlled trial and underwent 10 weeks of lower-body resistance training. Participants were randomly assigned to the Placebo (PLA), Soluble Milk Protein (SMP, with fast digestion rate) or Micellar Casein (MC, with slow digestion rate) group. During the 10-week training period, participants were instructed to take 30 g of the placebo or protein twice a day, or three times on training days. Tests were performed on quadriceps muscles at inclusion (PRE), after 4 weeks (MID) and after 10 weeks (POST) of training. They included muscle endurance (maximum number of repetitions during leg extensions using 70% of the individual maximal load), fatigue (decrease in muscle power after the endurance test), strength, power and muscle thickness.

Results: Muscle fatigue was significantly lower ($P < 0.05$) in the SMP group at MID and POST (-326.8 ± 114.1 W and -296.6 ± 130.1 W, respectively) as compared with PLA (-439.2 ± 153.9 W and -479.2 ± 138.1 W, respectively) and MC (-415.1 ± 165.1 W and -413.7 ± 139.4 W, respectively). Increases in maximal muscle power, strength, endurance and thickness were not statistically different between groups.

Conclusions: The present study demonstrated that protein composition has a large influence on muscular performance after prolonged resistance training. More specifically, as compared with placebo or micellar casein, soluble milk protein (fast digestible) appeared to significantly reduce muscle fatigue induced by intense resistance exercise.

Keywords: Muscle power, Endurance, Muscle thickness, Branched-chain amino acids

Background

Resistance training simultaneously stimulates catabolism and anabolism in active muscle fibers. The difference between these mechanisms is called net protein balance. When positive, the net protein balance favors increases in muscle mass, i.e., muscle hypertrophy. The effect of resistance training on net protein balance can persist up to 48 h [1]. In addition, any nutritional modification that could increase protein accretion in the muscle would maximize resistance training effects by enhancing muscle anabolism. In particular, it has now been well demonstrated that protein consumption after exercise shifts the balance in favor of muscle protein synthesis [2].

Composition of supplements may play a key role in influencing net protein balance since previous studies have revealed that only essential amino acids could stimulate muscle protein synthesis [3]. Furthermore, protein type, and not simply its amino acid composition, can

* Correspondence: nicolas.babault@u-bourgogne.fr
[1]National Institute for health and medical research (INSERM), unit 1093, Cognition, Action and sensorimotor plasticity, Dijon, France
[2]Centre for Performance Expertise, UFR STAPS, Dijon, France
Full list of author information is available at the end of the article

differentially modulate protein synthesis depending on digestion kinetics. For instance, milk contains two protein fractions, soluble proteins and micellar casein, with rapid and slow digestion rates, respectively [4]. As a consequence, muscle protein synthesis has been shown to be greater with soluble proteins such as whey when compared with casein [5].

In addition to increases in muscle mass, functional adaptations, such as strength increases, are also obtained after essential amino acid (EAA) supplementation [6]. For example, Vieillevoye et al. [7] found increases in lower body strength with EAA supplementation while no modification was obtained with placebo. Protein supplementation may also influence muscle fatigue. Indeed, previous authors [8] have reported an attenuation of fatigue during repeated bouts of dynamic contractions after four weeks of protein supplementation as a result of an increased muscle buffering capacity during endurance exercise. Other amino acids, such as branched-chain amino acids (BCAA; leucine, isoleucine and valine), might also reduce fatigue by lowering perceived exertion and favoring mental performance during prolonged exercise [9,10]. Taken altogether, these results seem to suggest that the effects of protein supplementation are largely dependent on their composition, and it can be hypothesized that supplementation with a rapidly-digesting protein would be more efficient to improve both strength and resistance to fatigue. Given that different amino acid compositions could easily be obtained from protein milk extraction, the aim of the present study was to compare the effects of two different formulations of milk protein supplementation, one fast (a soluble milk protein) and one slow (micellar casein), on muscle performance (endurance, fatigue, strength and power) during and after a 10-week resistance training program.

Methods

Participants

A total of 68 male participants were recruited for the study. All were practicing two to six hours of physical activity per week (<3 sessions a week). None were engaged in any physical activity aimed at increasing the size and strength of knee extensor muscles. All were healthy and free of injury in the three months preceding the study. The study excluded subjects who had previously received treatment with corticoids. Participants who were currently taking any dietary supplement, sports drink, or functional food intended to enhance performance or muscle mass, or had taken any of these in the previous month, were also excluded. Moreover, subjects with known hypersensitivity to any of the constituents of the products under study (milk protein or lactose) were excluded. Throughout the study, subjects maintained their usual training routines and diets. All gave their written informed consent after

being told about the experimental procedure. The study was conducted in accordance with the Helsinki Declaration and was approved by the local ethics committee (East I, number: 2011–38, 4 October 2011, AFSSAPS number: 2011-A00789-32).

After inclusion, participants were randomly divided into three experimental groups: 24 in the Placebo group (PLA), 22 in the Micellar protein group (MC), and 22 in the soluble milk protein group (SMP). Balanced randomization was made by blocks of four. The randomization code was not made available to anyone involved in conducting or evaluating the study and was released after the blind review and the freezing of the final database. The sample size was calculated *a priori* using Nquery Advisor software (ver. 6.01, Statistical solutions Ltd, Cork, Ireland) based on the primary criterion (muscle endurance) and allowing for a power > 90%. This statistical analysis indicated a minimum of 22 participants per experimental group.

Experimental procedure

The primary objective of this randomized, double-blind study, conducted with parallel arms, was to evaluate the effects of different milk protein supplements on muscle endurance and fatigue following a resistance training program. A soluble milk protein beverage was compared with a micellar casein beverage and placebo. Body composition, knee extensor muscle thickness, maximal strength, power and perceived exertion were also determined.

The experiment involved four testing sessions: one at inclusion (PRE), one at the middle of the training program (after 28 days; MID) and two at the end of the 10 weeks training program (POST and POST + 5) (Figure 1). Testing sessions were conducted on non-training days and always at the same time of day for a given subject. PRE, MID and POST sessions included measurements of (i) right vastus lateralis muscle thickness using ultrasonography, (ii) lower limb muscle power during vertical jumps, (iii) maximal strength on a leg extension machine (one repetition maximum, 1-RM), (iv) muscle power on the same leg extension machine at 70% of the 1-RM, (v) muscle endurance during an all-out test (maximum number of repetitions performed with a load corresponding to 70% of the session's 1-RM) and (vi) recovery, as determined by muscle power, immediately, 30 min and 60 min after the endurance test. Tests were always performed in the aforementioned order after a standardized warm-up. Warm-up consisted of light pedaling followed by submaximal voluntary contractions and vertical jumps in order to familiarize subjects with testing procedures. The POST + 5 session only consisted of an all-out endurance test performed with the same load as the one used at PRE, followed by recovery power measurements.

All subjects followed the same 10-week resistance training routines, three times per week with a rest day

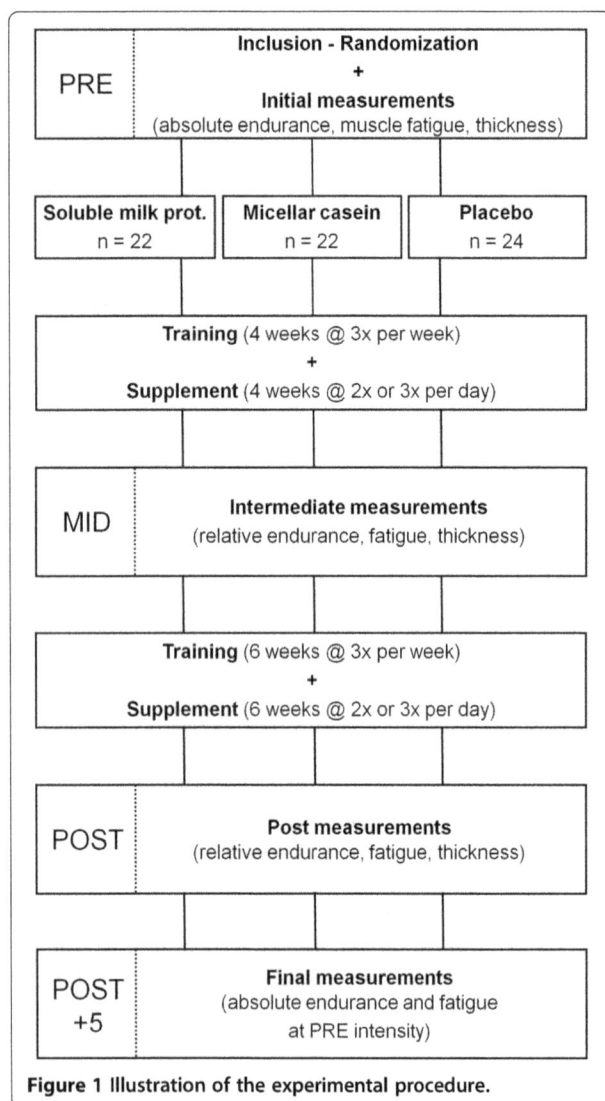

Figure 1 Illustration of the experimental procedure.

between sessions. The program was based on three exercises involving knee extensors (knee extension machine and horizontal leg press) and knee flexors (hamstring curl machine) (Technogym, Gambettola, Italy). Throughout the training program, sets number, repetition number and recovery between sets varied: from the first to seventh week, sets increased from three to five and repetition maximum (RM) number also increased from eight to 15. During weeks eight and nine, training consisted of four sets of 20 RM. During the last week, training consisted of five sets of six RM. Recovery beteween sets was 1–2 minutes. The load used for each exercise was regularly adapted depending on the 1-RM evaluated every two weeks. All training sessions were supervised by specialized teachers.

Dietary supplementation
The three products under study were presented as 30-g sachets to be diluted in 200 mL water. Once the powders

were diluted in cold water, drinks were of identical appearance, texture, taste, and all were isoenergetic (120 kcal per 30 g powder). Products were taken during the 10-weeks training period. On non-training days, protein intake was repeated twice, with the first in the morning after waking and the second during the afternoon. During training days, protein intake was repeated three times: in the morning and 30 min before and after the resistance training session. Protein supplementation was done either with Prolacta® or micellar casein.

Prolacta® (Lactalis, Retiers France) is a 90% soluble milk protein isolate. It is representative of native proteins in the non-casein phase of milk as it is a concentrate of native whey proteins extracted directly from skimmed cow milk by a soft membrane process (Lactalis Industry, Bourgbarré, France), and not from whey. Prolacta® is defined as a fast leucine-rich protein [4] differing from whey with a better amino acid composition. Moreover, Prolacta® has demonstrated larger postprandial protein retention than casein [11]. Each 30 g Prolacta® sachet contained 10 g of protein from Prolacta®, 10.5 g sucrose, 8.2 g maltodextrine, 0.3 g lactose and 1 g soy lecithin. Each 30 g micellar protein sachet (produced by Lactalis, Retiers France) contained 10 g of Micellar Casein, 10.5 g sucrose, 7.5 g maltodextrine, 1 g lactose and 1 g soy lecithin. The amino acid composition of each product is detailed in Table 1. Placebo composition was 10.5 g sucrose and 19.5 g maltodextrine and did not contain any protein.

Table 1 Amino acids composition (g) for 100 g of soluble milk protein (SMP) or micellar casein (MC)

	SMP	MC
Alanine	4.77	2.84
Arginine	2.25	3.50
Aspartic acid	11.34	6.44
Cystine	3.06	0.41
Glutamic acid	17.10	21.75
Glycine	1.98	1.74
Histidine	2.00	2.70
Isoleucine	5.04	4.92
Leucine	12.00	9.05
Lysine	9.63	7.39
Methionine	2.07	3.21
Phenylalanine	3.78	4.86
Proline	4.59	10.3
Serine	4.50	5.02
Threonine	5.04	3.67
Tryptophan	2.07	1.07
Tyrosine	3.42	5.03
Valine	5.13	6.22

Measurements

Muscle thickness

The right vastus lateralis muscle thickness was measured in real time using an ultrasound machine (AU5, Esaote Biomedica, Florence, Italy) coupled to a 50 mm probe at a 7.5 MHz frequency. Subjects were in the supine position with the knee flexed at a 45° angle. The probe was placed perpendicular to the skin surface in the middle of vastus lateralis muscle, i.e., 39% of thigh length measured from the superior border of the patella to the anterior superior iliac spine [12]. Thickness was calculated as the distance between superficial and deep aponeuroses measured at the ends and middle of each 3.8-cm-wide sonograph. Three images were independently obtained. The average value of these nine measures was calculated. Probe placement was carefully noted for reproduction during the other test sessions. Also, body composition (body weight, percent body fat) was quantified using a bio-impedance scale Fitness scale 7850 (Soehnle GmbH, Murrhardt, Germany).

Muscle strength

Subjects were seated on a leg extension machine (Multiform, La Roque d'Anthéron, France) with a 100° hip angle. The knee rotation axis was aligned with the machine rotation axis. The 1-RM was first determined after a standardized warm-up using five different loads and individually adjusted increments. Subjects were requested to lift each load only once. One minute of rest was permitted between trials. Care was taken to lift the load with a full range of motion (~100°). Range of motion was controlled using an electronic goniometer (Myotest, Sion, Switzerland).

Muscle endurance

Subjects were asked to lift a load corresponding to 70% of their 1-RM as many times as possible over a 100° range of motion. The test was stopped when subjects were unable to lift the load over a 80° range of motion during two consecutive repetitions. The number of repetitions was identified as subjects' "relative endurance" (PRE, MID and POST). Immediately after all endurance tests, the rating of perceived exertion was determined using a Borg scale [13]. The endurance test procedure was repeated five days after the end of the experimental period (POST + 5), but using the same load as the one used at inclusion (here called "absolute endurance").

Muscle fatigue and recovery

Muscle power and vertical jump performance were measured just before, immediately after, 30 min after and 60 min after the endurance tests, to evaluate muscle fatigue and recovery. Muscle power was measured using a linear encoder (Globus, Codogne, Italy) on the leg extension machine with the same load as during the endurance test

(70% of the 1-RM). Subjects were requested to lift the load as fast as possible (3 trials) throughout the 100° range of motion. The linear encoder measured the vertical velocity of the load being lifted and allowed measurements of muscle power during the entire range of motion. Peak power of the best repetition was considered for analyses. Immediately after muscle power assessments, subjects performed two counter movement jumps on an Optojump system (Optojump, Microgate, Bolzano, Italy), starting from a standing position, then squatting down to a 90° knee angle and extending the knees in one continuous movement. During these jumps, arms were kept close to the hips to minimize their contribution. The best jump height was retained for analyses.

Statistical analyses

Quantitative variables were presented as mean values and standard deviations (SD). Values were tested using a repeated measures analysis of variance. Groups (PLA, SMP and MC) were used as independent variables and time (PRE, MID, POST or POST + 5) was used as the dependent variable. A sensitivity analysis was also conducted and considered subjects with a muscle thickness at inclusion <22 mm (median value of study sample). Thirteen subjects were considered in both PLA and MC groups and 8 for SMP. In the case of significant main effects or interactions, Scheffé post-hoc tests were conducted. Qualitative variables (supplementation compliance or adverse effects) were presented as absolute and relative frequencies and were tested by using a Chi square test. Statistics were conducted using SAS software (Ver. 9.2, SAS Institute, Inc., Cary, NC, USA). $P < 0.05$ was taken as the level of statistical significance for all procedures.

Results

General observations

Initial values measured at PRE revealed comparable groups (Table 2). During the experimental protocol, compliance was evaluated by the percentage of products returned by subjects. The results show high average and comparable compliance between groups: 90.5%, 91.5% and 89.4% for PLA, MC and SMP groups, respectively ($P = 0.769$). In addition, tolerance to the three products under study was good and comparable in terms of frequency and nature. Of the 68 subjects who took products at least once, three subjects presented adverse events in each group. None of these events were due to the supplements ingested, but rather to personal convenience or injuries.

Muscle endurance

Absolute muscle endurance (Table 3), evaluated as the number of repetitions at 70% of the initial 1-RM, increased in all groups (+90.8 ± 58.8%, +81.2 ± 51.0%

Table 2 Main subjects' characteristics at inclusion (PRE)

	PLA	MC	SMP	ANOVA
Age (years)	22.0 ± 3.9	22.2 ± 3.9	22.5 ± 4.1	$P = 0.912$
BMI (Kg/m^2)	23.4 ± 3.7	23.7 ± 3.5	22.7 ± 2.4	P-0.546
Physical activity (hours/week)	4.1 ± 2.2	5.1 ± 2.4	5.4 ± 3.0	$P = 0.193$
Vastus lateralis thickness (mm)	21.0 ± 3.2	21.5 ± 3.1	21.5 ± 3.5	$P = 0.845$
Counter movement jump (cm)	32.4 ± 6.0	32.2 ± 4.1	32.6 ± 4.5	$P = 0.971$
1-RM (kg)	87.7 ± 16.7	86.6 ± 17.7	83.6 ± 16.0	$P = 0.702$
Number of repetitions	16.5 ± 4.0	16.8 ± 3.4	15.5 ± 3.9	$P = 0.527$
Perceived exertion	13.9 ± 2.1	14.3 ± 2.2	14.0 ± 1.9	$P = 0.820$

Data are mean values ± SD. PLA: placebo; MC: micellar casein; SMP: soluble milk protein; BMI: body mass index; 1-RM: maximum load lifted by leg extension.

and +73.7 ± 32.2% for SMP, MC and PLA, respectively) with no significant difference between groups ($P = 0.492$). However, when subjects with small muscle thickness were considered separately (thickness < 22 mm, sensitivity study), increases reached the significant level between SMP

Table 3 Changes of the main outcomes during and at the end of the experimental procedure

	PRE	MID	POST	POST + 5
Muscle endurance (number of repetitions)*				
SMP	15.5 ± 3.9	17.3 ± 4.7	19.2 ± 7.1	25.2 ± 13.7
MC	16.8 ± 3.4	19.3 ± 4.6	21.3 ± 6.0	25.8 ± 9.5
PLA	16.5 ± 4.0	18.5 ± 6.0	20.5 ± 7.0	25.2 ± 10.4
1-RM (kg)*				
SMP	83.5 ± 16.0	91.3 ± 13.7	96.1 ± 12.4	-
MC	86.6 ± 17.7	98.9 ± 18.2	98.9 ± 17.4	-
PLA	87.7 ± 16.7	100.3 ± 13.3	104.8 ± 11.3	-
Muscle thickness (mm)*				
SMP	21.5 ± 3.5	-	22.2 ± 3.5	-
MC	21.8 ± 3.1	-	22.1 ± 3.1	-
PLA	21.0 ± 3.2	-	22.0 ± 3.6	-
% body fat				
SMP	8.6 ± 2.2	8.5 ± 2.5	8.9 ± 2.6	-
MC	9.4 ± 4.3	9.8 ± 5.1	10.0 ± 4.6	-
PLA	9.9 ± 4.6	9.9 ± 4.5	10.3 ± 5.0	-
% body fat free mass				
SMP	48.2 ± 2.0	47.9 ± 2.0	47.9 ± 2.3	-
MC	47.1 ± 3.1	46.9 ± 3.5	46.7 ± 3.2	-
PLA	46.9 ± 3.4	47.4 ± 4.0	46.7 ± 3.4	-
Body mass (kg)				
SMP	70.8 ± 8.7	72.5 ± 8.1	72.2 ± 8.9	-
MC	77.7 ± 14.7	79.0 ± 15.1	79.2 ± 15.3	-
PLA	76.6 ± 13.3	77.7 ± 12.7	78.3 ± 13.2	-

Data are mean values ± SD. PLA: placebo; MC: micellar casein; SMP: soluble milk protein; BMI: body mass index; 1-RM: maximum load lifted by leg extension. *: significant effect ($P < 0.05$).

and PLA (+103.0 ± 61.1% and +65.0 ± 33.9%, respectively, $P < 0.05$). Similar results were obtained for relative endurance measured POST with a significant time effect but no differences between groups (Table 3). For all subjects, the 1-RM load was significantly increased after training (Table 3). No significant interaction was obtained for the rating of perceived exertion.

Muscle fatigue and recovery

Muscle fatigue, i.e. power reduction during the endurance test, was similar between groups at PRE. This decrease in power was significantly lower for SMP as compared with MC and PLA after four weeks (−326.8 ± 114.1 W, −415.1 ± 165.1 W and −439.2 ± 153.9 W, respectively; $P = 0.0483$) and after 10 weeks of training (−296.6 ± 130.1 W, −413.7 ± 139.4 W and −479.2 ± 138.1 W, respectively; $P = 0.0004$) (Figure 2). Accordingly, when comparing PRE and POST, fatigue was significantly reduced for SMP while it increased for MC and PLA (−35.9 ± 133.5 W, +89.3 ± 97.7 W and +64.8 ± 154.6 W, respectively; $P = 0.0125$).

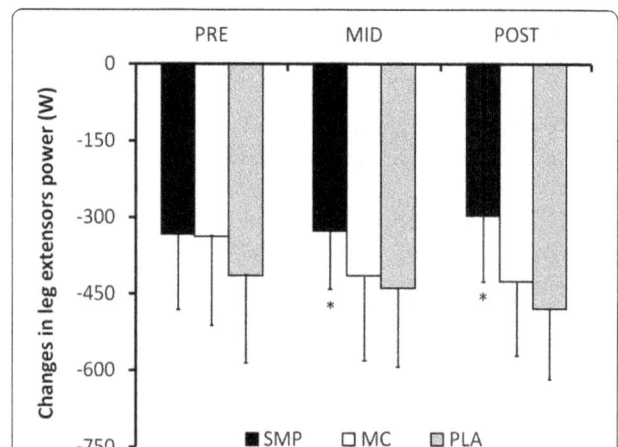

Figure 2 Muscle power decrease during the endurance test.
Mean (±SD) decreases in muscle power during the endurance test before the training period (PRE), after 4 weeks training (MID) and at the end of the training (POST). *: significant differences between groups ($P < 0.05$).

When considering PRE and POST + 5, slight between-groups differences were registered for counter movement jump height. For SMP, counter movement jump height measured immediately after the endurance test slightly increased while it decreased for MC and PLA (+0.9 ± 4.6 cm, −1.6 ± 2.3 cm and −0.7 ± 2.8 cm, respectively; P = 0.0686). A small difference was obtained for counter movement jump at POST + 5. As compared with baseline, 30 min after the endurance test, counter movement jump height significantly increased in SMP and PLA while it remained lower for MC (+1.9 ± 5.1 cm, +0.4 ± 2.1 cm and −0.6 ± 2.8 cm, respectively; P = 0.0965).

Muscle thickness

Muscle thickness and body composition changes are indicated in Table 3. While a significant increase in muscle thickness was obtained with time, no difference was registered between groups. Also, no significant difference was noticed for body mass, percent body fat or percent body fat free mass (Table 3).

Discussion

The present study aimed to test the hypothesis that supplementation with milk proteins of varying compositions, used in combination with resistance training, would have different effects on physical performance. The main results revealed enhanced muscle endurance (i.e., number of repetitions), reduced fatigue (i.e., muscle power loss) and slightly enhanced recovery (i.e., vertical jump height) with a supplement composed of fast-digesting protein (soluble milk protein) as compared with a slow-digesting protein (micellar casein) or with a placebo. It should be noted that differences between groups were larger when subjects with lower initial muscle thickness were considered.

Increased muscle endurance and reduced muscle fatigue were observed in the group with fast protein supplementation. Similar results have previously been obtained with acute intakes [14-16] and with chronic diets [17], while others failed to register any effects [18,19]. Three main mechanisms could be involved in the observed enhancement of muscle endurance and fatigue. The first may be related to glucose and glycogen availability. However, Falavigna et al. [17] concluded that chronic BCAA supplementation has no effect on glucose metabolism and could therefore be excluded. The second may originate from reduced exercise-induced muscle protein degradation. Indeed, Hoffman et al. [14] reported lower creatine kinase activity following resistance exercise with acute protein supplementation. Moreover, they also registered improved recovery 24 and 48 h post exercise. Such results may be attributable to an enhanced repair process through reduced protein breakdown and increased protein synthesis [15].

However, due to the widely different experimental designs, such a mechanism is unlikely when considering our muscle endurance results. A third mechanism, related to a reduced central fatigue, could also be possible. Indeed, BCAA intake may reduce the plasma ratio of free tryptophan/BCAA and therefore the transport of tryptophan into the brain. This would reduce the synthesis, concentration and release of 5-hydroxytryptamine that is directly related to the development of fatigue and to the consequent reduction of performance [10]. In humans, such an effect has mostly been evidenced by a reduced feeling of fatigue during exercise and also during cognitive tasks such as short-term memory [9]. In the present study, no difference was registered in perceived exertion at the end of the muscle endurance test but the number of repetitions was increased with SMP. Therefore, our results are in general accordance with the literature. In addition, SMP induced a reduction in muscle fatigue. Although unclear, such an increase in muscle endurance could be attributed to the protein composition and digestibility. Indeed, with rapid digestibility, whey has been shown to induce a transient and more pronounced rise in whole body protein synthesis than casein [1,4]. Therefore, it could be speculated that soluble milk protein, tested here, may reduce central fatigue as a result of this enhanced whole body protein synthesis. Moreover, the amino acid composition of the two tested protein beverages is different, which could have a significant impact on the reported outcomes [5]. For example, cysteine content is seven times greater in SMP as compared to MC. It is well known that cystine enhances glutathione synthesis [20], an endogenous muscle antioxidant. Using quite similar cysteine contents as in our study while comparing whey vs. casein, authors demonstrated the positive effects of daily cysteine supplementation on the augmentation of antioxidant defense and anaerobic cycling performance [21]. Similar positive results were obtained for fatigue and performance during various exercises [22,23] with increases in cystine, cysteine, and glutathione content as a result of N-acetylcysteine ingestion [22]. Therefore, beverages with various amino acid content and not only BCAA or leucine are beneficial during prolonged exercise.

Muscle strength, power and thickness, although improved after the experimental period, were not different between groups. Such results are quite surprising since both protein beverages should have enhanced muscle thickness and muscle strength increases as compared with the placebo. Indeed, protein and more particularly BCAA are well known to increase muscle protein synthesis. For example, leucine plays a major role in muscle protein synthesis [24-26] through the stimulation of the mammalian target of rapamycin signaling pathway [27]. The lack of differences in muscle thickness and strength between groups remains unclear but could be attributed to several factors such as the supplement characteristics, training type and training status.

Protein was supplemented twice on non-training days and three times on training days. On training days, protein was ingested before and after the exercise session. Although debated, such timing may appear as one of the most effective nutrient timing strategies for muscle protein synthesis [26]. As compared to a morning/evening intake group, Cribb and Hayes [28] observed larger muscle mass increases with protein intake before and after training. The best stimulus for protein synthesis appeared to be with protein feeding in close proximity to training sessions [29,30], with feeding recommended within the first two hours postexercise [31-33].

Protein quantity was 20 or 30 g.day^{-1} (non-training and training days, respectively) with 10 g before and 10 g after resistance training sessions. Prima facie, these doses seem unlikely to be responsible for the lack of difference between groups for muscle thickness or muscle strength. However, associated with the timing, a dose–response relationship for protein synthesis is generally obtained. For example, although the contents of EAA and BCAA used in the current study would be sufficient to stimulate the mammalian target of rapamycin signaling pathway, a dose twice as large seems more efficient [34]. In a recent review [35], Phillips recommended the ingestion of 20 g of high quality protein immediately after exercise to maximally stimulate protein synthesis; and several authors reported that consumption of 8 to 11.5 g of EAA containing 2 to 3 g of leucine after exercise may maximize the protein synthetic response [5,36,37]. Recently, authors have demonstrated that low doses of leucine (0.75 g) may stimulate muscle protein synthesis following resistance exercise in young healthy individuals [38]. Higher doses (3 g leucine), however, maintained muscle protein synthesis longer and may be more effective for anabolism after resistance exercise [38]. In our study, the suboptimal doses ingested after exercise might therefore have reduced the potential protein effects and the potential differences between groups for muscle strength and thickness. This dose–response relationship may also explain differences between groups for muscle endurance and fatigue. For example, Falavigna et al. [17] registered increased or reduced time to exhaustion during prolonged swimming in rats with low or high BCAA diets. Intakes should therefore be adequately chosen to obtain optimal adaptations.

It should be remembered that training and supplementation effects are potentiated in subjects exhibiting lower muscle thickness at inclusion. Such a result is not surprising since training is well known to have larger effects in untrained subjects. For example, greater increases in muscle cross-sectional area have been reported in subjects who had not previously engaged in resistance training in comparison with more accustomed subjects [39]. The effects of amino acids supply may also depend on training status, since greater disturbances in protein turnover (protein synthesis and degradation) are obtained following training in novice than in experienced athletes [40]. Moreover, the expected increase in protein synthesis following exercise appears to be smaller and shorter in trained athletes as compared with untrained subjects [41,42]. Thus, training status may influence muscle performance. Indeed, Vieillevoye et al. [7] found increases in lower body strength with an essential amino acid supplement while no modification was obtained with placebo. Surprisingly, in the same study, strength was similarly enhanced in both groups for the upper body. These authors concluded that supplementation and training adaptations seem to depend on the initial training status; the weaker the subjects, the larger the effect of protein supplementation on muscle strength. Moreover, the present study was conducted in physically active males. Hence, it is possible to speculate that, with untrained participants, differences between groups might have been revealed. Furthermore, a plateau, or 'ceiling effect', of the adaptive responses to training is generally observed for strength gains and the muscle protein synthetic response [40,43]. Hence, protein requirements and training stimulus are affected by training status and duration. For instance, greater protein intakes are required during the early stages of intensive bodybuilding training and more particularly in novices [44]. Modification of the training program might also have exacerbated differences between groups for all studied parameters. Training volume [45] concomitant with the load used in terms of 1-RM's percentage [46] are possible parameters.

Conclusions

In conclusion, the present experiment demonstrated that protein supplementation may enhance possible adaptations induced by resistance training. Our results suggest that the effects of protein supplementation depend on the protein composition. More specifically, it appears that soluble milk protein is particularly efficient to improve resistance to fatigue. Therefore, supplementation with soluble milk protein may be recommended in combination with to resistance training.

Abbreviations
BCAA: Branched-chain amino acids; MC: Micellar casein; MID: Testing in the middle; PLA: Placebo; PRE: Testing at inclusion; POST: Testing at the end; RM: Repetition maximum; SMP: Soluble milk protein.

Competing interests
Lactalis Recherche et Développement provided financial support to conduct the study. The funders have no role in data collection and analysis or preparation of the manuscript. PLR and FM, two authors, have an affiliation (employment) to the commercial funders of this research.

Authors' contributions
NB (corresponding author) was responsible for the study design, the execution of the measurements and the writing of the manuscript. GD participated in the study design and the writing of the manuscript. PLR and FM participated in the study design. FAA participated in the study design, the statistical analysis and the writing of the manuscript. All authors read and approved the final manuscript.

Acknowledgements
The authors would like to thank Mr. Jeremy Denuziller for helping with data collection.

Author details
[1]National Institute for health and medical research (INSERM), unit 1093, Cognition, Action and sensorimotor plasticity, Dijon, France. [2]Centre for Performance Expertise, UFR STAPS, Dijon, France. [3]Lactalis R&D, Retiers, France. [4]Chair of Medical Evaluation ESC, Dijon, France. [5]CEN Nutriment, Dijon, France. [6]Faculté des Sciences du Sport, Université de Bourgogne, BP 27877, 21078 Dijon, Cedex, France.

References
1. Burd NA, Tang JE, Moore DR, Phillips SM: **Exercise training and protein metabolism: Influences of contraction, protein intake, and sex-based differences.** *J Appl Physiol* 2009, **106**:1692–1701.
2. Rennie MJ, Wackerhage H, Spangenburg EE, Booth FW: **Control of the size of the human muscle mass.** *Annu Rev Physiol* 2004, **66**:799–828.
3. Tipton KD, Gurkin BE, Matin S, Wolfe RR: **Nonessential amino acids are not necessary to stimulate net muscle protein synthesis in healthy volunteers.** *J Nutr Biochem* 1999, **10**:89–95.
4. Boirie Y, Dangin M, Gachon P, Vasson MP, Maubois JL, Beaufrere B: **Slow and fast dietary proteins differently modulate postprandial protein accretion.** *Proc Natl Acad Sci U S A* 1997, **94**:14930–14935.
5. Tang JE, Moore DR, Kujbida GW, Tarnopolsky MA, Phillips SM: **Ingestion of whey hydrolysate, casein, or soy protein isolate: Effects on mixed muscle protein synthesis at rest and following resistance exercise in young men.** *J Appl Physiol* 2009, **107**(1985):987–992.
6. Cermak NM, Res PT, de Groot LC, Saris WH, van Loon LJ: **Protein supplementation augments the adaptive response of skeletal muscle to resistance-type exercise training: A meta-analysis.** *Am J Clin Nutr* 2012, **96**:1454–1464.
7. Vieillevoye S, Poortmans JR, Duchateau J, Carpentier A: **Effects of a combined essential amino acids/carbohydrate supplementation on muscle mass, architecture and maximal strength following heavy-load training.** *Eur J Appl Physiol* 2010, **110**:479–488.
8. Derave W, Ozdemir MS, Harris RC, Pottier A, Reyngoudt H, Koppo K, Wise JA, Achten E: **Beta-alanine supplementation augments muscle carnosine content and attenuates fatigue during repeated isokinetic contraction bouts in trained sprinters.** *J Appl Physiol* 2007, **103**:1736–1743.
9. Portier H, Chatard JC, Filaire E, Jaunet-Devienne MF, Robert A, Guezennec CY: **Effects of branched-chain amino acids supplementation on physiological and psychological performance during an offshore sailing race.** *Eur J Appl Physiol* 2008, **104**:787–794.
10. Blomstrand E: **A role for branched-chain amino acids in reducing central fatigue.** *J Nutr* 2006, **136**:544S–547S.
11. Gryson C, Walrand S, Giraudet C, Rousset P, Migne C, Bonhomme C, Le Ruyet P, Boirie Y: **"Fast proteins" With a unique essential amino acid content as an optimal nutrition in the elderly: Growing evidence.** *Clin Nutr*, in press.
12. Blazevich AJ, Gill ND, Zhou S: **Intra- and intermuscular variation in human quadriceps femoris architecture assessed in vivo.** *J Anat* 2006, **209**:289–310.
13. Borg G: **Perceived exertion as an indicator of somatic stress.** *Scand J Rehabil Med* 1970, **2**:92–98.
14. Hoffman JR, Ratamess NA, Tranchina CP, Rashti SL, Kang J, Faigenbaum AD: **Effect of a proprietary protein supplement on recovery indices following resistance exercise in strength/power athletes.** *Amino Acids* 2010, **38**:771–778.
15. Shimomura Y, Yamamoto Y, Bajotto G, Sato J, Murakami T, Shimomura N, Kobayashi H, Mawatari K: **Nutraceutical effects of branched-chain amino acids on skeletal muscle.** *J Nutr* 2006, **136**:529S–532S.
16. Blomstrand E, Hassmen P, Ekblom B, Newsholme EA: **Administration of branched-chain amino acids during sustained exercise–effects on performance and on plasma concentration of some amino acids.** *Eur J Appl Physiol Occup Physiol* 1991, **63**:83–88.
17. Falavigna G, Alves De Araujo J Jr, Rogero MM, Pires IS, Pedrosa RG, Martins E Jr, Alves de Castro I, Tirapegui J: **Effects of diets supplemented with branched-chain amino acids on the performance and fatigue mechanisms of rats submitted to prolonged physical exercise.** *Nutrients* 2012, **4**:1767–1780.
18. Kerksick CM, Rasmussen CJ, Lancaster SL, Magu B, Smith P, Melton C, Greenwood M, Almada AL, Earnest CP, Kreider RB: **The effects of protein and amino acid supplementation on performance and training adaptations during ten weeks of resistance training.** *J Strength Cond Res* 2006, **20**:643–653.
19. Davis JM, Welsh RS, De Volve KL, Davis JM, Welsh RS, De Volve KL, Alderson NA: **Effects of branched-chain amino acids and carbohydrate on fatigue during intermittent, high-intensity running.** *Int J Sports Med* 1999, **20**:309–314.
20. Mariotti F, Simbelie KL, Makarios-Lahham L, Huneau JF, Laplaize B, Tome D, Even PC: **Acute ingestion of dietary proteins improves post-exercise liver glutathione in rats in a dose-dependent relationship with their cysteine content.** *J Nutr* 2004, **134**:128–131.
21. Lands LC, Grey VL, Smountas AA: **Effect of supplementation with a cysteine donor on muscular performance.** *J Appl Physiol* 1999, **87**(1985):1381–1385.
22. Medved I, Brown MJ, Bjorksten AR, Murphy KT, Petersen AC, Sostaric S, Gong X, McKenna MJ: **N-acetylcysteine enhances muscle cysteine and glutathione availability and attenuates fatigue during prolonged exercise in endurance-trained individuals.** *J Appl Physiol* 2004, **97**(1985):1477–1485.
23. Pinheiro CH, Vitzel KF, Curi R: **Effect of n-acetylcysteine on markers of skeletal muscle injury after fatiguing contractile activity.** *Scand J Med Sci Sports* 2012, **22**:24–33.
24. Stock MS, Young JC, Golding LA, Kruskall LJ, Tandy RD, Conway-Klaassen JM, Beck TW: **The effects of adding leucine to pre and postexercise carbohydrate beverages on acute muscle recovery from resistance training.** *J Strength Cond Res* 2010, **24**:2211–2219.
25. Ispoglou T, King RF, Polman RC, Zanker C: **Daily l-leucine supplementation in novice trainees during a 12-week weight training program.** *Int J Sports Physiol Perform* 2011, **6**:38–50.
26. Stark M, Lukaszuk J, Prawitz A, Salacinski A: **Protein timing and its effects on muscular hypertrophy and strength in individuals engaged in weight-training.** *J Int Soc Sports Nutr* 2012, **9**:54.
27. Norton LE, Layman DK: **Leucine regulates translation initiation of protein synthesis in skeletal muscle after exercise.** *J Nutr* 2006, **136**:533S–537S.
28. Cribb PJ, Hayes A: **Effects of supplement timing and resistance exercise on skeletal muscle hypertrophy.** *Med Sci Sports Exerc* 2006, **38**:1918–1925.
29. Tipton KD, Elliott TA, Cree MG, Aarsland AA, Sanford AP, Wolfe RR: **Stimulation of net muscle protein synthesis by whey protein ingestion before and after exercise.** *Am J Physiol Endocrinol Metab* 2007, **292**:E71–E76.
30. Tipton KD, Rasmussen BB, Miller SL, Wolf SE, Owens-Stovall SK, Petrini BE, Wolfe RR: **Timing of amino acid-carbohydrate ingestion alters anabolic response of muscle to resistance exercise.** *Am J Physiol Endocrinol Metab* 2001, **281**:E197–E206.
31. Hartman JW, Tang JE, Wilkinson SB, Tarnopolsky MA, Lawrence RL, Fullerton AV, Phillips SM: **Consumption of fat-free fluid milk after resistance exercise promotes greater lean mass accretion than does consumption of soy or carbohydrate in young, novice, male weightlifters.** *Am J Clin Nutr* 2007, **86**:373–381.
32. Phillips SM, Tipton KD, Aarsland A, Wolf SE, Wolfe RR: **Mixed muscle protein synthesis and breakdown after resistance exercise in humans.** *Am J Physiol* 1997, **273**:E99–E107.
33. Rasmussen BB, Tipton KD, Miller SL, Wolf SE, Wolfe RR: **An oral essential amino acid-carbohydrate supplement enhances muscle protein anabolism after resistance exercise.** *J Appl Physiol* 2000, **88**:386–392.
34. Kakigi R, Yoshihara T, Ozaki H, Ogura Y, Ichinoseki-Sekine N, Kobayashi H, Naito H: **Whey protein intake after resistance exercise activates mtor**

signaling in a dose-dependent manner in human skeletal muscle.
Eur J Appl Physiol, **114**:735–742. in press.

35. Phillips SM: **Dietary protein requirements and adaptive advantages in athletes.** *Br J Nutr* 2012, **108**(Suppl 2):S158–S167.

36. Reidy PT, Walker DK, Dickinson JM, Gundermann DM, Drummond MJ, Timmerman KL, Fry CS, Borack MS, Cope MB, Mukherjea R, Jennings K, Volpi E, Rasmussen BB: **Protein blend ingestion following resistance exercise promotes human muscle protein synthesis.** *J Nutr* 2013, **143**:410–416.

37. Burke LM, Winter JA, Cameron-Smith D, Enslen M, Farnfield M, Decombaz J: **Effect of intake of different dietary protein sources on plasma amino acid profiles at rest and after exercise.** *Int J Sport Nutr Exerc Metab* 2012, **22**:452–462.

38. Churchward-Venne TA, Burd NA, Mitchell CJ, West DW, Philp A, Marcotte GR, Baker SK, Baar K, Phillips SM: **Supplementation of a suboptimal protein dose with leucine or essential amino acids: Effects on myofibrillar protein synthesis at rest and following resistance exercise in men.** *J Physiol* 2012, **590**:2751–2765.

39. Ahtiainen JP, Pakarinen A, Alen M, Kraemer WJ, Hakkinen K: **Muscle hypertrophy, hormonal adaptations and strength development during strength training in strength-trained and untrained men.** *Eur J Appl Physiol* 2003, **89**:555–563.

40. Phillips SM, Tipton KD, Ferrando AA, Wolfe RR: **Resistance training reduces the acute exercise-induced increase in muscle protein turnover.** *Am J Physiol* 1999, **276**:E118–E124.

41. Phillips SM, Parise G, Roy BD, Tipton KD, Wolfe RR, Tamopolsky MA: **Resistance-training-induced adaptations in skeletal muscle protein turnover in the fed state.** *Can J Physiol Pharmacol* 2002, **80**:1045–1053.

42. MacDougall JD, Gibala MJ, Tarnopolsky MA, MacDonald JR, Interisano SA, Yarasheski KE: **The time course for elevated muscle protein synthesis following heavy resistance exercise.** *Can J Appl Physiol* 1995, **20**:480–486.

43. Alway SE, Grumbt WH, Stray-Gundersen J, Gonyea WJ: **Effects of resistance training on elbow flexors of highly competitive bodybuilders.** *J Appl Physiol* 1992, **72**:1512–1521.

44. Lemon PW, Tarnopolsky MA, MacDougall JD, Atkinson SA: **Protein requirements and muscle mass/strength changes during intensive training in novice bodybuilders.** *J Appl Physiol* 1992, **73**:767–775.

45. Krieger JW: **Single vs. Multiple sets of resistance exercise for muscle hypertrophy: A meta-analysis.** *J Strength Cond Res* 2010, **24**:1150–1159.

46. Burd NA, West DW, Staples AW, Atherton PJ, Baker JM, Moore DR, Holwerda AM, Parise G, Rennie MJ, Baker SK, Phillips SM: **Low-load high volume resistance exercise stimulates muscle protein synthesis more than high-load low volume resistance exercise in young men.** *PLoS One* 2010, **5**:e12033.

12

The effect of turmeric (Curcumin) supplementation on cytokine and inflammatory marker responses following 2 hours of endurance cycling

Joseph N Sciberras[1][*], Stuart DR Galloway[2], Anthony Fenech[3], Godfrey Grech[5], Claude Farrugia[4], Deborah Duca[4] and Janet Mifsud[3]

Abstract

Background: Endurance exercise induces IL-6 production from myocytes that is thought to impair intracellular defence mechanisms. Curcumin inhibits NF-κB and activator protein 1, responsible for cytokine transcription, in cell lines. The aim of this study was to investigate the effect of curcumin supplementation on the cytokine and stress responses following 2 h of cycling.

Methods: Eleven male recreational athletes (35.5 ± 5.7 years; W_{max} 275 ± 6 W; 87.2 ± 10.3 kg) consuming a low carbohydrate diet of 2.3 ± 0.2 g/kg/day underwent three double blind trials with curcumin supplementation, placebo supplementation, and no supplementation (control) to observe the response of serum interleukins (IL-6, IL1-RA, IL-10), cortisol, c-reactive protein (CRP), and subjective assessment of training stress. Exercise was set at 95% lactate threshold (54 ± 7% W_{max}) to ensure that all athletes completed the trial protocol.

Results: The trial protocol elicted a rise in IL-6 and IL1-RA, but not IL-10. The supplementation regimen failed to produce statistically significant results when compared to placebo and control. IL-6 serum concentrations one hour following exercise were (Median (IQR): 2.0 (1.8-3.6) Curcumin; 4.8 (2.1-7.3) Placebo; 3.5 (1.9-7.7) Control). Differences between supplementation and placebo failed to reach statistical significance (p = 0.18) with the median test. Repeated measures ANOVA time-trial interaction was at p = 0.06 between curcumin supplementation and placebo. A positive correlation (p = 0.02) between absolute exercise intensity and 1 h post-exercise for IL-6 concentration was observed. Participants reported "better than usual" scores in the subjective assessment of psychological stress when supplementing with curcumin, indicating that they felt less stressed during training days (p = 0.04) compared to placebo even though there was no difference in RPE during any of the training days or trials.

Conclusion: The limitations of the current regimen and trial involved a number of factors including sample size, mode of exercise, intensity of exercise, and dose of curcumin. Nevertheless these results provide insight for future studies with larger samples, and multiple curcumin dosages to investigate if different curcumin regimens can lead to statistically different interleukin levels when compared to a control and placebo.

Keywords: Immunity, Interleukins, Natural polyphenols

* Correspondence: sciberras.n.joseph@gmail.com
[1]Sport Nutrition graduate from the University of Stirling, 74, San Anton Court, Pope John XXIII street, Birkirkara BKR1033, Malta
Full list of author information is available at the end of the article

Background

Research supports a role for nutritional interventions to maintain immune function in the post-exercise period [1-5] It is also widely recognized that endurance exercise stimulates an increase in circulating cytokines in the post-exercise period [6,7]. These cytokines include interleukin 1 beta (IL-1β), interleukin 6 (IL-6), interleukin 8 (IL-8), interleukin 10 (IL-10), and interleukin 1 receptor antagonist (IL1-RA). These cytokine responses following exercise do not mainly originate from circulating monocytes, but may influence secretion of other cytokines from cells which form part of the immune system [8,9]. The post-exercise rise in IL-6 is unrelated to muscle damage, but serves as a messenger from myocytes to increase hepatic glycogenolysis [10-12]. Interestingly, the release of IL-6 in the post-exercise period appears to be dependent upon carbohydrate availability [12].

IL-6 is a cell messenger which affects many cells and systems, such as lymphocytes, leads to the release of the anti-inflammatory hormone cortisol, and stimulates release of acute phase proteins and glucose from the liver [13] IL1-RA and IL-10 transcription are mediated by high IL-6 concentrations [14]. These immunomodulatory mechanisms result in a decreased amount of circulating Type 1 T-helper (Th1) cells [15]. This suggests that regular high volume exercise shifts the CD4 positive T lymphocyte profile from Th1 towards Th2. Th1 cells help neutralize intracellular infective agents like viruses and bacteria which are responsible for upper respiratory tract infections (URTI). Specific interleukins, involved in cellular immunity, are also inhibited by the increase in IL-6 [16]. Inhibition of IL-1 is mediated through IL1-RA, and IL-6 appears to blunt the effect of TNF-α, while the effects of interleukin 12 are countered by IL-10 [17]. Thus, factors that can modify the post-exercise cytokine response could assist in maintenance of immune function in athletes.

Cytokine transcription is mediated by the transcription factors NF-κB and activator protein 1 (AP-1) [18]. Activation of NF-κB is induced by several immunity mediators, cell signaling intermediates, and reactive oxygen species [19]. Curcumin found in the rhizome Curcuma longa (turmeric), is an anti-oxidant and anti-inflammatory, long used as a traditional herbal medicine [20-22]. It attenuates the activation of NF-κB and IκB kinase in cancer cell lines [23]. Researchers observed that curcumin inhibits the activity of IκB kinase and decreases the activity of NF-κB in intestinal epithelial cells [24]. Shisodia et al., reported that the activity of curcumin also affects the AP-1 pathway, and Akt signaling [25]. In a study on rats, curcumin was shown to reduce IL-6, IL-1β, and TNFα levels following eccentric exercise [26]. These authors concluded that curcumin may promote recovery following repeated strenuous activity. Curcumin has also been shown to affect numerous physiological pathways, including inflammation, and play important roles in pathological conditions, including diabetes and arthritis, as reviewed elsewhere [27-29].

These observations with curcumin in cell and animal models, leads us to hypothesize that curcumin supplementation in humans could reduce cytokine release following exercise. An acute blunting of the cytokine response to exercise may provide a strong basis for longer term studies examining a role for curcumin on immune function and recovery during periods of strenuous exercise training. The current study, therefore, aimed to observe the effects of curcumin supplementation on interleukin and other inflammatory marker responses following two hours of cycling in a low glycogen state.

Methods

Eleven recreationally active males (regular weekly aerobic activity during the last year for at least 3 h, mean age 35.5 ± 5.7 years; mean W_{max} 275 ± 56 W; mean weight 87.2 ± 10.3 kg; mean height 1.78 ± 0.07 m) volunteered to participate in the study. All of the participants gave their written informed consent to participate in the study which was approved by the ethics committees of the University of Stirling and University of Malta. Athletes were recruited from those attending talks held at sport clubs in Malta. Participants were screened for suitability prior to the experimental trials, including a medical visit by a licensed general practitioner. None reported a history of auto-immune disorders or medical conditions which could affect the results. Moreover they were not on medication or high dose vitamin C and/or vitamin E intake. Participants reported being free from infection for at least 4 weeks prior to the trial, and were in a steady period of endurance training. The number of participants needed was calculated by sample size testing based on literature review. Power was set at 80%, $p < 0.05$, with a difference in population means of 2 pg for interleukin 6, and standard deviation of 2 pg. This gave an approximate sample size of 8–10. The sample sizes and results obtained in studies listed in the review of Fischer, 2006 [30], on interleukins and exercise were also taken as a guide.

Participants were taught how to use diabetic nutritional exchanges to comply with the pre-trial prescribed diet. Preliminary measurement of lactate threshold and maximum workload were obtained together using a Computrainer lab ergometer (Racermate, Seattle, USA) and Lactate Scout (EKF-Diagnostics, Magdeburg, Germany). The Lactate Scout was validated prior to each test using the standard solution provided by the manufacturer. Lactate was measured by skin pricking every three minutes on the computrainer® lab; following which power was increased by 30 W. This continued until volitional fatigue or until the athlete was unable to maintain a cadence of 70 rpm. This was defined as the maximum workload.

Subjects were then allocated either to the curcumin supplement or placebo in a double blind randomized cross-over fashion. Subjects performed three trials in total (supplement/placebo and control) in which they exercised for 2 h at a power output equivalent to 95% of their lactate threshold, to ensure completion of the trial task. Supplement or placebo was taken for three days prior to the trial day, and finally on arrival at the clinic for the trial. Following a one week wash-out period the trial was repeated with supplementation/placebo accordingly. An identical further trial served as a control and was held following a further week without any supplementation. The control arm of the study was scheduled after the two experimental trials in an effort to minimize data loss from curcumin and placebo trials, through athlete drop out. In addition, participants undertook a supervised one hour interval training session on a cycle ergometer in the afternoon, two days prior to each trial, in an attempt to lower muscle glycogen stores. Participants were then assigned a diet containing 2.3 ± 0.2 g/kg carbohydrate, 1.0 ± 0.2 g/kg fat, and 1.3 ± 0.2 g/kg protein. This diet was aimed at minimising carbohydrate replenishment following training two days prior to the trial. Participants returned to their habitual diet immediately after the trial. Participants were requested to refrain from strenuous physical activity for 24 h prior to trials.

Upon arrival at the laboratory for the trials a cannula was inserted in an antecubital vein. Blood samples (20 ml, 4 serum and 2 EDTA tubes) were taken just before the exercise trial, immediately after completing the two hours cycling, and one hour following the cessation of exercise (Figure 1). A pedaling cadence of 70 rpm was maintained during trials using the Computrainer® ergometer, which was calibrated as per manufacturer's instructions. Prior to all training and trial sessions participants completed a daily analysis of life demands (DALDA) questionnaire to assess stress sources (part 1) and stress symptoms (part 2) [31].

Trials, conducted at St James Highway Clinic, commenced between 1 pm and 6 pm, at least 4 h following their last meal. Heart rate was measured using a Timex®

(Middlebury, USA) telemetry strap. Temperature and humidity, measured with a calibrated thermo-hygrometer (TFA-Dostmann, Mannheim, Germany), were maintained close to 20°C and 60% RH, respectively. Rating of perceived exertion was reported after 15 min into the trial and thereafter every 30 minutes. Only water was permitted during the trial. One athlete dropped out following the second trial, and did not complete the control trial. The curcumin supplement ("Meriva®") Curcumin) and corresponding identical placebo, together with respective certificate of analysis (CoA) were donated by Indena Spa. (Milan, Italy). Meriva® curcumin was chosen because of its superior bioavailability to other curcumin products. Researchers concluded that a single dosage of 376 mg of Meriva® curcumin was eighteen times superior to a standard curcumin dose of 2 g, giving a maximum plasma concentration of 207 ng/ml four hours following supplement ingestion [32]. Dosage for the present study subjects was a single dose of 500 mg of Meriva® curcumin (5 tablets) with midday meal for three days, and then 500 mg ingested just before exercise. Samples for plasma curcumin analysis were taken at the final blood sampling time only in this study, three hours post ingestion to coincide with assessment of post-exercise interleukin response.

Plasma and serum samples obtained after centrifuging were frozen at −80°C. Plasma samples for curcumin analysis were incubated for 4 hours with helix pomatia glucuronidase (Sigma Aldrich®, Delaware, USA) in a pH 5 sodium acetate buffer. This was followed by extraction with chloroform. The organic chloroform was dried under a nitrogen stream, and reconstituted in 4 ml curcumin spiked acetonitrile. These samples were then analysed for curcumin using a Waters HPLC (Milford, USA) using a method reported in literature [33]. The method was validated for identification and linearity using curcumin standard (Sigma Aldrich, Delaware, USA). Interleukins 6, 1RA, and 10 were assayed on all serum samples using ELISA kits supplied by R&D Systems Ltd (Minneapolis, USA). Haematocrit, haemoglobin concentration, white blood cell (WBC count), neutrophil proportion, cortisol concentration, and c-reactive protein concentration were

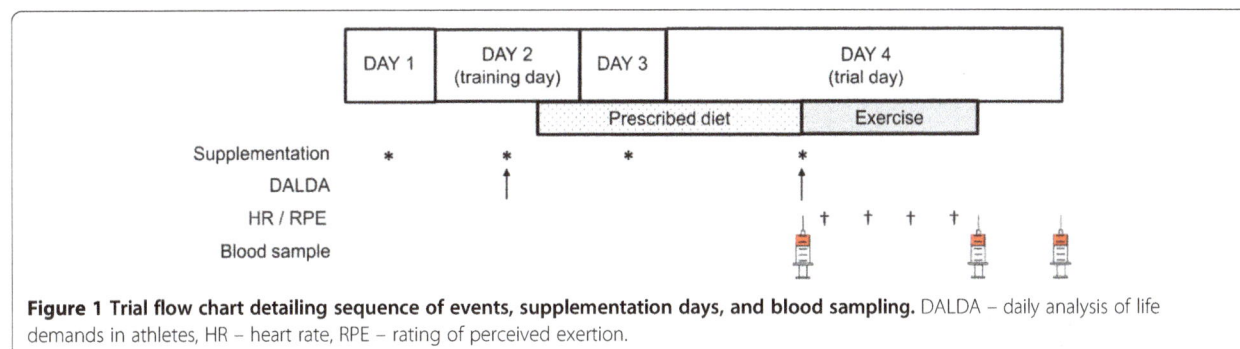

Figure 1 Trial flow chart detailing sequence of events, supplementation days, and blood sampling. DALDA – daily analysis of life demands in athletes, HR – heart rate, RPE – rating of perceived exertion.

all measured on blood taken immediately after exercise only (analyses were conducted by MLS laboratories, St James Hospital, Malta).

Repeated measures ANOVA was conducted with the values obtained for time, trial, and time x trial interactions. Any outliers in datasets were dealt with using Grubbs method [34]. Any significant within subject effects were then examined with the median test when data was not normally distributed (IL-6 conc.), otherwise student t-test was used. Ratings from the DALDA questionnaire were analysed with the wilcoxon test for paired non parametric data. Parametric results are tabulated as mean ± standard deviation, 95% confidence intervals are also given in brackets for Tables 1 and 2. Further results are graphically plotted as mean ± standard error of the mean. Median and inter-quartile range are reported when continuous data is not normally distributed. Spearman's correlation coefficient was calculated where associations were expected. The intra-assay coefficient of variation was 9.4% for IL-6; 6.4% for IL-1RA and 3.4% for the HPLC assay of curcumin.

Results

All participants undertook the trial at 95% lactate threshold. Relative to W_{max} the mean power output sustained during the 2 hour ride was $54 \pm 7\%$ of the mean maximum workload (range 39% to 63% of W_{max}). The humidity, temperature, and ergometer calibration values were all similar between trials (Table 1). Initial body mass and training volume were also not different between each trial (Table 1). None of the participants reported any adverse effect to supplementation or placebo ingestion. All participants reported adhering to their pre-trial diets on all trials. Participants completed all the trials in three weeks. Five participants started the trials with placebo and six with curcumin supplementation. HPLC analysis confirmed the presence of curcumin in plasma of all participants when taking the curcumin supplement. No curcumin was detected in plasma samples on other trials. Mean ± SD (range) curcumin concentration obtained was 79.7 ± 26.3 ng/ml (50.7 ng/ml to 125.5 ng/ml).

The reported perceived exertion increased significantly every 30 minutes during the 2 hour ride on all trials (mean (SD) RPE was: 9 ± 1; 10 ± 2; 11 ± 2 & 12 ± 2 at 15, 45, 75 and 105 minutes during exercise; $p < 0.01$). There were no significant differences in RPE ratings obtained during exercise between trials (11 ± 1; 11 ± 1; 11 ± 1 for curcumin, placebo and control trials, respectively). Mean (SD) heart rate during the exercise period was also not different between trials (118 ± 12; 117 ± 10; 117 ± 13 for curcumin, placebo and control trials, respectively). Whole blood analysis of the post-exercise samples revealed no differences in cortisol, c-reactive protein, haematocrit, haemoglobin, WBC, or neutrophil proportion between trials (Table 2).

Serum IL-6 data demonstrated a tendency for an interaction effect (time x trial interaction $p = 0.06$; $F = 4.03$) between curcumin and placebo trials (Figure 2). Curcumin only appeared to lower the concentration of IL-6 released one hour following exercise when compared to placebo, but this failed to reach statistical significance ($p = 0.18$; n = 10; 95% C.I. $1.63 \leq \times \leq 3.81$) (Figure 3). Estimation of size of effect proves difficult because one set of data is not normally distributed. Nonetheless Cohen's d is of 0.84 hinting at a possibly large effect (Figure 4). The correlation analysis revealed a significant association ($p = 0.02$) between IL-6 elevation and percentage W_{max} power output sustained during the exercise task (correlation coefficient rho 0.41 ($df = 30$)). No association was observed between attenuation of IL-6 response following exercise with the plasma concentration levels of curcumin ($p = 0.92$; correlation coefficient rho -0.04 ($df = 9$)). There was no difference between the trials for IL1-RA (time x trial interaction $p = 0.85$, ($F = 0.44$) when analysing the ANOVA for repeated measures. Correlation coefficient between percentage W_{max} power and change in IL1-RA concentration was 0.34 ($df = 30$), but failed to reach statistical significance ($p = 0.06$). There was no detectable increase in IL-10 on any of the trials.

The DALDA questionnaire (Table 3) revealed a higher number of "better than usual" results on the training day when ingesting curcumin compared to placebo and control. This was statistically significant between placebo

Table 1 Ambient conditions, ergometer calibration setting and initial body mass on the day of each trial

	Curcumin	Placebo	Control
Mean ambient humidity (% RH)	63 ± 6 (59–67)	62 ± 7 (58–66)	62 ± 6 (58–66)
Mean ambient temperature (°C)	19.9 ± 0.6 (19.5-20.3)	20.0 ± 0.4 (19.8-20.2)	20.1 ± 0.5 (19.8-20.4)
Calibration value of computrainer	2.7 ± 0.1 (2.6-2.8)	2.7 ± 0.1 (2.6-2.8)	2.8 ± 0.1 (2.7-2.9)
Body mass (kg)	86.7 ± 10.5 (80.5-92.9)	86.6 ± 10.4 (80.4-92.8)	87.5 ± 11.0 (80.7-94.3)
Training (Hours×Intensity)	11 ± 10 (5–17)	13 ± 9 (8–18)	13 ± 6 (9–17)

Habitual training load during the previous week was assessed using duration and intensity information. Training is reported in hours multiplied by intensity. Intensity was classified as low (1) medium (2) & high (3) Data are mean (± SD). Standard deviation and 95% confidence intervals are also reported following each value. No differences were noted between trials groups. Calibration value of the Computrainer is the value given to the ergometer as instructed by the manufacturer.

Table 2 Physiological parameters means (± SD) measured during trial, grouped by trial type

	Curcumin	Placebo	Control
Cortisol (nMol)	308 ± 200 (190–426)	266 ± 200 (148–384)	289 ± 228 (148–430)
C-Reactive protein (mg/l)	0.5 ± 0.3 (0.3-0.7)	0.9 ± 0.9 (0.4-1.4)	0.7 ± 0.6 (0.3-1.1)
Haematocrit (%)	43 ± 2 (42–44)	43 ± 3 (41–45)	43 ± 2 (42–43)
Haemoglobin (g/dl)	15.0 ± 0.7 (14.6-15.4)	14.0 ± 0.9 (13.5-14.5)	15.1 ± 0.8 (14.6-15.6)
WBC (10^9/L)	10.1 ± 2.7 (8.5-11.7)	9.6 ± 2.5 (8.1-11.1)	10.4 ± 2.6 (8.8-12.0)
Neutrophil (%)	61.9 ± 9.8 (56.1-67.7)	61.4 ± 9.2 (56.0-66.8)	63.5 ± 9.5 (57.6-69.4)

Confidence intervals 95% are also reported following each value.

Parameters show no significant difference between trials. These parameters were measured only at the end of exercise. Cortisol and C - reactive protein were measured to investigate any possible effects from the active compound curcumin. Haematocrit & Haemoglobin were measured to ensure that the athletes were in similar hydration status, while white blood cell and neutrophil percentage were needed to confirm that the athlete was not suffering from an infection at the time of the trial.

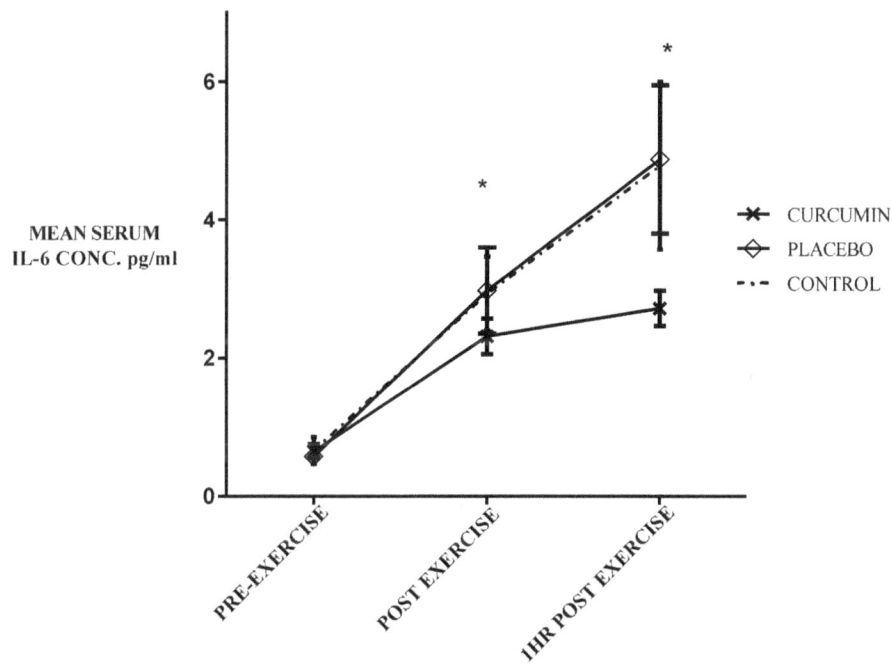

MEAN IL-6 VALUES DURING TRIALS

	CURCUMIN	PLACEBO	CONTROL
Serum IL-6 before exercise (pg/ml)	0.6±0.3 (0.4-0.8)	0.6±0.2 (±0.5-0.7)	0.7±0.6 (±0.3-1.1)
Serum IL- 6 post exercise (pg/ml)	2.3±0.8 (1.8-2.8)	3.0±2.1 (1.8-4.2)	3.0±1.7 (1.9-4.1)
Serum IL-6 1hr post exercise (pg/ml) (MEAN)	2.7±1.5 (1.8-3.6)	4.9±3.3 (2.8-7.0)	4.8±3.8 (2.4-7.2)
(MEDIAN)	2 (IQR 1.8-3.6)	4.8 (IQR 2.1-7.3)	3.5 (IQR 1.9-7.7)

Figure 2 Mean (±SEM) IL-6 concentration obtained before exercise, immediately after exercise, and one hour following exercise on each trial day. *indicates significant difference from pre-exercise on all trials. No statistical significant difference between interleukin 6 values was observed. Table shows mean cytokine levels, standard deviation, and 95% confidence intervals during trials. Median and interquartile range IQR are also shown for 1 hour post exercise.

MEAN IL1-RA VALUES DURING TRIALS

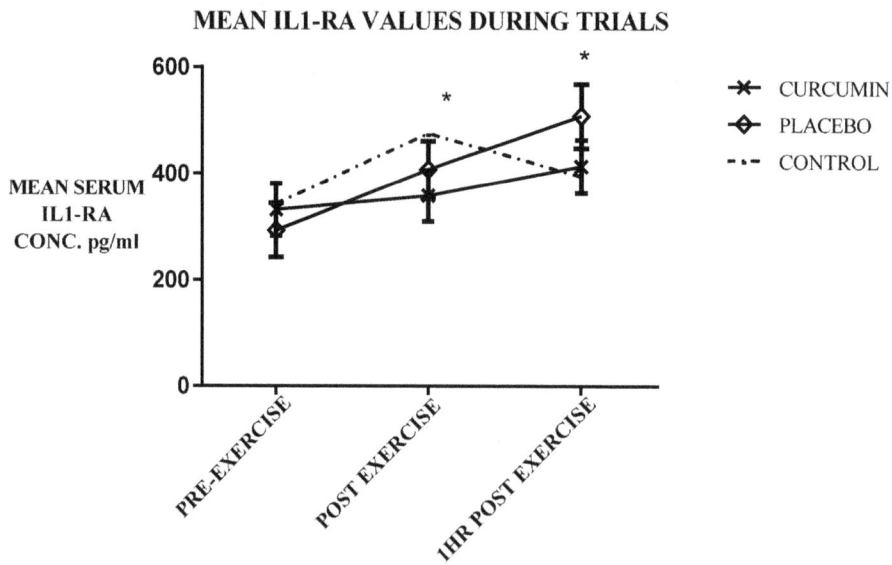

	CURCUMIN	PLACEBO	CONTROL
Serum IL1-RA before exercise (pg/ml)	332±162 (236-428)	293±170 (193-393)	343±95 (284-397)
Serum IL1-RA post exercise (pg/ml)	358±160 (263-453)	408±177 (303-513)	476±252 (327-625)
Serum IL1-RA 1hr post exercise (pg/ml)	414±158 (316-512)	508±200 (389-627)	395±131(314-476)

Figure 3 Mean (±SEM) IL1-RA concentration obtained before exercise, immediately after exercise, and one hour following exercise on each trial day. *indicates significant difference from pre-exercise. Table shows mean cytokine levels, standard deviation, and 95% confidence intervals during trials.

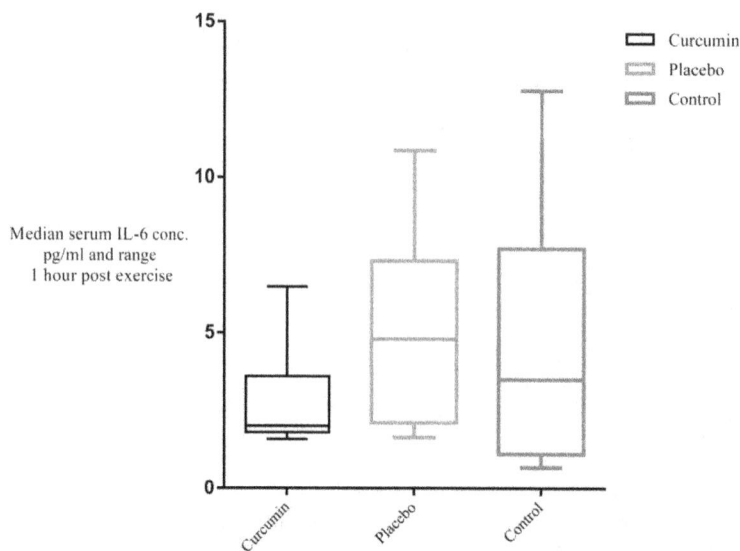

Figure 4 Median IL-6 concentration and range one hour post exercise for curcumin, placebo and control trials. Note curcumin dataset still positively skewed (towards low values) despite removing an outlier.

Table 3 DALDA (Daily Analysis of Life Demands on Athletes) questionnaire responses (median & range) for both training and trial days

	DALDA part 1 (training day) stress sources			DALDA (part 2 training day) stress symptoms		
RESPONSE	*A (Worse)*	*B (Same)*	*C (Better)*	*A (Worse)*	*B (Same)*	*C (Better)*
CURCUMIN (n = 11)	0 (0–3)	4 (4–9)	3 (0–5)[†]	1 (0–4)	21(4–25)	3 (0–19)†
PLACEBO (n = 11)	1 (0–5)	7 (2–9)	1 (0–6)	2 (0–7)	20 (8–25)	2 (0–15)
CONTROL (n = 10)	2 (0–3)	6 (2–9)	0 (0–7)	2 (0–9)	22 (5–25)	2 (0–18)
	DALDA part 1 (trial day) stress sources			**DALDA part 2 (trial day) stress symptoms**		
RESPONSE	*A (Worse)*	*B (Same)*	*C (Better)*	*A (Worse)*	*B (Same)*	*C (Better)*
CURCUMIN (n = 11)	2 (0–4)	6 (2–9)	1 (0–7)	2 (0–5)	22 (5–25)	1 (0–20)
PLACEBO (n = 11)	1 (0–5)	8 (2–9)	0 (0–6)	1 (0–6)	23 (5–25)	0 (0–18)
CONTROL (n = 10)	2 (0–3)	7 (3–9)	0 (0–6)	3 (0–8)	22 (4–25)	1 (0–19)

Data is grouped according to trial type. A – Worse than usual; B – Same as usual; C – Better than usual. [†]indicates statistical significant difference between curcumin and placebo trials, p-value in both parts between curcumin and placebo is 0.04 using Wilcoxon signed ranks.

and supplementation in both stress sources (Part 1, p = 0.04) and stress symptoms (Part 2, p = 0.04). The number of "better than usual" results obtained between curcumin and control on the training day was also higher but not statistically significant (Part 1,p = 0.06; and Part 2, p = 0.14). There were no differences in scoring on Part 1 or Part 2 of the DALDA questionnaire between treatments on the trial days.

Discussion

The current study has not revealed a statistically significant difference between the supplementation with curcumin vs. placebo or control. However these results suggest that a positive inhibitory effect of curcumin on IL-6 production/release or an enhanced uptake *in vivo could occur at* higher supplementation doses, and under different trial conditions (suggested underneath). These observations, although again not statistically significant, lend some support to the previous cell and animal model data, and suggest that further studies in humans may be warranted. The lack of statistical significance in our dataset suggests that sample size, mode of exercise, intensity of exercise, dose of curcumin, or sample collection times are interesting issues for discussion and further investigation.

Sample size estimates using the mean difference 1 hr post-exercise, and standard deviation, from the present study indicate that adequate power could be obtained with 26 participants. Given the large variance in response of IL-6 post-exercise within the current study it would be of interest to analyse responses in a similar trial on a group who may provide a more homogeneous response. The recruitment of cyclists also may have limited our ability to observe any possible effect of curcumin on post-exercise cytokine concentration, due to the absence of eccentric contractions or weight bearing impact during the exercise task. A two hour long exercise regimen was chosen because duration of exercise is considered a better predictor of serum interleukin elevation than intensity. Running is associated with a higher rise in cytokine concentration post-exercise than observed following cycling [30], and may therefore be a mode of choice in future studies.

Despite the light exercise intensity examined in the present study a response in IL-6 and IL1-RA was still elicited, primarily because the exercise was of sufficient duration. We deliberately adopted a low carbohydrate diet in an attempt to exacerbate the cytokine response to prolonged cycling exercise [12], and this seems to have been effective. Participants whose trial was at a higher workload intensity relative to their maximum workload capacity had a greater increase in IL1-RA and IL-6 concentration one hour after exercise. This was statistically significant for IL-6, and close to statistical significance for IL1-RA. It is important to note that some studies observing higher cytokine responses employed a performance time/distance trial following a period of cycling at a submaximal steady state intensity [12]. This type of protocol would enhance the cytokine response post-exercise, and indicates that higher intensity bouts may be of most interest in future studies examining curcumin effects on cytokine response.

Although our data indicate no statistically significant effect of curcumin supplementation on IL-6 and IL1-RA response to exercise, this could be due to the curcumin dose and plasma curcumin response. Cuomo and colleagues previously indicated that serum micro-molar concentrations of curcumin would likely be necessary for pharmacological *in vivo* effects [32]. Indeed, it is possible that a significant effect on post-exercise interleukin concentrations would have been achieved with a higher plasma curcumin concentration in the present study. The curcumin concentration achieved in the present study was almost 80 ng/ml (0.22 µmoles/L). A recent paper observed an effect of curcumin on plasma oxidative stress markers following exertion in humans when plasma curcumin concentration was elevated to around 100 ng/ml [35]. Recent work [36] has demonstrated that intraperitoneal injection of curcumin counteracts muscle atrophy in rats possibly also through anti-oxidant actions. It is unclear if such effects can be demonstrated in a human model and what dose of curcumin would be required to achieve this, but translation to a human model could provide relevant outcomes for sport or clinical practice. It is, therefore, recommended that future studies quantify the plasma concentration of curcumin required to achieve significant clinically relevant outcomes and investigate any possible association with anti-oxidant activity. Furthermore, blood sampling after 2, 16, & 24 hours following exercise would have provided further data on cortisol, C-reactive protein, and interleukin 10 responses which are known to be influenced by circulating IL-6 concentration, but at a later time than the last blood sample taken in our study.

Ratings of perceived exertion significantly increased throughout the exercise period on all trials. Given the prior glycogen depleting exercise during the training day, and prescribed low carbohydrate diet, it is likely that glycogen depletion contributed towards increased ratings of exertion during the exercise period. The DALDA results indicate that participants felt better on the second day of curcumin supplementation (the training day). The number of "better than usual" responses was higher than placebo and control on the second day of supplementation. It is important to note that DALDA is a retrospective tool of psychological causes and symptoms [31], while that ratings of perceived exertion (RPE) is a prospective tool assessing the extent of exercise difficulty. The study was aimed to provide the same repeatable exercise stressor every time the trial was repeated conducted with curcumin, placebo, and control. The fact that the RPE has did not changed to the extent of its sensitivity, between experimental variables provides evidence that the study managed to reproduce similar exercise conditions in all trials. A study on patients suffering from osteoarthritis taking 1 g of curcumin supplementation for eight months showed less pain and better movement reported by patients taking the supplementation versus placebo [37]. Moreover our views are supported by a recent study on curcumin supplementation and delayed muscle onset soreness (DOMS). This study has demonstrated that, participants taking 400 mg curcumin supplementation for 2 days, report less DOMS than participants taking placebo [38]. The authors suggest that potentially acute curcumin supplementation may be of use to help participants with higher intensity training workloads.

Interestingly, researchers have recently described significant anti-inflammatory effects of curcumin, and have confirmed that curcumin acts to inhibit lipopolysaccharide stimulated NF-κB, reduce IL-6, and reduce PMA induced reactive oxygen species (ROS) production, in human neutrophils [39]. Furthermore, others [40] have noted a significant attenuation in skeletal muscle IL-6 mRNA during exercise with anti-oxidant vitamin supplementation (vitamin C and E); and lead to significantly decreased plasma IL-6 concentration. Starkie and colleagues note a significant reduction in plasma IL-6 but not in skeletal muscle IL-6 mRNA following carbohydrate intake [41]. These observations suggest that measurement of early events in cytokine production are important to monitor in future human studies, and that concurrent supplementation of carbohydrate alongside an anti-oxidant like curcumin might have a superior effect to that of carbohydrate on its own on attenuation of cytokine response following exercise. It must be noted that subjects in our study were glycogen depleted, and that further studies are needed to confirm or refute similar findings or trends in athletes who are carbohydrate replete. As such the usefulness of curcumin supplementation during competition or training needs to be studied separately.

The present study also included a control arm, intended to identify any placebo effects, especially in subjective measures and to help confirm any trends observed with curcumin supplementation. No statistical difference between placebo and control values was found for any variables and no difference was observed from control in those who commenced the study with either curcumin supplementation, or placebo supplementation. This suggests both that the washout period was sufficiently long between trials with our present protocol and that trial stress was adequately reproduced.

Conclusion

There is considerable debate concerning the impact of blunting cytokine and inflammatory marker responses to exercise on the adaptive stimulus to exercise [42], and further work is required to determine the effects of blunting cytokine and inflammatory marker responses to exercise on incidence of infection, and training adaptation in athletes. Given that the limited bioavailability of the polyphenol curcumin has been now improved with new preparations as used in the present study, it would seem prudent to direct more research towards athletic and clinical populations. In conclusion, the results from the present study did not reveal any statistical difference between intervention and placebo. However our interpretation based on the findings presented in this paper does not exclude the possibility of an attenuating effect on IL-6 by curcumin. This is supported by the results obtained in this study and corroborated by findings in other published studies. We conclude that the effect of curcumin supplementation on interleukins and other inflammatory markers needs to be further investigated with observations in a larger sample including examination of exercise mode, intensity effects, and curcumin dose effects.

Competing interests

The authors declare that they have no competing interests.

Authors' contributions

JNS designed the study including trials & analysis, collected, analysed samples & data, prepared the manuscript; SG designed the study, supervised, reviewed data, & prepared manuscript; AF designed and supervised analysis & reviewed manuscript, GG supervised cytokine analysis, CF supervised HPLC analysis, DD designed and supervised HPLC analysis & JM supervised the study and reviewed manuscript. All authors read and approved the final manuscript.

Acknowledgements

Analysis was carried out at the department of pharmacology and therapeutics, and department of chemistry laboratories. The help of the respective laboratory officers is acknowledged. A special thanks to Dr. Bridgette Ellul, Dr. Neville Calleja, Dr. Christian Saliba, Pro-Rector Richard Muscat & Professor Roger Ellul Micallef for their support and mentorship. Many thanks to Dr. Gregory Attard & St James Highway Clinics This study was aided by a grant from the Maltese Sports Council.

Author details

[1]Sport Nutrition graduate from the University of Stirling, 74, San Anton Court, Pope John XXIII street, Birkirkara BKR1033, Malta. [2]Health and Exercise Sciences Research Group, School of Sport, University of Stirling, Stirling, Scotland. [3]Department of Clinical Pharmacology and Therapeutics, University of Malta, Msida, Malta. [4]Department of Chemistry, University of Malta, Msida, Malta. [5]Department of Pathology, University of Malta, Msida, Malta.

References

1. Nehlsen-Cannarella SL, Fagoaga OR, Nieman DC, Henson DA, Butterworth DE, Schmitt RL, et al. Carbohydrate and the cytokine response to 2.5 h of running. J Appl Physiol. 1997;82:1662–7.
2. Gleeson M, Blannin AK, Walsh NP, Bishop NC, Clark AM. Effect of low and high carbohydrate diets on the plasma glutamine and circulating leukocyte responses to exercise. Int J Sport Nutr Exerc Metab. 1998;8:49–59.
3. Mitchell JB, Pizza FX, Paquet A, Davis BJ, Forrest MB, Braun WA. Influence of carbohydrate status on immune responses before and after endurance exercise. J Appl Physiol. 1998;84:1917–25.
4. Nieman DC. Immunonutrition support for athletes [review]. Nutr Rev. 2008;66(6):310–20. DOI:10.1111/j.1753-4887.2008.00038.x.
5. Walsh NP, Gleeson M, Pyne DB, Niema D, Dhabhar FS, Shephard R, et al. Position statement part two: maintaining immune health. Exerc Immunol Rev. 2011;17:64–103.
6. Northoff H, Berg A. Immmunologic mediators as parameters of the reaction to strenuous exercise. Int J Sports Med. 1991;12(1):S9–S15.
7. Ostrowski K, Rohde T, Asp S, Schjerling P, Pedersen BK. Chemokines are elevated in plasma after strenuous exercise in humans. Eur J Appl Physiol. 2000;84(3):244–5.
8. Lancaster GL, Khan Q, Drysdale PT, Wallace F, Jeukendrup AE, Drayson MT, et al. Effect of prolonged strenuous exercise and carbohydrate ingestion on type 1 and type 2 T lymphocyte intracellular cytokine production in humans. J Appl Physiol. 2005;98:565–71. doi:10.1152/japplphysiol.00754.2004.
9. Starkie RL, Rolland J, Angus DJ, Anderson MJ, Febbraio MA. Circulating monocytes are not the source of the elevations in plasma IL-6 and TNF-α levels after prolonged running. Am J Physiol Cell Physiol. 2007;280:C769–74.
10. Ostrowski K, Rohde T, Zacho M, Asp S, Pedersen BK. Evidence that interleukin 6 is produced in human skeletal muscle during prolonged running. J Physiol. 1998;508(3):889–94.
11. Steensberg A, van Hall G, Osada T, Sacchetti M, Bengt S, Pedersen BK. Production of interleukin 6 in contracting human skeletal muscles can account for the exercise induced increase in plasma interleukin 6. J Physiol. 2000;529(1):237–42.
12. Bishop NC, Walsh NP, Haines DL, Richards DE, Gleeson M. Pre-exercise carbohydrate status and immune responses to prolonged cycling II: effect on plasma cytokine concentration. Int J Sport Nutr Exerc Metab. 2001;11:503–12.

13. Papanicolaou DA, Wilder RL, Manolagas SC, Chrousos GP. The pathophysiological roles of interleukin 6 in human disease [NIH Conference]. Ann Intern Med. 1998;128(2):128–37.
14. Steensberg A, Fischer CP, Keller C, Moller K, Pedersen BK. IL-6 enhances plasma IL1-RA, IL-10, and cortisol in humans. Am J Physiol Endocrinol Metab. 2003;285:E433–7.
15. Blannin AK. Acute exercise and the innate immune function. In: Gleeson M, editor. Immune Function in Sport and Exercise. 1st ed. Edinburgh, UK: Churchill Livingstone; 2006. p. 67–91.
16. Lakier SL. Overtraining, excessive exercise, and altered immunity, is this a T-helper-1 versus T-helper-2 lymphocyte response? Sports Med. 2003;33 (5):347–65.
17. Lancaster GL. Exercise and cytokines. In: Gleeson M, editor. Immune Function in Sport and Exercise. 2006th ed. Edinburgh, UK: Churchill Livingstone; 2006. p. 205–21.
18. Tak PP, Firestein GS. NF-κB a key role in inflammatory diseases. J Clin Investig. 2001;107(1):7–11.
19. Gloire G, Legrand-Poels S, Piette J. NF-κB activation by reactive oxygen species: fifteen years later. Biochem Pharmacol. 2006;72:1493–505. doi:10.1016/j.bcp.2006.04.011.
20. Anand P, Sherin TG, Kunnumakkara AB, Sundaram C, Harikumar KB, Sung B, et al. Biological activities of curcumin and its analogues & congeners) made by man and Mother Nature. Biochem Pharmacol. 2008;76:1590–611.
21. Pfeiffer E, Hoehle SI, Walch SG, Riess A, Solyom AM, Metzler M. Curcuminoids Form Reactive Glucuronides In Vitro. J Agric Food Chem. 2007;55:538–44.
22. Somparn P, Phisalaphong C, Nakornchai S, Unchern S, Phumala N, Morales NP. Comparative Antioxidant Activities of Curcumin and Its Demethoxy and Hydrogenated Derivatives. Biol Pharm Bull. 2007;1:74–8.
23. Bharti AC, Donato N, Singh S, Aggarwal B. Curcumin (diferuloylmethane) down-regulates the constitutive activation of nuclear factor -kB and IkBa kinase in human multiple myeloma cells, leading to suppression of proliferation and induction of apoptosis. Blood. 2003;101:1053–62. doi:10.1182/blood-2002-05-1320.
24. Jobin C, Bradham CA, Russo MP, Juma B, Narula AS, Brenner DA, et al. Curcumin blocks cytokine mediated NF-κB activation and pro-inflammatory gene expression by inhibiting inhibitory factor I-κB kinase activity. J Immunol. 1999;163:3474–83.
25. Shisodia S, Singh T, Chaturvedi MM. Modulation of transcription factors by curcumin. In: Aggarwal BB, Surh Y, Shisodia S, editors. The Molecular Targets and Therapeutic Uses of Curcumin in Health and Disease. 1st ed. New York, USA: Springer; 2007. p. 127–49.
26. Davis JM, Murph, EA, Carmichael MD, Zielinski MR, Groschwitz CM, Brown, AS, Gangemi JD, Ghaffer A, Mayer EP. Curcumin effects on inflammation and performance recovery following eccentric exercise-induced muscle damage. American Journal of Physiology - Regulatory, Integrative and Comparative Physiology 2007, 292: R2168-R2173. doi:10.1152/ajpregu.00858.2006
27. Aggarwal BB, Harikumar KB. Potential Therapeutic Effects of Curcumin, the Anti-inflammatory Agent, Against Neurodegenerative, Cardiovascular, Pulmonary, Metabolic, Autoimmune and Neoplastic Diseases. Int J Biochem Cell Biol. 2008;41(1):40–59. doi:10.1016/j.biocel.2008.06.010.
28. Kawanishi N, Kato K, Takahashi M, Mizokami T, Otsuka T, Imaizumi T, et al. Curcumin attenuates oxidative stress following downhill running-induced muscle damage. Biochem Biophys Res Commun. 2013;22:573–8.
29. Akazawa N, Choi Y, Miyakia A, Tanabe Y, Sugawara J, Ajisaka R, et al. Curcumin ingestion and exercise training improve vascular endothelial function in postmenopausal women. Nutr Res. 2012;32(10):795–9. doi:10.1016/j.nutres.2012.09.002.
30. Fischer CP. Interleukin-6 in acute exercise and training: what is the biological relevance? Exerc Immunol Rev. 2006;12:6–33.
31. Rushall BS. A tool for measuring stress tolerance in elite athletes. J Appl Sport Psychol. 1990;2:51–66.
32. Cuomo J, Appendino G, Dern AS, Schneider E, McKinnon TP, Brown MJ, et al. Comparative absorption of a standardized curcuminoid mixture and its lecithin formulation. J Nat Prod. 2011;74:664–9.
33. Hao K, Zhao XP, Liu XQ, Wang GJ. LC determination of curcumin in dog plasma for a pharmacokinetic study. Chromatographia. 2006;64(9/10):531–5.
34. Grubbs FE. Procedures for detecting outlying observations in samples. Technometrics. 1969;11(1):1–21. doi:10.1080/00401706.1969.10490657.
35. Takahashi M, Suzuki K, Kim HK, Otsuka Y, Imaizumi A, Miyashita M, Sakamoto S. Effects of curcumin supplementation on exercise-induced oxidative stress

in humans. Int J Sports Med 2013, Published online. doi:https://dx.doi.org/10.1055/s-0033-1357185

36. Vitadello M, Germinario E, Ravara B, Dalla Libera L, Danieli-Betto D, Gorsza L. Curcumin counteracts loss of force and atrophy of hindlimb unloaded rat soleus by hampering neuronal nitric oxide synthase untethering from sarcolemma. J Physiol. 2014;592:2637–52.

37. Belcaro G, Cesarone MR, Dugall M, Pellegrini L, Ledda A, Grossi MG, et al. Efficacy and safety of Meriva®, a curcumin-phoshatidylcholine complex, during extended administration in osteoarthritis patients. Altern Med Rev. 2008;15(4):337–44.

38. Drobnic F, Riera J, Appendino G, Togni S, Franceschi F, Valle X, et al. Reduction of delayed onset muscle soreness by a novel curcumin delivery system (Meriva®): a randomised, placebo-controlled trial. J Int Soc Sports Nutr. 2014;11:31. doi:10.1186/1550-2783-11-31.

39. Antoine F, Simard J, Girard D. Curcumin inhibits agent-induced human neutrophil functions in vitro and lipopolysaccharide-induced neutrophilic infiltration in vivo. Int Immunopharmacol. 2013;17:1101–7. http://dx.doi.org/10.1016/j.intimp.2013.09.024.

40. Fischer CP, Hiscock NJ, Penkowa M, Basu S, Vessby B, Kallner A, et al. Supplementation with vitamins C and E inhibits the release of interleukin 6 from contracting human skeletal muscle. J Physiol. 2004;558(2):633–45.

41. Starkie RL, Arkinstall MJ, Koukoulas I, Hawley JA, Febbraio MA. Carbohydrate ingestion attenuates the rise in plasma interleukin-6, but not skeletal muscle interleukin-6 mRNA during exercise in humans. J Physiol. 2001;533(2):585–91.

42. Peternelj T, Coombs JS. Antioxidant supplementation during exercise training: beneficial or detrimental? Sports Med. 2011;41(12):1043–69.

13

Amino acid supplementation and impact on immune function in the context of exercise

Vinicius Fernandes Cruzat[1*], Maurício Krause[2] and Philip Newsholme[1*]

Abstract

Moderate and chronic bouts of exercise may lead to positive metabolic, molecular, and morphological adaptations, improving health. Although exercise training stimulates the production of reactive oxygen species (ROS), their overall intracellular concentration may not reach damaging levels due to enhancement of antioxidant responses. However, inadequate exercise training (i.e., single bout of high-intensity or excessive exercise) may result in oxidative stress, muscle fatigue and muscle injury. Moreover, during the recovery period, impaired immunity has been reported, for example; excessive-inflammation and compensatory immunosuppression. Nutritional supplements, sometimes referred to as immuno-nutrients, may be required to reduce immunosuppression and excessive inflammation. Herein, we discuss the action and the possible targets of key immuno-nutrients such as L-glutamine, L-arginine, branched chain amino acids (BCAA) and whey protein.

Keywords: Immunonutrition, L-glutamine, L-arginine, L-leucine, Oxidative stress

Introduction

Elite athletes competing in national and international events are required to engage in multiple strenuous exercise training sessions to improve their performance. Although regular practice and moderate intensity exercise, for the general population, is essential to reduce the risk of chronic inflammatory diseases, athletes engaged in intense, prolonged or exhaustive physical exercise are more susceptible to the adverse effects from high-intensity exercise. Such effects include high rates of protein catabolism, a pro-inflammatory profile, accompanied by muscle damage, soreness, chronic oxidative stress [1] and immune suppression [2,3]. A large number of studies have reported the harmful side effects (overtraining syndrome) and increased upper respiratory tract infection (URTI) promoted by exhaustive physical exercise [2,4,5].

Although a balanced diet with high quality and sufficient quantity of nutrients is essential, there is growing evidence that some non-synthetic supplements can assist optimal nutrition. In fact, the use of nutritional supplements especially the provision of amino acids, has grown year-on-year [6]. There are few articles in the literature to address the topic of nutritional supplementation and immune consequences, from a metabolic and molecular standpoint. The use of proteins and amino acids for supplementation deserves special attention, since these molecules are critical for anti-oxidant and fuel provision, participating in the whole-body energy homeostasis, growth, development, recovery and immune responses. The key targets for immunonutrition may include provision of key metabolites for immune cells *per se*, the inflammatory response and cytokine release, the production of chaperone proteins such as the heat shock proteins (HSPs), redox balance (including glutathione, GSH metabolism), and protection of skeletal muscle mass (Figure 1).

The evolution of immunonutrition

Key considerations that motivate athletes to consume nutritional supplements include: i) to improve their performance, ii) to strengthen immune function and, iii) to minimise the exercise recovery period [7]. The most widely used supplements are vitamins and minerals. Many studies have described the use of proteins, such as whey for supplements or isolated amino acids [8,9]. Although the use of nutritional ergogenic aids in sports is topical, how and which nutrients may impact health and immune defense are interesting to the clinical nutrition field.

* Correspondence: vinifc@usp.br; philip.newsholme@curtin.edu.au
[1]CHIRI Biosciences Research Precinct, Faculty of Health Sciences, School of Biomedical Sciences, Curtin University, GPO Box U1987, Perth, Western Australia, Australia
Full list of author information is available at the end of the article

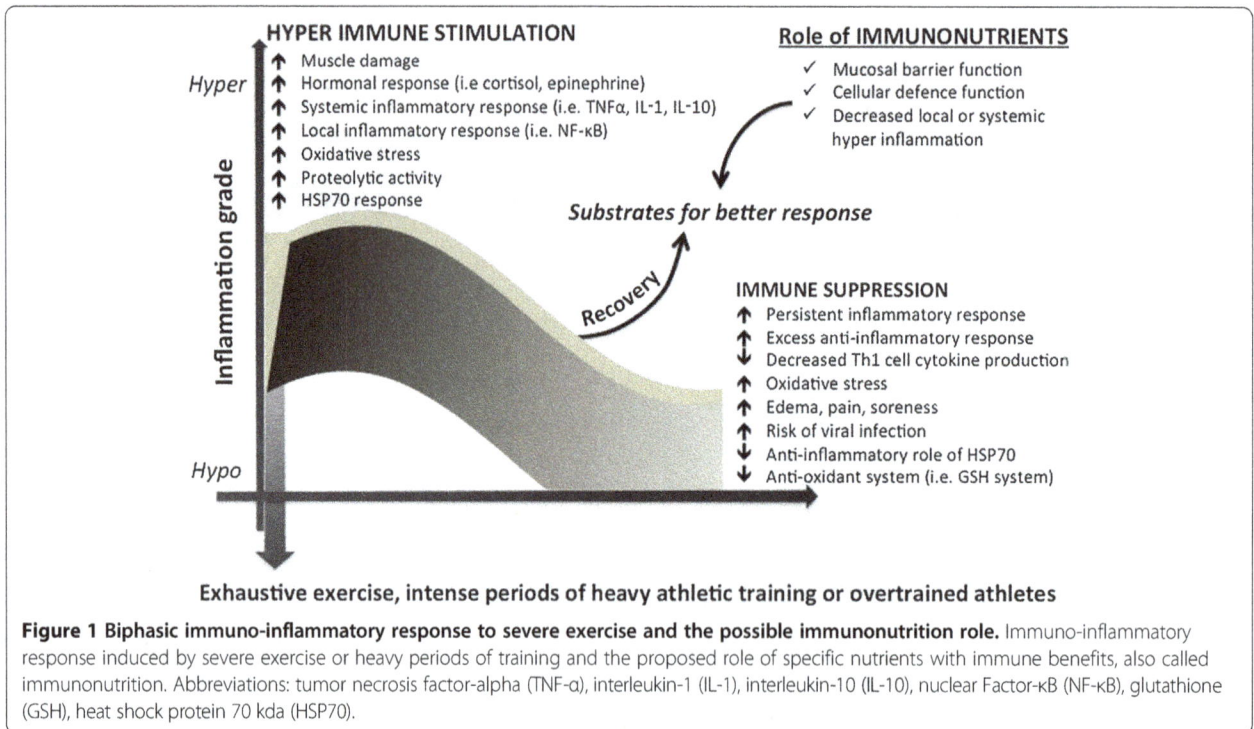

Figure 1 Biphasic immuno-inflammatory response to severe exercise and the possible immunonutrition role. Immuno-inflammatory response induced by severe exercise or heavy periods of training and the proposed role of specific nutrients with immune benefits, also called immunonutrition. Abbreviations: tumor necrosis factor-alpha (TNF-α), interleukin-1 (IL-1), interleukin-10 (IL-10), nuclear Factor-κB (NF-κB), glutathione (GSH), heat shock protein 70 kda (HSP70).

The role of nutritional support for immune function can be traced to 1810, when J. F. Menkel described that malnourished people in England presented with thymus atrophy. Other reports from the early 1900s, describe vitamin intervention studies [10] and reports exist from Ghetto physicians during World War II as to the poor health outcomes due to malnutrition [11]. More recently, positive outcomes related to total parenteral nutrition (TPN) administration, required during intensive medical care, have been described. These developments subsequently resulted in the formulation of products that could potentially modulate immune system activity, described as "immunonutrition" products. These interventions became popular for use with patients after 1990.

Most of the recent studies clearly demonstrate the importance of nutrients for trauma and surgical patients, as well as the frail elderly. Hence, strategies that include specific nutrients for enhanced immune function are frequently used in clinical nutrition therapy (e.g., for patients with burns, sepsis, cancer, HIV) and post-surgical situations using enteral or TPN routes. However, the concept of immunonutrition may be more widely applied, since the specific nutritional substrates for immune response can act on alternative targets, such as the gut mucosal barrier. Since athletes are at increased risk of upper respiratory tract infection (URTI), overtraining syndrome, chronic inflammatory response and oxidative stress [4], during and after periods of heavy exercise [12], immunonutritional approaches may be

considered for future recommendations in the sport science field (Figure 1).

Exercise-induced changes in the immune system: an overview

Changes in cytokine profile

Regular practice of moderate-intensity physical exercise has been shown to efficiently and positively impact physiological imbalances caused by different pathological situations. Exercise has been prescribed as a complementary therapeutic strategy in different modes of immunological dysfunction [13]. It has been clearly demonstrated that exercise induces considerable changes in immune function related to physiological responses to both metabolic and hormonal exercise-related alterations (Figure 1). Most of the exercise responses on the immune system are mediated by hormones such as adrenalin, cortisol, growth hormone (GH), and pro- and anti-inflammatory cytokines. The immunological changes are dependent on exercise intensity, type, and duration. For instance, cytokine production is modulated by a range of physiological stimuli that accompany exercise, such as stress hormones, energy crisis and oxidative stress [14]. In turn, exercise-induced cytokine effects depend on the type of mediator involved and the balance between pro-inflammatory cytokines (IL-1, TNF-α, IFNα, IFNγ, TNF-β, IL-2, IL-12, and MCP-1) and anti-inflammatory ones (IL-4, IL-10, IL-13, IL-12p40, IL-1ra).

During moderate intensity exercise, pro-inflammatory cytokine production is downregulated and anti-inflammatory cytokines, such as IL-1 receptor antagonist (IL-1ra), IL-10 and IL-6, are upregulated [15-17]. Strenuous and prolonged exercise induces increases in circulating TNF-α, IL-1β and IL-6 levels. This is counterbalanced by cytokine inhibitors (IL-1ra, sTNF-r1 and sTNF-r2) and the anti-inflammatory cytokine IL-10 [18]. The magnitude of the changes differs markedly depending on the cytokine being examined. For instance, plasma concentrations of IL-1 and TNF-α increase one-to two fold, whereas IL-6 has been reported to increase over 100-fold after prolonged exercise [18].

A large number of studies have reported increased plasma concentrations of anti-inflammatory cytokines, such as IL-1ra, IL-4 and IL-10, after various forms of exercise including brief maximal exercise [19], resistance exercise [19,20], downhill running [21,22], intense eccentric cycling [23], and endurance running and cycling [19,24,25]. Increased production of anti-inflammatory cytokines during exercise may serve to restrict pro-inflammatory reactions to exercise-induced muscle damage [23] and may also limit the production of pro-inflammatory cytokines associated with the development of ill states [26]. Conversely, increased production of anti-inflammatory cytokines during severe exercise may result in enhanced susceptibility to infections via alteration in the pro- vs. anti-inflammatory cytokine balance favoring an anti-inflammatory response [25].

Importantly, exercise induces robust increases in production and release of IL-6 [27,28] from skeletal muscle. IL-6 then stimulates the appearance, in the circulation, of the anti-inflammatory cytokines IL-1ra and IL-10, and inhibits the production of the pro-inflammatory cytokine TNF-α [18,26]. Hence, moderate exercise may decrease pro-inflammatory cytokine production while increasing anti-inflammatory cytokine production and action, which may induce a very strong anti-inflammatory cytokine response. The main modulator of these responses is likely the appearance of IL-6 in the circulation.

Another immune-regulatory protein that is now receiving considerable attention is HSP72. Studies have demonstrated HSP72 participation in conditions associated with inflammation such as type 1 (T1DM) and type 2 diabetes mellitus (T2DM), aging, and obesity [29-32]. HSP72 can induce different inflammatory responses according to its location (intra vs. extracellular) positioning this protein as a master regulator for the fine-tuned control of the immune system: while iHSP70 has anti-inflammatory effects, eHSP70 induce the opposite. Physical exercise is a very well known inductor of HSP70 expression [30,33,34]. Interestingly, some studies have demonstrated that exercise is a physiological stimulus that promotes an increase in the eHSP70 concentration [35,36]. Both intensity and duration of exercise have effects as determined in plasma [37] and muscle samples [33,34]. The rise in circulating levels of eHSP70 precedes any gene or protein expression changes in HSP70 in skeletal muscle [27,34]. Additionally, acute exercise induces transient changes in the numbers and response of circulating lymphocytes which are considered a major eHSP70 source (nearly 100% of total eHSP70 release from the immune system) [38,39].

Muscle damage, oxidative stress and inflammation

Activation of immune responses and adaptations after an acute exercise bout is related to muscle damage. Skeletal muscle damage that normally occurs after an acute and intense exercise bout is followed by a local inflammatory response that is "dose-dependent" on the intensity and duration of the exercise [40]. Moderate local inflammation is essential for the adaptation of the muscle, bone, and connective tissues [41]. The subsequent inflammation that occurs in response to the muscle damage is induced and intensified by the production of reactive oxygen and nitrogen species (ROS and RNS, respectively). Additionally, several cytokines (most pro-inflammatory), and molecules (histamine, serotonin and prostaglandins) are released, causing edema, pain and further inflammation until resolution and muscle recovery occurs [42-44]. Local inflammatory reactions may be induced during muscle cell apoptosis or necrosis by activated macrophages and by inflammatory cytokines [45].

The sources of ROS in exercise are many, for example, the activation of the superoxide generating NADPH-oxidase from immune cells that infiltrate the damaged area [46]. Elevated metabolism or enhanced mitochondrial activity (i.e. exercise), can continuously subject many tissue specific cells to insult from ROS and RNS. Intracellular O_2^- may combine with NO to generate peroxynitrite, which may cause inhibition of activity of number of key signal transducing or metabolic enzymes [1]. Overproduction of ROS or a failure in intracellular defenses against ROS may stimulate molecular events resulting in disease [1]. There is a direct relation between muscle damage, neutrophil infiltration and ROS generation during the inflammatory process [43]. The free radical production during exercise has an essential role for signal transduction, the induction of cell damage, and for the initiation of the inflammatory response. Although the training results in a reduction of ROS through adaptations of the antioxidant systems, inadequate exercise training may result in changes in the redox status, oxidative stress [34,44], muscle fatigue, and muscle injury [1,47,48]. In addition, during certain types of exercise (especially those involving eccentric contractions), there is a significant release of Fe^{2+} ions that may aggravate the oxidative stress due to chemical reactivity, culminating in muscle fatigue and damage [43].

Several muscle proteins, including actin, myosin, Ca^{2+} and K^+ pumps are sensitive to the redox state, thus changes in ROS or RNS production can directly affect muscle contraction [49]. ROS and RNS can induce rises in intracellular Ca^{2+} (through interaction with Ca^{2+} channels) and also inactivation of several enzymes from anaerobic and aerobic metabolism, leading to muscle fatigue [50]. Since oxidative stress and excessive inflammation are related to the loss of muscle function, several strategies have been used to improve the muscle and immune cell redox status, using nutritional and anti-oxidant interventions [41].

Redox status: the target for immunonutrition?

Additionally to the previously cited redox-sensitive proteins, nuclear factor-κB (NF-κB) is extremely sensitive to the redox status of the cells [51]. This protein is a ubiquitous transcription factor originally discovered in B-lymphocytes, which is essential for inflammatory responses to a variety of signals, immune function, endothelial cell activation, and the control of cell growth. NF-κB is normally located in the cytoplasm in an inactive form bound to an inhibitory IκB protein. A wide variety of inflammatory stimuli (such as excessive ROS and RNS) can utilize specific signal transducing pathways to enable phosphorylation of IκB by IκB kinase (IKK) and thus ensure its proteasomal degradation [52]. IκB degradation will release NF-κB, allowing it to translocate to the nucleus and induce pro-inflammatory gene expression. In this way, our cells have very sensitive and responsive control mechanisms for regulating redox status and thus NF-κB activation, to regulate the optimal level of inflammation. The most important intracellular non-enzymatic antioxidants are GSH and its oxidative form GSSG (oxidized glutathione) [1,53].

GSH (γ-glutamyl-cysteinyl-glycine) is the predominant low-molecular-weight thiol (0.5-10 mmol/L) in animal cells. It is now well accepted that many forms of thiol oxidation (disulphide formation, gluathionylation and S-nitrosylation) are reversible and can provide a mechanism used by skeletal muscle cells in the regulation of metabolic signaling and transcriptional processes, including in muscle adaptation after exercise and training [1,54]. Since the cellular redox state is crucial for several molecular pathways, and glutathione seems to be the key regulator/sensor for redox status, strategies aiming at improving GSH synthesis are now being studied. The synthesis of GSH from glutamate, cysteine, and glycine is catalyzed sequentially by two key cytosolic enzymes, γ-glutamylcysteine synthetase (GCS) and GSH synthetase (Figure 2). GCS is the key regulatory enzyme, activated by several types of stress including oxidative and nitrosative stress, inflammation, heat stress, and others [55]. It is therefore reasonable to speculate that amino acid and protein supplementation, may provide intracellular GSH precursors - an essential strategy to improve GSH synthesis and redox protection, leading also to better control of the inflammatory status and muscle recovery [56].

However, although antioxidant supplementation may at first be considered as beneficial, the consequent reduction of ROS/RNS could actually have negative effects in non-athletes. Muscle redox state may be best improved by providing skeletal muscle cells with the key natural precursors for GSH synthesis and allowing the cells to synthesize what they actually require. Exercise-induced ROS is not detrimental to human health, thus endogenous antioxidants may be sufficient to protect against exercise-induced oxidative damage, however this may not be applicable for elite athletes.

In addition to GSH metabolism, the levels of iHSP72 may also be involved in the control of exercise-induced muscle inflammation and adaptation [57]. Their expression has been shown to be induced by a wide range of stressors such as oxidative stress, thermal stress, hypoxia, viral infection, heavy metal contamination, ischemia, exercise metabolic stress and many others [33,53]. As molecular chaperones, the HSP70 family can interact with other proteins (unfolded, in non-native state and/or stress-denatured conformations) to avoid inappropriately interactions, formation of protein aggregates and degradation of damaged proteins, helping the correct refolding of proteins. Other HSP functions include protein translocation, anti-apoptosis, and also anti-inflammatory response [58]. The anti-inflammatory role of the HSP70 is mediated by its interaction with the proteins involved in the activation of the NF-κB, blocking its translocation to the nucleus and slowing of the inflammatory process [51,58]. Interestingly, specific amino acid supplementation has been shown to induce HSP70 and GSH in many cells, as will be described below.

Immune mediating effects of L-glutamine

L-glutamine is probably the most widely recognized immuno-nutrient since it can be used as an oxidizable fuel, a substrate for nucleotide synthesis, a modulator of intermediary metabolism of amino acids [59,60], HSP expression [33] and a component of GSH-mediated antioxidant defense (Figure 2) [44,61], thus serving as a key substrate for cell survival, maintenance and proliferation. The use of L-glutamine as a nutritional supplement for sport and exercise increased in the 90's, based on several clinical nutritional studies, that found benefits in attenuate the dramatic decrease in plasma and tissues L-glutamine levels [62], as well as immune cell function, including lymphocytes [8,61] and neutrophils [59,63]. Several important publications have described the importance of L-glutamine in clinical nutrition [59,62,64].

Oral L-glutamine supplementation (0.1 g/kg body wt) for athletes appeared to have a beneficial effect by attenuating the exercise-induced decrease in plasma L-glutamine

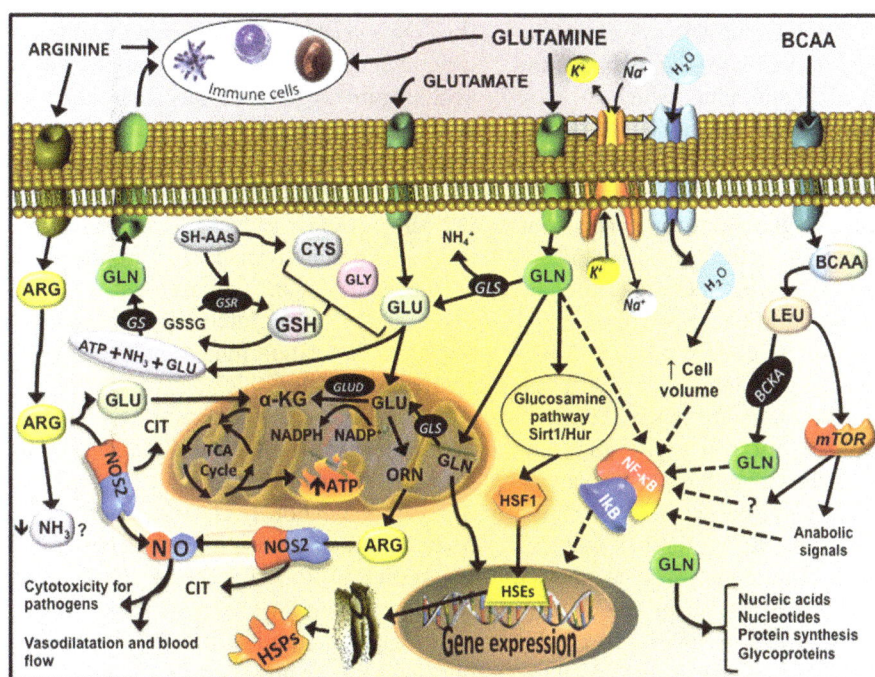

Figure 2 Immune, antioxidant and inflammatory targets that L-glutamine, L-arginine and BCAA are involved. From L-glutamine, glutamate (GLU) is produced through glutaminase activity (GLS), releasing ammonium ion (NH_4^+). Inside of mitochondria or in the cytosol, glutamate from L-glutamine, L-leucine (LEU) or L-arginine (ARG) is an important fuel (ATP) and/or precursor for the synthesis of intermediate metabolism of amino acids such as ornithine (ORN), antioxidant defenses such as glutathione (GSH), anabolic signals through mTOR cascade, and cell repair system such the as the heat shock proteins (HSPs). HSPs are modulated by the heat shock factor 1, which is activated by the glucosamine pathway, sirtuin 1 (Sirt1) and human antigen R (Hur), also known as nutrient sensors. De novo L-glutamine synthesis can occur through L-glutamine synthetase (GS), using glutamate, ATP and ammonia (NH_3). L-glutamine is transported inside the cell trough active transport with sodium (Na^+) potassium (K^+) ATPase, which augment the absorption of water, altering the volume of the cell and stimulate the resistance to damage. L-arginine availability is important to NO production through nitric oxide synthase 2 (NOS2) and citrulline (CIT). Other Abbreviations: heat shock elements (HSEs); oxidized GSH (GSSG); GSH-S reductase (GSR); glutamate dehydrogenase (GLUD); alpha-ketoglutarato (α-KG).

levels [4,65], the decreased number of lymphocytes, and eventually the risk of URTI's [66]. Nevertheless, the efficacy of L-glutamine supplementation has raised many doubts and controversies, as subsequent studies with fixed (20–30 g/day) or variable (0.3 - 0.5 g/kg body wt) doses, or even in association with other macronutrients, such carbohydrates, did not report similar outcomes [12,67,68]. Possibly, for these reasons the last consensus statement in 2011 did not recommend L-glutamine supplements for sports and exercise [69].

The divergences between the clinical and sport nutrition data resulted on the idea that, perhaps, L-glutamine stores within the body cannot be sufficiently depleted by exercise [69]. Although, the evidences that L-glutamine is a direct modulator of the glutathione (antioxidant properties) and HSPs (with chaperone function and inflammatory control) synthesis (Figure 2) deserve some consideration. Furthermore, when L-glutamine is provided by oral or enteral ways in its free form, the amino acid is highly metabolized by the gut, fact that may explain the lower effect in other tissues and circulating cells, such as the immune cells. A possible alternative way is the exogenous administration

of L-glutamine chemically attached to another amino acid (e.g. L-alanine), usually as a dipeptide, such L-alanyl-L-glutamine.

In humans [66] and animal models [70], acute oral L-glutamine supplementation, in its free form or as a dipeptide, is able to increase the plasma L-glutamine concentration between 30 to 120 minutes after ingestion. However, L-glutamine containing dipeptides are highly soluble and stable in solution, often used in enteral nutrition and TPN, and achieve high L-glutamine and L-alanine into the circulation. This effect has been attributed to the glycopeptide transport protein (PepT-1) in the intestinal cells (enterocytes), which have a more efficient transport mechanism for the absorption of dipeptides and tripeptides than for the absorption of free amino acids [71]. In this manner, L-glutamine from dipeptide administration can avoid metabolism by enterocytes, proceeding directly to the systemic circulation [47,72], therefore increasing its availability to immune cells and other tissues [61]. In the dipeptide or in its free form, L-alanine can spare L-glutamine metabolism allowing the latter to be used by high-demand tissues [61].

In vivo studies have shown that L-glutamine supplements (free along with L-alanine and glutamine containing dipeptides) are able to increase the hepatic and muscular concentration of L-glutamine, which in turns increases the tissue concentration of GSH, attenuating the oxidative stress induced by long duration physical exercise [44]. This antioxidant effect is attributed to the supply of L-glutamate from L-glutamine, especially from plasma to immune cells and skeletal muscles [59,60]. When transported inside the cell, L-glutamine simultaneously promotes the uptake of water, an increase in sodium ion Na^+ uptake and the release of potassium ions (K^+), which increase the cell hydration state and volume, which is important in the resistance to injury (Figure 2) [73]. L-glutamine availability increase neutrophil and lymphocyte activity and function [74], for example, generating NADPH for the NADPH oxidase enzyme [63], stimulating intermediary metabolism, and preventing apoptosis by maintaining mitochondrial function [8,74,75]. In fact, L-glutamine supplementation may attenuate muscle damage and inflammation (e.g. levels of TNF-α and PgE$_2$) induced by exhausting exercise [47].

More recently, several studies have reported glutamine-enhanced stimulation of the HSP response induced by acute or chronic inflammation [34,61]. L-glutamine activates intracellular nutrient sensors such as the sirtuins. Specifically sirtuin 1 (SIRT1)/human antigen R (HUR) may be activated through glucosamines [76] leading to activation of the heat shock transcription factor, HSF-1, and the heat shock elements (HSEs) in the nucleus [61], promoting cell survival [76]. SIRT1 acts on many substrates, including histones, forkhead box O (FOXO), NFκB and p53 [77]. Moreover, L-glutamine availability is a limiting step for mTOR complex 1 (mTORC1) activation pathway, a major regulator of cell size and tissue mass in both normal and diseased states [78]. Considering the highly evolutionarily conserved HSF-1-HSP70 response (known as the Stress Response), then the tight integration between metabolic (e.g., intermediary amino acid metabolism) and immune signaling leading to optimal responses against pathogens should not be unexpected. In summary, growing evidence in support of the immune mediating effects of L-glutamine, has resulted in an increase in interest for use in supplementation. More studies in athletes are required to determine optimal supplementation strategies, including the use of dipeptides with and without free amino acids.

L-arginine- NO pathway

Nitric Oxide (NO) plays an important role in many functions in the body regulating vasodilatation and blood flow, inflammation and immune system activation, insulin secretion and sensitivity [79,80], mitochondrial function and neurotransmission. The amino acid L-arginine is the main precursor of NO via nitric oxide synthase (NOS) activity, thus the availability of this amino acid may modulate NO production in conditions of competition for this amino acid (Figure 2) [81]. Dietary L-arginine and L-citrulline supplements may increase levels of NO metabolites. Although the effects of L-arginine supplementation has shown positive effects in many conditions such as diabetes [82] and cardiovascular diseases [83], this response has not been directly related to an improvement in performance related to sport and exercise [84]. Many of the positive aspects of L-arginine supplementation are related to improved circulation (due to increased NO levels) in sedentary individuals.

L-arginine supplementation in exercise training has not resulted in clearly defined outcomes. The high variability seems to be attributed to: i) human *vs.* animal models; ii) healthy *vs.* non-healthy subjects; iii) differences in body composition among subjects; iv) individual training status; v) duration of the supplementation and vi) type of exercise.

Although L-arginine can be produced by the adult human body (synthesized from L-glutamine, glutamate, and proline via the intestinal-renal axis in humans and most other mammals) [85], this amino acid is considered as a "conditionally essential" under conditions such as diabetes, additional ingestion may be required to normalize the plasma levels. L-arginine is a known powerful amino acid-based secretagogue for insulin, growth hormone (GH), glucagon and adrenaline [86]. Since this amino acid plays a critical role in cytoplasmic and nuclear protein synthesis, it has been used and suggested as an inductor of muscle growth and immune protection. L-arginine supplementation is known to increase the levels of both GH and IGF-1 in the blood but reduce IGFBP-3 protein levels [84]. However, most human studies have failed to show that L-arginine can provide improvements in performance in the sport and exercise context [87-90].

An increase in NO may result in improved blood flow and this could potentially be beneficial for individuals engaged in exercise training [90], by increasing nutrient delivery and/or waste-product removal from exercising skeletal muscles [90]. However, L-arginine, NO donors and NOS inhibitors induce effects on blood pressure, heart rate, and blood flow at rest conditions [83], several studies have shown that these agents have no effect on these variables during exercise in humans [83,91]. Even though L-arginine supplementation increases blood flow in basal conditions, the amino acid does not change this variable during exercise. This could indicate that during exercise, other mechanisms of vasodilation in the microcirculation system of active muscles may be involved. There is evidence that vasodilatory prostanoids [92] may be important in determining responses to acetylcholine (Ach) in both diabetic [93] and non-diabetic subjects

[94,95], their effects mediated through an increase in cyclic AMP.

L-arginine supplementation may improve maximal (VO_{2max} test) exercise capacity in patients with cardiovascular disease [92,96]. However, in healthy subjects, L-arginine-α-ketoglutarate did not influence body composition, muscular strength endurance, or aerobic capacity [97]. The finding that L-arginine-α-ketoglutarate supplementation did not improve aerobic capacity supports earlier studies that L-arginine improves VO_{2max} in various disease populations but not in healthy individuals [98]. In addition, L-arginine failed to improve muscular performance and recovery, independently of the training status [90].

Inadequate intake of dietary L-arginine may impair NO synthesis by both constitutive and inducible NOS in mammals [99], indicating a role for L-arginine in immune function. The effects of L-arginine supplementation on lymphocyte count has been reported [100], in a study which determined whether the transient hyperammonemia induced by high-intensity exercise (HI) could influence white blood cell distribution, and whether L-arginine could affect this parameter. Thirty-nine male jiu-jitsu practitioners were submitted to an acute bout of HI exercise using placebo or L-arginine (100 mg·kg-1 of body mass·day-1). Increases in lymphocyte number and ammonia were simultaneously reduced by L-arginine supplementation. Since the authors did not measure the pre-supplementation levels of L-arginine, it is difficult to know if the effect was induced by the higher levels of the amino acid or only by the correction of lower levels among the athletes.

In conclusion, it is clear that L-arginine supplementation improves exercise capacity and blood flow in conditions associated with endothelial dysfunction, such reduced basal NO production. However, in healthy individuals with normal levels of circulating NO, L-arginine supplementation has little or no effect.

Multiple aspects of BCAA

From the nine amino acids nutritionally classified as essentials, three of these compounds are the branched chain amino acids (BCAA; L-valine, L-leucine and L-isoleucine). Mostly protein foods, such as meat, poultry, fish, eggs, milk and cheese can containing on average 15 to 20 grams of BCAA per 100 g of protein [101]. The presence of BCAA in the most primitive organisms that existed before the complex cellular evolution of higher organisms shows the importance this compounds to the metabolic evolution. BCAA are predominantly metabolized in the skeletal muscle, which means that they escape from liver metabolism and, after ingestion; they rapidly increase their concentration in plasma. Although the liver cannot directly metabolize BCAA, this tissue has an active system for the degradation of the α-branched-chain-keto acids (BCKA)

derived from the corresponding BCAA [102] through the branched-chain α-keto acid dehydrogenase (BCKD), which contribute to gluconeogenesis [76].

Oxidative stress may be one of the underlying links between chronic inflammatory response and skeletal muscle wasting [102,103], a fact that may negatively impact on macrophage and neutrophil function [74], as well as on lymphocyte proliferation [3]. Skeletal muscle cells have high activity of BCAA transaminases and L-glutamine synthetase, key enzymes in the synthesis of L-glutamine and other intermediary amino acids [12]. In this regard, when BCAA is present in the culture medium, lymphocyte proliferation capacity is increased; however, this most likely reflects an inability to synthesize sufficient amino acids and protein required for proliferation [104], which reinforces the important role of skeletal muscle in immune regulation. In animal [105] and human studies [106-108] under catabolic situations, such as infection or malnutrition, BCAA are crucial for the maintenance of immune function [104]. However, in catabolic but non-deficient situations, such as in elite athletes involved in heavy endurance or resistance training, the effects of BCAA administration is still not clear. When a large amount of protein is consumed, typically by athletes, an abundance of dietary BCAA will be available for metabolic and immune requirements (high-quality protein sources range from approximately 18-26% BCAA [109]).

In one study, acute and chronic BCAA supplementation (about 6 g/d) to *endurance* athletes resulted in attenuation of the fall in the plasma L-glutamine concentration and also modified the immune suppression promoted by the exercise [107]. Once stimulated through the supplementation of BCAA, cellular L-leucine uptake may enhance the synthesis and availability of L-glutamine by providing glutamate in the intracellular environment. Hence, it is believed that the immune effects of BCAA may be dependent on L-glutamine metabolism in the tissues, such as the skeletal muscle. In fact, in hyper-catabolic situations, such as burning, sepsis and malnutrition, BCAA administration can modulate inflammation through the L-glutamine pathway [110]. However, considering the effects of exercise, this pathway deserves some considerations. When lymphocytes are maintained *in vitro* in a low level of L-glutamine, identical to the lowest plasma L-glutamine concentration measured post-exercise (300 - 400 μM), these cells perform equally well [59] as when L-glutamine is added at a higher concentration similar to the resting plasma level (600 μM) [12]. Consequently, BCAA effects for sports and exercise with regard to immune function, may occur independently of L-glutamine synthesis and stimulation.

Some studies have reported that BCAA administration may attenuate higher inflammatory responses and muscle soreness induced by severe exercise. Prior to resistance squat exercise, BCAA supplementation (100 mg/kg body weight) was able to reduce the delayed-onset muscle soreness (DOMS) [111]. This effect is due to BCAA oxidation in tissues via generation of BCKA's, such α-ketoisocaproate, α-keto-β-methylvalerate and α-ketoisovalerate derived from L-leucine, L-isoleucine and L-valine, respectively, and L-glutamine synthesis. BCAA supply and oxidation can inhibit the activity of pyruvate dehydrogenase, a key regulatory site between glycolysis and the citric acid cycle, a mechanism that favors the deviation of pyruvate to the formation of L-alanine which, after release, acts as a precursor in hepatic gluconeogenesis [112]. In fact, in animal studies, chronic supplementation with BCAA promoted a higher hepatic and muscle glycogen synthesis, even after an exhaustive exercise test [112]. L-leucine improved protein synthesis [105] through mTOR stimulation, hVpS34 and calcium-related proteins (Figure 2) [113], not during but after exercise activity [108]. This effect can limit the excessive activation of NF-κB, attenuating the uncontrolled inflammation and its effects, which include the DOMS.

Another possible protective mechanism of BCAA may be mediated through the antioxidant system. It has been shown that BCAA supplementation increased the expression of genes involved in the antioxidant defense, such superoxide dismutase (SOD) 1 and 2, catalase (CAT) and glutathione peroxidase 1 (GPx1) in trained middle-aged mice. Moreover, the same work reported reductions in oxidative stress in cardiac and skeletal muscle [110]. This led to the idea that redox balance can be a target for the potential benefits promoted by BCAA administration. In fact, BCAA and BCAA along with other sulphur-containing amino acids, such L-taurine, attenuated the DOMS and muscle damage induced by eccentric exercise [114].

The multiple aspects of BCAA, particularly L-leucine has shed light on their possible roles in metabolic disease. Of the BCAA only L-leucine has potent effects upon protein turnover (i.e. stimulates protein synthesis and inhibits protein degradation) via mTOR downstream pathways, thus inadequate ingestion of L-leucine may decrease relative concentrations of L-valine and L-isoleucine. This effect negatively impacts on protein turnover and is called L-leucine paradox, which may be explained by an imbalance of BCAA oxidation in the tricarboxylic acid cycle (TCA) via BCKD complex and anaplerosis reactions. The close relationship between BCAA and its participation in cell bioenergetics and oxidative metabolism may promote an insulinotropic effect in pancreatic β-cells [76]. Conversely, BCAA catabolism is associated with decreased insulin sensitivity in obese patients, fact that corroborates with animal models with excess intake of BCAA and lipids. In this scenario, BCAA catabolism, especially in muscle and liver would result in increased propionyl

and succinyl CoA synthesis, leading to incomplete oxidation of fatty acids. In conclusion, while progress has been made, more studies are needed to establish the crosstalk between lipids and BCAA, as well as BCAA roles in metabolic dysfunctions [115].

Whey proteins as an amino acid source

The constituents of milk have become recognized as functional foods, with direct impact on human health. Milk has two primary 'fractions' of proteins: caseins and whey. Whey is the liquid portion that represents ~ 20% of the total protein content of bovine milk [116]. The advances in food processing, such ultrafiltration and microfiltration have resulted in the development of different whey protein products from dairy plants worldwide. The most well known whey proteins are: concentrate (about 80-95% of protein, with or without lactose), isolate (about 90-95% of protein, normally without carbohydrates), hydrolysed (smaller peptide fractions, reduce immunological reactions, such allergy) and non-denatured (native protein structures) [117]. Furthermore, whey proteins with casein, albumin and/or soy protein, commonly called blend products can be found in retail stores. For more details see Marshall [117] and Luhovyy, Akhavan [118].

Although whey proteins are considered as nutritional supplements, which means extra to the diet, the amino acid composition is very similar to that found in the skeletal muscles, providing almost all of the amino acids in approximate proportion to their ratios [119,120]. Hence, these products are incorporated in the diet and not provided extra to the meal protein composition (e.g. meats plus whey). Accordingly, whey proteins it's more likely a complement, than a supplement. Moreover, the components of whey include beta-lactoglobulin, alpha-lactalbumin, bovine serum albumin, lactoferrin, immunoglobulins (e.g. IgA), lactoperoxidase enzymes, glycomacropeptides, vitamins such as vitamin D, and minerals such as Ca^{2+} [117,121]. Lactoferrin and lactoferricin, demonstrate anti-microbial activity; lysosome, lactoperoxidase and diverse globulins and peptides provide a synergistic protective "cocktail" activity against viral and bacterial organisms [121]. In some chronic diseases with high inflammatory profile and adiposity, whey proteins have been used as adjuvant therapy acting in calcitropic hormones, such parathyroid hormone and 1,25 dihydroxycholecalciferol (1,25 - (OH 2)-D) [121]. Alone or combined with an exercise intervention whey studies demonstrate enhancements in energy loss through faecal fat excretion [122], regulation of glucose homeostasis [123] and adipogenesis [121], resulting in an anti- inflammatory effect (Figure 3) [124].

Whey protein supplements are considered also as a cocktail of amino acids, since they contain up to 26% of BCAA, plus L-arginine, L-lysine, L-glutamine, among others. Thus, the effects of whey protein in the immune

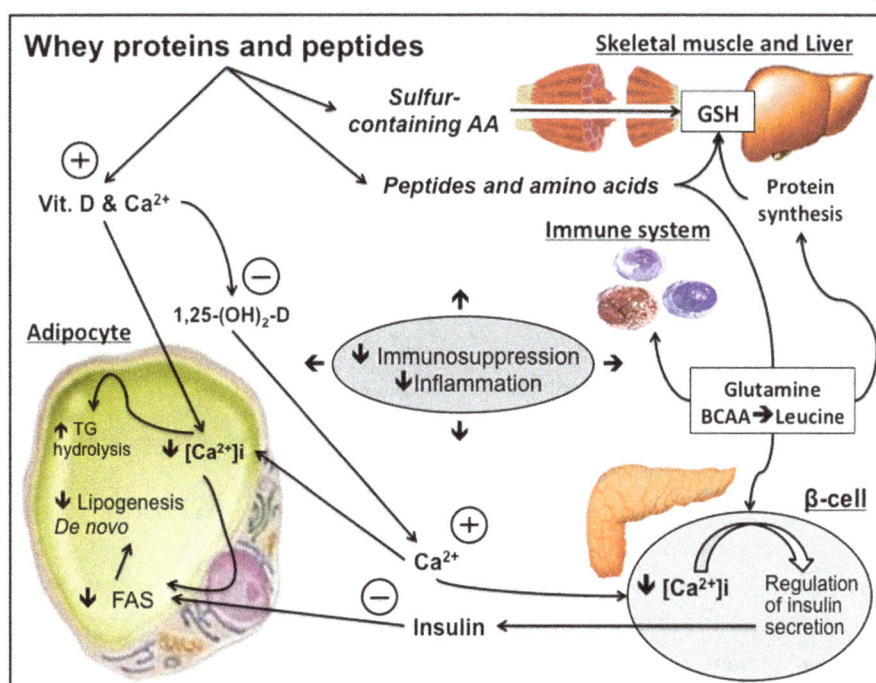

Figure 3 Mechanisms involving whey proteins as a source of different immuno-nutrients. Whey proteins can influence lipid metabolism, muscle protein synthesis/breakdown, antioxidant system, mediated by GSH. Abbreviations: Calcium (Ca^{2+}), 1,25 Hydroxycholecalciferol (1,25-$(OH)_2$-D), intracellular Calcium concentration ($[Ca^{2+}]i$), Fatty Acid Synthase (FAS), Triacylglycerols (TGs).

system may represent the effect of particular amino acids *per se*. Moreover, whey proteins are rapidly digested and absorbed, resulting postprandial muscle protein synthesis [125,126]. Several studies observed changes in muscle growth and performance increments with the chronic ingestion of whey protein supplements [121,127,128]. In one study, triathletes subjected to exhaustive exercise, exhibited a decreased mitochondrial transmembrane potential in both lymphocytes and neutrophils, which leads to apoptotic death and DNA fragmentation [8]. When whey protein enriched with L-glutamine is supplemented, this scenario is reversed, especially in lymphocytes [8], essential for the response against viral infections, such as URTI. On the other hand, the rapid absorption of whey products from the gut, and the hyperaminoacidemia is not the only critical characteristic for maximizing muscle protein synthesis. The time that amino acids are maintained in plasma is also important for the muscle protein turnover, providing gains in muscle mass. There are few studies comparing protein mixtures. Reidy, Walker [129] showed that a blend of whey and soy protein prolonged the elevation in blood amino acid levels after ingestion, when compared to whey protein alone, promoting a greater total muscle protein synthesis measured by the protein fractional synthetic rate (FSR). This is in agreement with other works, which found higher nitrogen retention, and less oxidation with whey blends combined with slowly digested

protein, such as casein [130]. Stimulating post-exercise muscle protein synthesis and amino acid concentration maintenance, may also contribute to immune function however, more studies are needed.

The amino acid profile of whey protein supplements also includes sulphur-containing amino acids, such cysteine and taurine [121]. The high proportion of amino donors of sulfhydryl groups may attenuate the reduction of intracellular GSH concentration induced by intensive exercise [128]. Since immune cells, such as lymphocytes can be sensitive to a range of intracellular sulfhydryl compounds, such GSH and cysteine (Figure 2), whey supplementation may not only attenuate the oxidative stress induced by exercise but also help the maintenance of the redox status in immune cells. Experimental evidence support this mechanistic effect [117]. In a recent study, it was observed that the fall in the GHS content, in trained subjects submitted to an intense exercise program (4 weeks), have occurred in parallel with a decline in lymphocytes number. However, this scenario was reversed by N-acetyl-cysteine supplementation [131]. Furthermore, whey protein can act as an immune modulator through other mechanisms, such as L-glutamine, which is critical for the L-glutamine-GSH axis (Figure 3). Collectively, whey proteins via provision of an amino acid cocktail, exert per se an immune function through redox regulations pathways, and this seems particularly important in individuals engaged in intense and exhaustive exercise training programs, such elite athletes.

Conclusion

Immunonutrition for clinical applications to sports activities represents an emerging area for health, especially regarding supply of proteins and amino acids, since they are required for the optimal synthesis and concentration of a variety of immune related proteins (including cytokines and antibodies). Amino acids will feed into and impact on the regulation of key metabolic pathways in immune cells and the cellular oxidative stress response. At the anti-inflammatory molecular level, new findings have been reported such as enhancement of HSP levels, NO synthesis, and GSH/GSSG regulation, all essential for optimal immune function and recovery from intense periods of training.

Competing interest
The authors declare that they have no competing interest.

Authors' contribution
This review was designed by VFC; manuscript preparation and written were undertaken by VFC, MK and PN; figures preparation were made by VFC; supervision of the manuscript was made by PN and MK. All authors approved the final version of the paper.

Acknowledgments
The authors thank the School of Biomedical Sciences, Curtin University, Perth, Western Australia for provision of excellent research facilities and the Brazilian National Council for Scientific and Technological Development (CNPq - Science Without Borders Programme, process 245562/2012-5).

Author details
[1]CHIRI Biosciences Research Precinct, Faculty of Health Sciences, School of Biomedical Sciences, Curtin University, GPO Box U1987, Perth, Western Australia, Australia. [2]Laboratory of Cellular Physiology, Department of Physiology, Institute of Basic Health Sciences, Federal University of Rio Grande do Sul, Porto Alegre, RS, Brazil.

References
1. Finaud J, Lac G, Filaire E: Oxidative stress: relationship with exercise and training. *Sports Med* 2006, **36**:327–358.
2. Gleeson M: Immune function in sport and exercise. *J Appl Physiol* 2007, **103**:693–699.
3. Tanskanen M, Atalay M, Uusitalo A: Altered oxidative stress in overtrained athletes. *J Sports Sci* 2010, **28**:309–317.
4. Gleeson M, Nieman DC, Pedersen BK: Exercise, nutrition and immune function. *J Sports Sci* 2004, **22**:115–125.
5. Kreher JB, Schwartz JB: Overtraining syndrome: a practical guide. *Sports Health* 2012, **4**:128–138.
6. Zelig R, Rigassio Radler D: Understanding the properties of common dietary supplements: clinical implications for healthcare practitioners. *Nutr Clin Pract* 2012, **27**:767–776.
7. Nieper A: Nutritional supplement practices in UK junior National track and field athletes. *Br J Sports Med* 2005, **39**:645–649.
8. Cury-Boaventura MF, Levada-Pires AC, Folador A, Gorjao R, Alba-Loureiro TC, Hirabara SM, Peres FP, Silva PR, Curi R, Pithon-Curi TC: Effects of exercise on leukocyte death: prevention by hydrolyzed whey protein enriched with glutamine dipeptide. *Eur J Appl Physiol* 2008, **103**:289–294.
9. Nogiec CD, Kasif S: To supplement or not to supplement: a metabolic network framework for human nutritional supplements. *PLoS One* 2013, **8**:e68751.
10. Crook EM, Hopkins FG: Further observations on the system ascorbic acid-glutathione-ascorbic acid-oxidase. *Biochem J* 1938, **32**:1356–1363.
11. Satyaraj E: Emerging paradigms in immunonutrition. *Top Companion Anim Med* 2011, **26**:25–32.
12. Hiscock N, Pedersen BK: Exercise-induced immunodepression– plasma glutamine is not the link. *J Appl Physiol* 2002, **93**:813–822.
13. Costa Rosa LF: Exercise as a time-conditioning effector in chronic disease: a complementary treatment strategy. *Evid Based Complement Alternat Med* 2004, **1**:63–70.
14. Cannon JG: Inflammatory cytokines in nonpathological States. *News Physiol Sci* 2000, **15**:298–303.
15. Drenth JP, Van Uum SH, Van Deuren M, Pesman GJ, Van der Ven-Jongekrijg J, Van der Meer JW: Endurance run increases circulating IL-6 and IL-1ra but downregulates ex vivo TNF-alpha and IL-1 beta production. *J Appl Physiol* 1995, **79**:1497–1503.
16. Nieman DC, Pedersen BK: Exercise and immune function. Recent developments. *Sports Med* 1999, **27**:73–80.
17. Rohde TMD, Richter EA, Kiens B, Pedersen BK: Prolonged submaximal eccentric exercise is associated with increased levels of plasma IL-6. *Am J Physiol* 1997, **273**:E85–E91.
18. Ostrowski K, Rohde T, Asp S, Schjerling P, Pedersen BK: Pro- and anti-inflammatory cytokine balance in strenuous exercise in humans. *J Physiol* 1999, **515**(Pt 1):287–291.
19. Brenner IK, Natale VM, Vasiliou P, Moldoveanu AI, Shek PN, Shephard RJ: Impact of three different types of exercise on components of the inflammatory response. *Eur J Appl Physiol Occup Physiol* 1999, **80**:452–460.
20. Smith LL, Anwar A, Fragen M, Rananto C, Johnson R, Holbert D: Cytokines and cell adhesion molecules associated with high-intensity eccentric exercise. *Eur J Appl Physiol* 2000, **82**:61–67.
21. Malm C: Exercise immunology: the current state of man and mouse. *Sports Med* 2004, **34**:555–566.
22. Petersen EW, Ostrowski K, Ibfelt T, Richelle M, Offord E, Halkjaer-Kristensen J, Pedersen BK: Effect of vitamin supplementation on cytokine response and on muscle damage after strenuous exercise. *Am J Physiol Cell Physiol* 2001, **280**:C1570–C1575.
23. Toft AD, Jensen LB, Bruunsgaard H, Ibfelt T, Halkjaer-Kristensen J, Febbraio M, Pedersen BK: Cytokine response to eccentric exercise in young and elderly humans. *Am J Physiol Cell Physiol* 2002, **283**:C289–C295.
24. Nieman DC, Henson DA, McAnulty SR, McAnulty LS, Morrow JD, Ahmed A, Heward CB: Vitamin E and immunity after the Kona Triathlon World Championship. *Med Sci Sports Exerc* 2004, **36**:1328–1335.
25. Suzuki K, Nakaji S, Kurakake S, Totsuka M, Sato K, Kuriyama T, Fujimoto H, Shibusawa K, Machida K, Sugawara K: Exhaustive exercise and type-1/type-2 cytokine balance with special focus on interleukin-12 p40/p70. *Exerc Immunol Rev* 2003, **9**:48–57.
26. Petersen AM, Pedersen BK: The anti-inflammatory effect of exercise. *J Appl Physiol* 2005, **98**:1154–1162.
27. Febbraio MA, Steensberg A, Walsh R, Koukoulas I, van Hall G, Saltin B, Pedersen BK: Reduced glycogen availability is associated with an elevation in HSP72 in contracting human skeletal muscle. *J Physiol* 2002, **538**:911–917.
28. Pedersen BK, Steensberg A, Schjerling P: Muscle-derived interleukin-6: possible biological effects. *J Physiol* 2001, **536**:329–337.
29. Krause M, Keane K, Rodrigues-Krause J, Crognale D, Egan B, De Vito G, Murphy C, Newsholme P: Elevated levels of extracellular heat-shock protein 72 (eHSP72) are positively correlated with insulin resistance in vivo and cause pancreatic beta-cell dysfunction and death in vitro. *Clin Sci* 2014, **126**:739–752.
30. Krause M, Rodrigues-Krause Jda C: Extracellular heat shock proteins (eHSP70) in exercise: possible targets outside the immune system and their role for neurodegenerative disorders treatment. *Med Hypotheses* 2011, **76**:286–290.
31. Hooper PL, Balogh G, Rivas E, Kavanagh K, Vigh L: The importance of the cellular stress response in the pathogenesis and treatment of type 2 diabetes. *Cell Stress Chaperones* 2014, **19**(4):447–464.
32. Krause Mda S, de Bittencourt PI Jr: Type 1 diabetes: can exercise impair the autoimmune event? The L-arginine/glutamine coupling hypothesis. *Cell Biochem Funct* 2008, **26**:406–433.
33. Heck TG, Scholer CM, de Bittencourt PI: HSP70 expression: does it a novel fatigue signalling factor from immune system to the brain? *Cell Biochem Funct* 2011, **29**:215–226.

34. Petry ER, Cruzat VF, Heck TG, Leite JS, Homem de Bittencourt PI Jr, Tirapegui J: Alanyl-glutamine and glutamine plus alanine supplements improve skeletal redox status in trained rats: involvement of heat shock protein pathways. Life Sci 2014, 94:130–136.

35. Ziemann E, Zembron-Lacny A, Kasperska A, Antosiewicz J, Grzywacz T, Garsztka T, Laskowski R: Exercise training-induced changes in inflammatory mediators and heat shock proteins in young tennis players. J Sports Sci Med 2013, 12:282–289.

36. Gibson OR, Dennis A, Parfitt T, Taylor L, Watt PW, Maxwell NS: Extracellular Hsp72 concentration relates to a minimum endogenous criteria during acute exercise-heat exposure. Cell Stress Chaperones 2014, 19:389–400.

37. Fehrenbach E, Niess AM, Voelker K, Northoff H, Mooren FC: Exercise intensity and duration affect blood soluble HSP72. Int J Sports Med 2005, 26:552–557.

38. Hunter-Lavin C, Davies EL, Bacelar MM, Marshall MJ, Andrew SM, Williams JH: Hsp70 release from peripheral blood mononuclear cells. Biochem Biophys Res Commun 2004, 324:511–517.

39. Ireland HE, Leoni F, Altaie O, Birch CS, Coleman RC, Hunter-Lavin C, Williams JH: Measuring the secretion of heat shock proteins from cells. Methods 2007, 43:176–183.

40. Sorichter S, Koller A, Haid C, Wicke K, Judmaier W, Werner P, Raas E: Light concentric exercise and heavy eccentric muscle loading: effects on CK, MRI and markers of inflammation. Int J Sports Med 1995, 16:288–295.

41. Bryer SC, Goldfarb AH: Effect of high dose vitamin C supplementation on muscle soreness, damage, function, and oxidative stress to eccentric exercise. Int J Sport Nutr Exerc Metab 2006, 16:270–280.

42. Peake JM, Nosaka K, Muthalib M, Suzuki K: Systemic inflammatory responses to maximal versus submaximal lengthening contractions of the elbow flexors. Exerc Immunol Rev 2006, 12:72–85.

43. Niess AM, Simon P: Response and adaptation of skeletal muscle to exercise-the role of reactive oxygen species. Front Biosci 2007, 12:4826–4838.

44. Cruzat VF, Tirapegui J: Effects of oral supplementation with glutamine and alanyl-glutamine on glutamine, glutamate, and glutathione status in trained rats and subjected to long-duration exercise. Nutrition 2009, 25:428–435.

45. Pedersen BKOK, Rohde T, Bruunsgaard H: The cytokine response to strenuous exercise. Can J Physiol Pharmacol 1998, 76:505–511.

46. Rodrigues-Krause J, Krause M, Cunha Gdos S, Perin D, Martins JB, Alberton CL, Schaun MI, De Bittencourt PI Jr, Reischak-Oliveira A: Ballet dancers cardiorespiratory, oxidative and muscle damage responses to classes and rehearsals. Eur J Sport Sci 2014, 14:199–208.

47. Cruzat VF, Rogero MM, Tirapegui J: Effects of supplementation with free glutamine and the dipeptide alanyl-glutamine on parameters of muscle damage and inflammation in rats submitted to prolonged exercise. Cell Biochem Funct 2010, 28:24–30.

48. Palazzetti S, Richard MJ, Favier A, Margaritis I: Overloaded training increases exercise-induced oxidative stress and damage. Can J Appl Physiol 2003, 28:588–604.

49. Reid MB: Free radicals and muscle fatigue: of ROS, canaries, and the IOC. Free Radic Biol Med 2008, 44:169–179.

50. Duhamel TA, Green HJ, Perco JG, Ouyang J: Metabolic and sarcoplasmic reticulum Ca2+ cycling responses in human muscle 4 days following prolonged exercise. Can J Physiol Pharmacol 2005, 83:643–655.

51. Silveira EM, Rodrigues MF, Krause MS, Vianna DR, Almeida BS, Rossato JS, Oliveira LP Jr, Curi R, de Bittencourt PI Jr: Acute exercise stimulates macrophage function: possible role of NF-kappaB pathways. Cell Biochem Funct 2007, 25:63–73.

52. Pillon NJ, Bilan PJ, Fink LN, Klip A: Cross-talk between skeletal muscle and immune cells: muscle-derived mediators and metabolic implications. Am J Physiol Endocrinol Metab 2013, 304:E453–E465.

53. Krause MS, Oliveira LP Jr, Silveira EM, Vianna DR, Rossato JS, Almeida BS, Rodrigues MF, Fernandes AJ, Costa JA, Curi R, De Bittencourt PI Jr: MRP1/GS-X pump ATPase expression: is this the explanation for the cytoprotection of the heart against oxidative stress-induced redox imbalance in comparison to skeletal muscle cells? Cell Biochem Funct 2007, 25:23–32.

54. Ji LL: Modulation of skeletal muscle antioxidant defense by exercise: Role of redox signaling. Free Radic Biol Med 2008, 44:142–152.

55. Wu G, Fang YZ, Yang S, Lupton JR, Turner ND: Glutathione metabolism and its implications for health. J Nutr 2004, 134:489–492.

56. Newsholme P, Krause M, Newsholme EA, Stear SJ, Burke LM, Castell LM: BJSM reviews: A to Z of nutritional supplements: dietary supplements, sports nutrition foods and ergogenic aids for health and performance–part 18. Br J Sports Med 2011, 45:230–232.

57. Rodrigues-Krause J, Krause M, O'Hagan C, De Vito G, Boreham C, Murphy C, Newsholme P, Colleran G: Divergence of intracellular and extracellular HSP72 in type 2 diabetes: does fat matter? Cell Stress Chaperones 2012, 17:293–302.

58. Homem de Bittencourt PI Jr, Lagranha DJ, Maslinkiewicz A, Senna SM, Tavares AM, Baldissera LP, Janner DR, Peralta JS, Bock PM, Gutierrez LL, Scola G, Heck TG, Krause MS, Cruz LA, Abdalla DS, Lagranha CJ, Lima T, Curi R: LipoCardium: endothelium-directed cyclopentenone prostaglandin-based liposome formulation that completely reverses atherosclerotic lesions. Atherosclerosis 2007, 193:245–258.

59. Newsholme P: Why is L-glutamine metabolism important to cells of the immune system in health, postinjury, surgery or infection? J Nutr 2001, 131:2515S–2522S. discussion 2523S-2514S.

60. Curi R, Newsholme P, Procopio J, Lagranha C, Gorjao R, Pithon-Curi TC: Glutamine, gene expression, and cell function. Front Biosci 2007, 12:344–357.

61. Cruzat VF, Pantaleao LC, Donato J Jr, de Bittencourt PI Jr, Tirapegui J: Oral supplementations with free and dipeptide forms of L-glutamine in endotoxemic mice: effects on muscle glutamine-glutathione axis and heat shock proteins. J Nutr Biochem 2014, 25:345–352.

62. Wernerman J: Clinical use of glutamine supplementation. J Nutr 2008, 138:2040S–2044S.

63. Pithon-Curi TC, Schumacher RI, Freitas JJ, Lagranha C, Newsholme P, Palanch AC, Doi SQ, Curi R: Glutamine delays spontaneous apoptosis in neutrophils. Am J Physiol Cell Physiol 2003, 284:C1355–C1361.

64. Roth E: Nonnutritive effects of glutamine. J Nutr 2008, 138:2025S–2031S.

65. Hiscock N, Petersen EW, Krzywkowski K, Boza J, Halkjaer-Kristensen J, Pedersen BK: Glutamine supplementation further enhances exercise-induced plasma IL-6. J Appl Physiol 2003, 95:145–148.

66. Castell LM, Newsholme EA: The effects of oral glutamine supplementation on athletes after prolonged, exhaustive exercise. Nutrition 1997, 13:738–742.

67. Castell LM, Poortmans JR, Leclercq R, Brasseur M, Duchateau J, Newsholme EA: Some aspects of the acute phase response after a marathon race, and the effects of glutamine supplementation. Eur J Appl Physiol Occup Physiol 1997, 75:47–53.

68. Krzywkowski K, Petersen EW, Ostrowski K, Kristensen JH, Boza J, Pedersen BK: Effect of glutamine supplementation on exercise-induced changes in lymphocyte function. Am J Physiol Cell Physiol 2001, 281:C1259–C1265.

69. Walsh NP, Gleeson M, Pyne DB, Nieman DC, Dhabhar FS, Shephard RJ, Oliver SJ, Bermon S, Kajeniene A: Position statement. Part two: maintaining immune health. Exerc Immunol Rev 2011, 17:64–103.

70. Rogero MM, Tirapegui J, Pedrosa RG, Pires ISD, de Castro IA: Plasma and tissue glutamine response to acute and chronic supplementation with L-glutamine and L-alanyl-L-glutamine in rats. Nutr Res 2004, 24:261–270.

71. Nässl A-M, Rubio-Aliaga I, Fenselau H, Marth MK, Kottra G, Daniel H: Amino acid absorption and homeostasis in mice lacking the intestinal peptide transporter PEPT1. Am J Physiol Gastrointest Liver Physiol 2011, 301:G128–G137.

72. Rogero MM, Tirapegui J, Pedrosa RG, de Castro IA, Pires ISD: Effect of alanyl-glutamine supplementation on plasma and tissue glutamine concentrations in rats submitted to exhaustive exercise. Nutrition 2006, 22:564–571.

73. Usher-Smith JA, Huang CLH, Fraser JA: Control of cell volume in skeletal muscle. Biol Rev Camb Philos Soc 2009, 84:143–159.

74. Pithon-Curi TC, Trezena AG, Tavares-Lima W, Curi R: Evidence that glutamine is involved in neutrophil function. Cell Biochem Funct 2002, 20:81–86.

75. Cury-Boaventura MF, Peres FP, Levada-Pires AC, Silva PRS, Curi R, Pithon-Curi TC: Effect of supplementation with hydrolyzed whey protein enriched with glutamine dipeptide on performance of triathletes. Med Sci Sport Exer 2008, 40:S102–S103.

76. Newsholme P, Cruzat V, Arfuso F, Keane K: Nutrient regulation of insulin secretion and action. J Endocrinol 2014, 221:R105–R120.

77. Kotas ME, Gorecki MC, Gillum MP: Sirtuin-1 is a nutrient-dependent modulator of inflammation. Adipocyte 2013, 2:113–118.

78. Nicklin P, Bergman P, Zhang B, Triantafellow E, Wang H, Nyfeler B, Yang H, Hild M, Kung C, Wilson C, Myer VE, MacKeigan JP, Porter JA, Wang YK, Cantley LC, Finan PM, Murphy LO: Bidirectional transport of amino acids regulates mTOR and autophagy. Cell 2009, 136:521–534.

79. Krause M, Rodrigues-Krause J, O'Hagan C, De Vito G, Boreham C, Susta D, Newsholme P, Murphy C: Differential nitric oxide levels in the blood and skeletal muscle of type 2 diabetic subjects may be consequence of adiposity: a preliminary study. *Metabolism* 2012, **61**:1528–1537.

80. Krause MS, McClenaghan NH, Flatt PR, de Bittencourt PI, Murphy C, Newsholme P: L-arginine is essential for pancreatic beta-cell functional integrity, metabolism and defense from inflammatory challenge. *J Endocrinol* 2011, **211**:87–97.

81. Newsholme P, Homem De Bittencourt PI, OH C, De Vito G, Murphy C, Krause MS: Exercise and possible molecular mechanisms of protection from vascular disease and diabetes: the central role of ROS and nitric oxide. *Clin Sci (Lond)* 2009, **118**:341–349.

82. Lucotti P, Setola E, Monti LD, Galluccio E, Costa S, Sandoli EP, Fermo I, Rabaiotti G, Gatti R, Piatti P: Beneficial effects of a long-term oral L-arginine treatment added to a hypocaloric diet and exercise training program in obese, insulin-resistant type 2 diabetic patients. *Am J Physiol Endocrinol Metab* 2006, **291**:E906–E912.

83. Fayh AP, Krause M, Rodrigues-Krause J, Ribeiro JL, Ribeiro JP, Friedman R, Moreira JC, Reischak-Oliveira A: Effects of L-arginine supplementation on blood flow, oxidative stress status and exercise responses in young adults with uncomplicated type I diabetes. *Eur J Nutr* 2013, **52**:975–983.

84. Zajac A, Poprzecki S, Zebrowska A, Chalimoniuk M, Langfort J: Arginine and ornithine supplementation increases growth hormone and insulin-like growth factor-1 serum levels after heavy-resistance exercise in strength-trained athletes. *J Strength Cond Res* 2010, **24**:1082–1090.

85. Newsholme P, Stenson L, Sulvucci M, Sumayao R, Krause M: *Amino Acid Metabolism*. Secondth edition. Elsevier; 2011.

86. McConell GK: Effects of L-arginine supplementation on exercise metabolism. *Curr Opin Clin Nutr Metab Care* 2007, **10**:46–51.

87. Alvares TS, Conte CA, Paschoalin VM, Silva JT, Meirelles Cde M, Bhambhani YN, Gomes PS: Acute l-arginine supplementation increases muscle blood volume but not strength performance. *Appl Physiol Nutr Metab* 2012, **37**:115–126.

88. Greer BK, Jones BT: Acute arginine supplementation fails to improve muscle endurance or affect blood pressure responses to resistance training. *J Strength Cond Res* 2011, **25**:1789–1794.

89. Tang JE, Lysecki PJ, Manolakos JJ, MacDonald MJ, Tarnopolsky MA, Phillips SM: Bolus arginine supplementation affects neither muscle blood flow nor muscle protein synthesis in young men at rest or after resistance exercise. *J Nutr* 2011, **141**:195–200.

90. Wax B, Kavazis AN, Webb HE, Brown SP: Acute L-arginine alpha ketoglutarate supplementation fails to improve muscular performance in resistance trained and untrained men. *J Int Soc Sports Nutr* 2012, **9**:17.

91. Bradley SJ, Kingwell BA, McConell GK: Nitric oxide synthase inhibition reduces leg glucose uptake but not blood flow during dynamic exercise in humans. *Diabetes* 1999, **48**:1815–1821.

92. Cheng JW, Baldwin SN: L-arginine in the management of cardiovascular diseases. *Ann Pharmacother* 2001, **35**:755–764.

93. Poston L, Taylor PD: Glaxo/MRS Young Investigator Prize. Endothelium-mediated vascular function in insulin-dependent diabetes mellitus. *Clin Sci (Lond)* 1995, **88**:245–255.

94. Kilbom A, Wennmalm A: Endogenous prostaglandins as local regulators of blood flow in man: effect of indomethacin on reactive and functional hyperaemia. *J Physiol* 1976, **257**:109–121.

95. Cowley AJ, Stainer K, Rowley JM, Wilcox RG: Effect of aspirin and indomethacin on exercise-induced changes in blood pressure and limb blood flow in normal volunteers. *Cardiovasc Res* 1985, **19**:177–180.

96. Nagaya N, Uematsu M, Oya H, Sato N, Sakamaki F, Kyotani S, Ueno K, Nakanishi N, Yamagishi M, Miyatake K: Short-term oral administration of L-arginine improves hemodynamics and exercise capacity in patients with precapillary pulmonary hypertension. *Am J Respir Crit Care Med* 2001, **163**:887–891.

97. Campbell B, Roberts M, Kerksick C, Wilborn C, Marcello B, Taylor L, Nassar E, Leutholtz B, Bowden R, Rasmussen C, Greenwood M, Kreider R: Pharmacokinetics, safety, and effects on exercise performance of L-arginine alpha-ketoglutarate in trained adult men. *Nutrition* 2006, **22**:872–881.

98. Abel T, Knechtle B, Perret C, Eser P, von Arx P, Knecht H: Influence of chronic supplementation of arginine aspartate in endurance athletes on performance and substrate metabolism - a randomized, double-blind, placebo-controlled study. *Int J Sports Med* 2005, **26**:344–349.

99. Flynn NE, Meininger CJ, Haynes TE, Wu G: The metabolic basis of arginine nutrition and pharmacotherapy. *Biomed Pharmacother* 2002, **56**:427–438.

100. Goncalves LC, Bessa A, Freitas-Dias R, Luzes R, Werneck-de-Castro JP, Bassini A, Cameron LC: A sportomics strategy to analyze the ability of arginine to modulate both ammonia and lymphocyte levels in blood after high-intensity exercise. *J Int Soc Sports Nutr* 2012, **9**:30.

101. Burke LM, Castell LM, Stear SJ, Rogers PJ, Blomstrand E, Gurr S, Mitchell N, Stephens FB, Greenhaff PL: A-Z of nutritional supplements: dietary supplements, sports nutrition foods and ergogenic aids for health and performance Part 4. *Br J Sports Med* 2009, **43**:1088–1090.

102. Nicastro H, da Luz CR, Chaves DF, Bechara LR, Voltarelli VA, Rogero MM, Lancha AH Jr: Does branched-chain amino acids supplementation modulate skeletal muscle remodeling through inflammation modulation? Possible mechanisms of action. *J Nutr Metab* 2012, **2012**:136937.

103. Tisdale MJ: Is there a common mechanism linking muscle wasting in various disease types? *Curr Opin Support Palliat Care* 2007, **1**:287–292.

104. Li P, Yin YL, Li D, Kim SW, Wu G: Amino acids and immune function. *Br J Nutr* 2007, **98**:237–252.

105. Donato J Jr, Pedrosa RG, Cruzat VF, Pires IS, Tirapegui J: Effects of leucine supplementation on the body composition and protein status of rats submitted to food restriction. *Nutrition* 2006, **22**:520–527.

106. Frexes-Steed M, Lacy DB, Collins J, Abumrad NN: Role of leucine and other amino acids in regulating protein metabolism in vivo. *Am J Physiol* 1992, **262**:E925–E935.

107. Bassit RA, Sawada LA, Bacurau RF, Navarro F, Martins E Jr, Santos RV, Caperuto EC, Rogeri P, Costa Rosa LF: Branched-chain amino acid supplementation and the immune response of long-distance athletes. *Nutrition* 2002, **18**:376–379.

108. Blomstrand E, Saltin B: BCAA intake affects protein metabolism in muscle after but not during exercise in humans. *Am J Physiol Endocrinol Metab* 2001, **281**:E365–E374.

109. Phillips SM: Dietary protein requirements and adaptive advantages in athletes. *Br J Nutr* 2012, **108**(Suppl 2):S158–S167.

110. D'Antona G, Ragni M, Cardile A, Tedesco L, Dossena M, Bruttini F, Caliaro F, Corsetti G, Bottinelli R, Carruba MO, Valerio A, Nisoli E: Branched-chain amino acid supplementation promotes survival and supports cardiac and skeletal muscle mitochondrial biogenesis in middle-aged mice. *Cell Metab* 2010, **12**:362–372.

111. Shimomura Y, Inaguma A, Watanabe S, Yamamoto Y, Muramatsu Y, Bajotto G, Sato J, Shimomura N, Kobayashi H, Mawatari K: Branched-chain amino acid supplementation before squat exercise and delayed-onset muscle soreness. *Int J Sport Nutr Exerc Metab* 2010, **20**:236–244.

112. de Araujo JA, Falavigna G, Rogero MM, Pires ISO, Pedrosa RG, Castro IA, Donato J, Tirapegui J: Effect of chronic supplementation with branched-chain amino acids on the performance and hepatic and muscle glycogen content in trained rats. *Life Sci* 2006, **79**:1343–1348.

113. Gulati P, Gaspers LD, Dann SG, Joaquin M, Nobukuni T, Natt F, Kozma SC, Thomas AP, Thomas G: Amino acids activate mTOR complex 1 via Ca2 +/CaM signaling to hVps34. *Cell Metab* 2008, **7**:456–465.

114. Ra SG, Miyazaki T, Ishikura K, Nagayama H, Suzuki T, Maeda S, Ito M, Matsuzaki Y, Ohmori H: Additional effects of taurine on the benefits of BCAA intake for the delayed-onset muscle soreness and muscle damage induced by high-intensity eccentric exercise. *Adv Exp Med Biol* 2013, **776**:179–187.

115. Newgard CB: Interplay between lipids and branched-chain amino acids in development of insulin resistance. *Cell Metab* 2012, **15**:606–614.

116. Ranchordas MK, Burd NA, Godfrey RJ, Senchina DS, Stear SJ, Burke LM, Castell LM: A-Z of nutritional supplements: dietary supplements, sports nutrition foods and ergogenic aids for health and performance: Part 43. *Br J Sports Med* 2013, **47**:399–400.

117. Marshall K: Therapeutic applications of whey protein. *Altern Med Rev* 2004, **9**:136–156.

118. Luhovyy BL, Akhavan T, Anderson GH: Whey proteins in the regulation of food intake and satiety. *J Am Coll Nutr* 2007, **26**:704S–712S.

119. Maughan RJ: Quality assurance issues in the use of dietary supplements, with special reference to protein supplements. *J Nutr* 2013, **143**:1843S–1847S.

120. Hoppe C, Andersen GS, Jacobsen S, Mølgaard C, Friis H, Sangild PT, Michaelsen KF: The Use of Whey or Skimmed Milk Powder in Fortified Blended Foods for Vulnerable Groups. *J Nutr* 2008, **138**:145S–161S.

121. Ha E, Zemel MB: **Functional properties of whey, whey components, and essential amino acids : mechanisms underlying health benefits for active people (review).** *J Nutr Biochem* 2003, **14**:251–258.

122. Soares MJ, Murhadi LL, Kurpad AV, Chan She Ping-Delfos WL, Piers LS: **Mechanistic roles for calcium and vitamin D in the regulation of body weight.** *Obes Rev* 2012, **13**:592–605.

123. Gaudel C, Nongonierma AB, Maher S, Flynn S, Krause M, Murray BA, Kelly PM, Baird AW, FitzGerald RJ, Newsholme P: **A whey protein hydrolysate promotes insulinotropic activity in a clonal pancreatic β-cell line and enhances glycemic function in ob/ob mice.** *J Nutr* 2013, **143**:1109–1114.

124. Josse AR, Atkinson SA, Tarnopolsky MA, Phillips SM: **Increased consumption of dairy foods and protein during diet- and exercise-induced weight loss promotes fat mass loss and lean mass gain in overweight and obese premenopausal women.** *J Nutr* 2011, **141**:1626–1634.

125. Burd NA, Yang Y, Moore DR, Tang JE, Tarnopolsky MA, Phillips SM: **Greater stimulation of myofibrillar protein synthesis with ingestion of whey protein isolate v. micellar casein at rest and after resistance exercise in elderly men.** *Br J Nutr* 2012, **108**:958–962.

126. Tang JE, Moore DR, Kujbida GW, Tarnopolsky MA, Phillips SM: **Ingestion of whey hydrolysate, casein, or soy protein isolate: effects on mixed muscle protein synthesis at rest and following resistance exercise in young men.** *J Appl Physiol* 2009, **107**:987–992.

127. Burke DG, Chilibeck PD, Davidson KS, Candow DG, Farthing J, Smith-Palmer T: **The effect of whey protein supplementation with and without creatine monohydrate combined with resistance training on lean tissue mass and muscle strength.** *Int J Sport Nutr Exerc Metab* 2001, **11**:349–364.

128. Lands LC, Grey VL, Smountas AA: **Effect of supplementation with a cysteine donor on muscular performance.** *J Appl Physiol* 1999, **87**:1381–1385.

129. Reidy PT, Walker DK, Dickinson JM, Gundermann DM, Drummond MJ, Timmerman KL, Fry CS, Borack MS, Cope MB, Mukherjea R, Jennings K, Volpi E, Rasmussen BB: **Protein blend ingestion following resistance exercise promotes human muscle protein synthesis.** *J Nutr* 2013, **143**:410–416.

130. Hartman JW, Tang JE, Wilkinson SB, Tarnopolsky MA, Lawrence RL, Fullerton AV, Phillips SM: **Consumption of fat-free fluid milk after resistance exercise promotes greater lean mass accretion than does consumption of soy or carbohydrate in young, novice, male weightlifters.** *Am J Clin Nutr* 2007, **86**:373–381.

131. Kinscherf R, Fischbach T, Mihm S, Roth S, Hohenhaus-Sievert E, Weiss C, Edler L, Bartsch P, Droge W: **Effect of glutathione depletion and oral N-acetyl-cysteine treatment on CD4+ and CD8+ cells.** *FASEB J* 1994, **8**:448–451.

14

28 days of creatine nitrate supplementation is apparently safe in healthy individuals

Jordan M Joy[1,2], Ryan P Lowery[1], Paul H Falcone[2], Matt M Mosman[2], Roxanne M Vogel[2], Laura R Carson[2], Chih-Yin Tai[2], David Choate[3], Dylan Kimber[3], Jacob A Ormes[1], Jacob M Wilson[1] and Jordan R Moon[2,4*]

Abstract

Background: Creatine monohydrate has become a very popular nutritional supplement for its ergogenic effects. The safety of creatine monohydrate has previously been confirmed. However with each novel form of creatine that emerges, its safety must be verified. Therefore, the purpose of this study was to examine the safety of a novel form of creatine, creatine nitrate (CN), over a 28 day period.

Methods: 58 young males and females (Pooled: 24.3 ± 3.9 years, 144.9 ± 8.0 cm, 74.2 ± 13.0 kg) participated in this study across two laboratories. Subjects were equally and randomly assigned to consume either 1 g ($n = 18$) or 2 g ($n = 20$) of CN or remained unsupplemented ($n = 20$). Blood draws for full safety panels were conducted by a trained phlebotomist prior to and at the conclusion of the supplementation period.

Results: Pooled data from both laboratories revealed significant group x time interactions for absolute lymphocytes and absolute monocytes ($p < 0.05$). Analysis of the 1 g treatment revealed lab x time differences for red blood cell distribution width, platelets, absolute monocytes, creatinine, blood urea nitrogen (BUN):creatinine, sodium, protein, and alanine aminotransferase (ALT) ($p < 0.05$). Analysis of the 2 g treatment revealed lab x time differences for BUN:creatinine and ALT ($p < 0.05$). BUN and BUN:creatinine increased beyond the clinical reference range for the 2 g treatment of Lab 2, but BUN did not reach statistical significance.

Conclusion: Overall, CN appears to be safe in both 1 g and 2 g servings daily for up to a 28 day period. While those with previously elevated BUN levels may see additional increases resulting in post-supplementation values slightly beyond normal physiological range, these results have minor clinical significance and are not cause for concern. Otherwise, all hematological safety markers remained within normal range, suggesting that CN supplementation has no adverse effects in daily doses up to 2 g over 28 days and may be an alternative to creatine monohydrate supplementation.

Keywords: Creatine, Nitrate, Safety, Health, Hematology, Immunity, Immune system

Introduction

In regards to ergogenic supplementation, creatine's effects have been researched in humans since the early 1990's. Earnest and colleagues examined supplemental creatine's effects on both body composition and muscular performance [1]. After supplementing with creatine for only 2 weeks, subjects were tested with three 30s Wingate sprints, 1 repetition maximum in the bench press, and repetitions to failure at 70% 1RM. They discovered that creatine supplementation improved repeated sprint performance, bench press strength, fatigue resistance, body weight, and relative lifting volume. They also observed an insignificant trend for fat free mass. Creatine has since been verified as a potent supplement for each of these and more variables on numerous occasions [2-5].

Creatine supplementation's ergogenic effects are largely explained by increasing intramuscular phosphocreatine (PCr) stores [6]. The increase in PCr allows

* Correspondence: jordan@musclepharm.com
[2]MusclePharm Sports Science Institute, MusclePharm Corp., Denver, CO, USA
[4]Department of Sports Exercise Science, United States Sports Academy, Daphne, AL, USA
Full list of author information is available at the end of the article

adenosine diphosphate (ADP) to be readily rephosphorylated to adenosine triphosphate (ATP) [7,8], which is depleted rapidly during strenuous exercise. Thus, increasing the amount of PCr through creatine supplementation increases the capacity to rephosphorylate ADP to ATP, and this allows the athlete to resist fatigue and maintain a higher level of performance [6,9-11].

This increase in fatigue resistance created by creatine supplementation allows for increased training volume. As demonstrated by several laboratories, creatine supplementation is able to increase repetitions to failure [1,12]. Therefore, many athletes have adopted creatine use during pre-season and/or off-season training for the cumulative effects of increased training volume [13], and they are not using creatine exclusively for acute performance benefits. In addition to chronic performance benefits, creatine aids those seeking to increase muscle mass [2-5,14]. Muscle mass increases can be explained in part by creatine increasing training volume [1], but it is also partially explained by other factors. Saremi et al. [5] confirmed creatine's effects on increasing lean body mass after chronic resistance training, and in addition, they observed decreased levels of myostatin in the creatine supplemented group. Olsen and colleagues have demonstrated increased myonuclei and muscle fiber area after 16 weeks of concurrent resistance training and creatine supplementation [15]. Additionally, 12 weeks creatine supplementation has been demonstrated to increase myogenic regulatory factor expression and myogenin, both of which initiate transcription and regulate gene expression, which likely contribute to the anabolic effects of creatine [16].

Similarly, dietary nitrate has been receiving more attention for its effects on energy efficiency and work capacity. Nitrate supplementation, typically in the form of foods or juices high in inorganic nitrate such as beet root juice, has primarily been demonstrated to decrease oxygen cost despite maintaining work load [17-21]. This has led to improved performance [22,23] and increased muscle contractile efficiency by decreasing the ATP cost of muscle contraction [17,24]. Despite health benefits of nitrate supplementation [25,26], concerns have been raised over nitrosamines [27,28], and consumers may still be weary of consumption. It is also possible that healthcare practitioners may not fully understand the role of nutritional supplements, nutrition, and exercise, and therefore, they may raise unfounded safety concerns.

Because of the ergogenic effects of creatine and phosphocreatine and the ATP sparing effects of nitrate [17], the two supplements have been combined efficaciously along with other ingredients [29]. While both nitrates and creatine should help enhance performance similar to taking both ingredients alone, little is known about the safety of creatine bound to a nitrate when ingested regularly. Therefore, the purpose of this study was to examine the safety of a novel form of creatine, creatine nitrate (CN). We hypothesized that CN supplementation would not produce abnormal changes in hematological safety markers.

Methods

Experimental design

In a randomized design, a total of 58 subjects were recruited for this study across two laboratories. Subjects were randomly divided into control (CRL), 1 serving (G1), or 2 serving (G2) groups. Wherein, the CRL group did not supplement and G1 and G2 consumed 1 serving (1 g) and 2 servings (2 g) of CN (Iron Cre3™, MusclePharm Inc., Denver, CO), respectively, every day for 28 days in an unblinded manner. In addition to the CN, the supplement contained 1 g of carbohydrate, 500 mg of vitamin C, 500 IU of Vitamin E, 18 mg of Calcium, and 800 mg of a proprietary blend consisting of taurine, coconut water powder, and L-glutamine per serving. Supplement containers were weighed prior to and following the supplementation period and supplement consumption logs were completed by each participant to ensure compliance. Blood draws were conducted prior to and at the conclusion of the supplementation period. MusclePharm Sports Science Institute (Lab 1) received approval from the MusclePharm Sports Science Institute IRB, and the University of Tampa Human Performance and Nutrition Laboratory (Lab 2) received approval from the University of Tampa IRB. Each subject was provided written informed consent prior to participation in the study.

Participants

Forty-two subjects (25.2 ± 4.9 years, 173.8 ± 10.2 cm, 77.2 ± 16.7 kg, CRL n = 20, G1 n = 10, G2 n = 12) were recruited by Lab 1, while Lab 2 recruited the remaining 16 (21.9 ± 1.1 yrs, 68.9 ± 2.3 cm, 66.4 ± 3.2 kg, G1 n = 8, G2 n = 8). Subjects were required to be at least recreationally active (≥ 3 days/week of moderate to vigorous intensity exercise), free of any disease or disorder which may produce confounding results, non-smokers, and have abstained from creatine or nitrate supplementation for the month immediately prior to beginning CN supplementation, as assessed by pre-participation health history, exercise, and supplementation questionnaires.

Measurements

All measurements were taken prior to and at the conclusion of the 28-day supplementation period. Following a 10-hour fast, all subjects submitted a blood sample for analysis in the morning to prevent diurnal variations. All blood draws were performed via venipuncture by a trained phlebotomist. Samples were analyzed for complete metabolic panels and complete blood counts by an external laboratory (Laboratory Corporation of America, Denver, CO; ANY LAB TEST NOW, Tampa, FL). All collected samples were analyzed for the following markers: white blood cell count (WBC), red blood cell count (RBC), hemoglobin, hematocrit, mean corpuscular volume (MCV), mean corpuscular hemoglobin (MCH), mean corpuscular hemoglobin concentration (MCHC), red blood cell distribution width (RDW), platelets (percent and absolute), neutrophils (percent and absolute), lymphocytes (percent and absolute), monocytes (percent and absolute), eosinophils (percent and absolute), basophils (percent and absolute), serum glucose, blood urea nitrogen (BUN), creatinine, estimated glomerular filtration rate (eGFR), BUN:creatinine, sodium, potassium, chloride, carbon dioxide, calcium, protein, albumin, globulin, albumin:globulin, bilirubin, alkaline phosphatase, aspartate aminotransferase (AST), and alanine aminotransferase (ALT). Intra-test Coefficient of Variation (CV) for Lab 2 blood measurements were all under 3%. Inter-test reliability results from 12 men and women measures up to one week apart from Lab 1 resulted in no significant differences from day-to-day (p > 0.05) and an average inter-test %CV of 6.9%.

Statistical analyses

Pooled data was analyzed using a 3x2 repeated measures ANCOVA model for all group, time, and group by time interactions with the pre value as the covariate. A bonferroni post-hoc analysis was used to locate differences. Shapiro-Wilk tests were used to determine normality of the data. The Minimal Difference (MD) needed to be considered real was determined using the method previously described by Weir [30]. Data are presented as mean ± standard deviation. All data were analyzed using Statistica software (Statsoft, 2011).

Results

Pooled

Significant group by time interactions were present for absolute lymphocytes (p < 0.05). Wherein, G1 increased to a lesser extent than CRL, G2 decreased significantly relative to CRL, and G2 significantly decreased from pre to post. Absolute lymphocytes had a normal distribution at baseline (p = 0.55), yet the distribution was negatively skewed (p < 0.05) after the supplementation period. Significant group by time interactions were present for absolute monocytes (p < 0.05). G1 increased relative to CRL and G2 increased to a lesser extent than G1. Absolute monocytes was positively skewed at both time points (p < 0.05). All data is presented in Additional file 1: Table S1.

Inter-laboratory comparisons: one serving

Significant group by time interactions were present for RDW (p < 0.05). Lab 2 observed greater increases in RDW relative to Lab 1 and significantly increased from pre to post. Significant group by time interactions were observed for platelets (p < 0.05). Lab 1 observed a significant decrease in platelets relative to CRL, and Lab 2 observed a significant increase in platelets compared to decrements in both CRL and Lab 1. Platelets were normally distributed at baseline (p = 0.17), and negatively skewed (p < 0.05) at post. Significant group by time interactions existed for absolute monocytes (p < 0.05). Wherein, Lab 2 observed significant increases compared to Lab 1 and CRL. Significant group by time interactions were present for creatinine (p < 0.05). Lab 2 observed significant decrements relative to CRL. A significant group by time interaction was present for BUN:creatinine (p < 0.05). Wherein, Lab 2 observed significant increases pre to post. A significant group by time interaction was observed for sodium (p < 0.05). Lab 2 observed a significant increase over CRL. A significant interaction was observed for serum protein (p <0.05). Lab 2 observed a significant increase relative to CRL. Significant group by time interactions were observed for ALT (p < 0.05). Lab 2 observed greater decrements relative to CRL and Lab 1. ALT was positively skewed at baseline (p < 0.05), but it was normally distributed (p = 0.52) at post. RDW, platelets, absolute monocytes, creatinine, BUN:creatinine, sodium, and serum protein were either normally distributed, negatively skewed, or positively skewed at baseline without a change in skewness at post. With the exception of BUN:creatinine, all of these markers remained within clinical reference ranges, indicating clinical insignificance. All data is presented in Additional file 2: Table S2.

Inter-laboratory comparisons: two serving

Significant group by time interactions were present for BUN:creatinine (p < 0.05). Lab 2 observed significant increases relative to CRL and Lab 1 as well as within group differences pre to post. BUN:creatinine was positively skewed at baseline (p < 0.05), and at post, it became normally distributed (p = 0.16). Significant group by time interactions were observed for ALT (p < 0.05). Wherein, Lab 1 and Lab 2 observed greater decrements than CRL. ALT was positively skewed at baseline (p < 0.05), yet it was normally distributed at post (p = 0.93). All data is presented in Additional file 3: Table S3.

Discussion

The results of the present study confirm our hypothesis that CN supplementation will not cause abnormal changes in hematological safety markers. When analyzing the pooled data from both laboratories, significant interactions were observed only for absolute lymphocytes and monocytes, yet these remained within the accepted physiological range and not clinically significant. Also, percent lymphocytes and monocytes were unchanged. While remaining within range, we observed unusual effects between groups. For lymphocytes, the CRL group had a greater change than G1, and for monocytes, G1 increased to a greater extent than G2. These results suggest a natural variation for these markers. Alternatively, data was collected during the winter months, and subjects may have experienced these unusual outcomes as an effect of weather. Although significant interactions were observed concerning Lab 2 in the one serving treatment, it must be mentioned that many of these differences were not observed in the two serving treatment, and the CRL sample was represented solely from Lab 1. Thus, some of the differences are not likely due to CN supplementation, and variations between subjects may be due to variations in climate between Denver, CO and Tampa, FL [31]. However, the difference in absolute monocytes may have influenced the significance observed for absolute monocytes in the pooled sample. In the analysis of both the one and two serving treatments, significant interactions were observed for ALT, yet CN supplementation appeared to lower ALT relative to control, which is not a cause for concern. When analyzing the data between laboratories, BUN:creatinine from Lab 2 increased beyond the acceptable range for the two serving treatment (Additional file 3: Table S3). This was likely due to a large, yet insignificant ($p = 0.40$), increase in BUN, which was also slightly outside the acceptable range after the supplementation period. However, subjects were already at the high end of the acceptable range, and the magnitude of change was attenuated when examining a larger sample (Additional file 1: Table S1).

Analysis of clinical significance at the individual level was conducted using the MD statistic that calculates the (biological and reliability) error needed to be exceeded in order for an individual measurement to be considered real as described by Weir [30]. If a subject exceeded the MD, the change was considered a true change. Variables that were significantly different at the group level were evaluated at the individual level and subjects with changes that exceeded MD were evaluated to determine clinical significance. Clinical significance at the individual level was reached when a score that exceeded the MD crossed the upper or lower limits for each variable. In the pooled analysis, one subject in G2 experienced a decrease in absolute monocytes, bringing them within the clinical reference range, and two subjects from G1 equally increased, entering the clinical reference range, and decreased, exiting the reference range. In both cases, the supplement does not appear to be causing specific,

directional changes in absolute monocytes. In the 1 serving inter-laboratory comparison, 2 subjects from Lab 2 demonstrated increases in RDW, which caused them to surpass the upper limit of the clinical reference range. One subject from Lab 2 decreased, leaving the accepted range, for creatinine. One subject from Lab 2 increased, leaving the accepted range, for BUN:Cr. From Lab 1, one subject experienced a decrease in ALT, entering the accepted range. In the 2-serving comparison, 4 subjects from Lab 2 increased; 2 started in and remained outside the range, and 2 exited the range. All subjects remained within 3 standard deviations of the mean and exceeded the MD. It is also worthy to note that 8 subjects in the CRL group experienced changes in at least one variable that exceeded the MD and was outside the accepted range. Collectively, individual analyses supports our hypothesis and also supports the notion of variability. Additionally, absolute lymphocytes in the pooled analysis, platelets and ALT in the 1 serving inter-laboratory analysis, and BUN:creatinine and ALT in the 2 serving inter-laboratory analysis were distributed differently from pre to post, increasing the probability for type 1 statistical error [32].

The present findings generally agree with previous literature. The safety of creatine has been confirmed on several occasions [33], including several clinical populations [34,35]. Shelmadine et al. [36] examined the safety of a multi-ingredient supplement containing creatine, ingredients known to influence the nitrate/nitric oxide pathway, and other ingredients over an identical time period of 28 days. These researchers observed no change in clinical serum or whole blood chemistry markers, and they concluded that the supplement was safe for consumption for this duration. Other multi-ingredient supplements containing creatine have confirmed its safety for a period of up to nine weeks [37,38].

While creatine monohydrate is recognized as safe, the nitrate component of CN may still be troublesome to athletes or practitioners. Concerns over nitrate and other nitrosamines began as early as 1970. Lijinsky and Epstein [28] published a manuscript identifying dietary nitrosamines as carcinogens. However, more recent evidence suggests that dietary nitrate is safe for human consumption [39]. Moreover, dietary nitrate has been reported to reduce blood pressure [19,21,25]. Webb et al. [40] provided subjects with beetroot juice high in nitrates and observed lower systolic blood pressure after only one hour, while diastolic blood pressure and mean arterial pressure remained significantly lower after 24 hours. These findings identify nitrate as possibly beneficial to long-term health. In a review of nitrate supplementation, Hoon and colleagues [41] reported no major health consequences of nitrate supplementation, and only one minor adverse event, the discoloration of urine, which is attributed to those studies which supplemented with beet-root juice. However, provided that creatine's safety has been so thoroughly investigated, any health complication from CN is likely due to the nitrate component.

This is the first study to examine the safety of CN. From the present results, we can conclude that CN in doses of up to 2 g are safe for human consumption for a duration of 28 days. All measured variables remained within the normal range across groups, with the exception of BUN which was not statistically significant when the groups were compared. Therefore, CN supplementation may be contraindicated for those already high in BUN. Additionally while the differences observed for absolute monocytes and lymphocytes appear to be due to variability and remained within range, CN may be unadvisable for daily consumption for those with a weakened immune system. In the present study, CN was supplemented for only 28 days, and future research may be interested in examining CN for a longer trial period to confirm its safety. Moreover, future studies are required to determine the efficacy of CN, as the combined effects of nitrates and creatine on both longitudinal and acute changes in performance and body composition are currently unknown.

Additional files

Additional file 1: Table S1. Pooled data from Lab 1 and Lab 2. All data are presented as mean ± standard deviation. * denotes significantly different from CRL, [a] denotes significantly different from pre value, and [b] denotes significantly different from G1.

Additional file 2: Table S2. Data comparison between Lab 1 and Lab 2 for the 1 serving treatment. All data are presented as mean ± standard deviation. * denotes significantly different from CRL, [a] denotes significantly different from pre value, and [b] denotes significantly different from Lab 1.

Additional file 3: Table S3. Data comparison between Lab 1 and Lab 2 for the 2 serving treatment. All data are presented as mean ± standard deviation. * denotes significantly different from CRL, [a] denotes significantly different from pre value, and [b] denotes significantly different from Lab 1.

Abbreviations

PCr: Phosphocreatine; ADP: Adenosine diphosphate; ATP: Adenosine triphosphate; CN: Creatine nitrate; Lab 1: MusclePharm Sports Science Institute; Lab 2: University of Tampa Human Performance and Sports Nutrition Laboratory; WBC: White blood cell; RBC: Red blood cell; MCV: Mean corpuscular volume; MCH: Mean corpuscular hemoglobin; MCHC: Mean corpuscular hemoglobin concentration; RDW: Red blood cell distribution width; BUN: Blood urea nitrogen; eGFR: Estimated glomerular filtration rate; AST: Aspartate aminotransferase; ALT: Alanine aminotransferase; MD: Minimal difference.

Competing interests

JJ, PF, CT, MM, LC, and JM are employees of the funding source, MusclePharm corporation. However, the remaining authors have no financial interests concerning the outcome of this investigation. Additionally, this publication should not be viewed as endorsement by the investigators, the United States Sports Academy, the University of Tampa, or MusclePharm corporation.

Authors' contributions

JJ, PF, CT, MM, LC, DK, DC, and JM participated in data collection for Lab 1. JJ, RP, and JW participated in data collection for Lab 2. All authors contributed to the conception of the experimental design, drafting of the manuscript, and interpretation of data. All authors have read and approved the final manuscript.

Acknowledgements

We would like to thank Dr. Michael P. Kim and all of the participants as well as MusclePharm corporation for supplying product and funding the investigation.

Author details

[1]Department of Health Sciences and Human Performance, The University of Tampa, Tampa, FL, USA. [2]MusclePharm Sports Science Institute, MusclePharm Corp., Denver, CO, USA. [3]Metropolitan State University, Denver, CO, USA. [4]Department of Sports Exercise Science, United States Sports Academy, Daphne, AL, USA.

References

1. Earnest CP, Snell PG, Rodriguez R, Almada AL, Mitchell TL: The effect of creatine monohydrate ingestion on anaerobic power indices, muscular strength and body composition. *Acta Physiol Scand* 1995, **153**:207–209.
2. Vandenberghe K, Goris M, Van Hecke P, Van Leemputte M, Vangerven L, Hespel P: Long-term creatine intake is beneficial to muscle performance during resistance training. *J Appl Physiol* 1997, **83**:2055–2063.
3. Kreider RB, Ferreira M, Wilson M, Grindstaff P, Plisk S, Reinardy J, Cantler E, Almada AL: Effects of creatine supplementation on body composition, strength, and sprint performance. *Med Sci Sports Exerc* 1998, **30**:73–82.
4. Becque MD, Lochmann JD, Melrose DR: Effects of oral creatine supplementation on muscular strength and body composition. *Med Sci Sports Exerc* 2000, **32**:654–658.
5. Saremi A, Gharakhanloo R, Sharghi S, Gharaati MR, Larijani B, Omidfar K: Effects of oral creatine and resistance training on serum myostatin and GASP-1. *Mol Cell Endocrinol* 2010, **317**:25–30.
6. Harris RC, Soderlund K, Hultman E: Elevation of creatine in resting and exercised muscle of normal subjects by creatine supplementation. *Clin Sci* 1992, **83**:367–374.
7. Chanutin A: The fate of creatine when administered to man. *J Biol Chem* 1926, **67**:29–41.
8. Hultman E, Bergstrom J, Spriet LL, Soderlund K: *Energy Metabolism and Fatigue*. Champaign, IL: Human Kinetics; 1990.
9. Greenhaff PL, Bodin K, Soderlund K, Hultman E: Effect of oral creatine supplementation on skeletal muscle phosphocreatine resynthesis. *Am J Physiol* 1994, **266**:E725–E730.
10. Greenhaff PL, Casey A, Short AH, Harris R, Soderlund K, Hultman E: Influence of oral creatine supplementation of muscle torque during repeated bouts of maximal voluntary exercise in man. *Clin Sci* 1993, **84**:565–571.
11. Hultman E, Soderlund K, Timmons JA, Cederblad G, Greenhaff PL: Muscle creatine loading in men. *J Appl Physiol* 1996, **81**:232–237.
12. Warber JP, Tharion WJ, Patton JF, Champagne CM, Mitotti P, Lieberman HR: The effect of creatine monohydrate supplementation on obstacle course and multiple bench press performance. *J Strength Cond Res* 2002, **16**:500–508.
13. Rawson ES, Volek JS: Effects of creatine supplementation and resistance training on muscle strength and weightlifting performance. *J Strength Cond Res* 2003, **17**:822–831.
14. Tarnopolsky MA, Mahoney DJ, Vajsar J, Rodriguez C, Doherty TJ, Roy BD, Biggar D: Creatine monohydrate enhances strength and body composition in Duchenne muscular dystrophy. *Neurology* 2004, **62**:1771–1777.
15. Olsen S, Aagaard P, Kadi F, Tufekovic G, Verney J, Olesen JL, Suetta C, Kjaer M: Creatine supplementation augments the increase in satellite cell and myonuclei number in human skeletal muscle induced by strength training. *J Physiol* 2006, **573**:525–534.
16. Willoughby DS, Rosene JM: Effects of oral creatine and resistance training on myogenic regulatory factor expression. *Med Sci Sports Exerc* 2003, **35**:923–929.

17. Bailey SJ, Fulford J, Vanhatalo A, Winyard PG, Blackwell JR, DiMenna FJ, Wilkerson DP, Benjamin N, Jones AM: **Dietary nitrate supplementation enhances muscle contractile efficiency during knee-extensor exercise in humans.** *J Appl Physiol* 2010, **109:**135–148.

18. Bailey SJ, Winyard P, Vanhatalo A, Blackwell JR, Dimenna FJ, Wilkerson DP, Tarr J, Benjamin N, Jones AM: **Dietary nitrate supplementation reduces the O2 cost of low-intensity exercise and enhances tolerance to high-intensity exercise in humans.** *J Appl Physiol* 2009, **107:**1144–1155.

19. Larsen FJ, Weitzberg E, Lundberg JO, Ekblom B: **Effects of dietary nitrate on oxygen cost during exercise.** *Acta Physiol* 2007, **191:**59–66.

20. Larsen FJ, Weitzberg E, Lundberg JO, Ekblom B: **Dietary nitrate reduces maximal oxygen consumption while maintaining work performance in maximal exercise.** *Free Radic Biol Med* 2010, **48:**342–347.

21. Vanhatalo A, Bailey SJ, Blackwell JR, DiMenna FJ, Pavey TG, Wilkerson DP, Benjamin N, Winyard PG, Jones AM: **Acute and chronic effects of dietary nitrate supplementation on blood pressure and the physiological responses to moderate-intensity and incremental exercise.** *Am J Physiol Regul Integr Comp Physiol* 2010, **299:**R1121–R1131.

22. Cermak NM, Gibala MJ, van Loon LJ: **Nitrate supplementation's improvement of 10-km time-trial performance in trained cyclists.** *Int J Sport Nutr Exerc Metab* 2012, **22:**64–71.

23. Lansley KE, Winyard PG, Bailey SJ, Vanhatalo A, Wilkerson DP, Blackwell JR, Gilchrist M, Benjamin N, Jones AM: **Acute dietary nitrate supplementation improves cycling time trial performance.** *Med Sci Sports Exerc* 2011, **43:**1125–1131.

24. Fulford J, Winyard PG, Vanhatalo A, Bailey SJ, Blackwell JR, Jones AM: **Influence of dietary nitrate supplementation on human skeletal muscle metabolism and force production during maximum voluntary contractions.** *Pflugers Archiv* 2013, **465:**517–528.

25. Kapil V, Milsom AB, Okorie M, Maleki-Toyserkani S, Akram F, Rehman F, Arghandawi S, Pearl V, Benjamin N, Loukogeorgakis S, Macallister R, Hobbs JA, Webb AJ, Ahluwalia A: **Inorganic nitrate supplementation lowers blood pressure in humans: role for nitrite-derived NO.** *Hypertension* 2010, **56:**274–281.

26. Carlstrom M, Persson AE, Larsson E, Hezel M, Scheffer PG, Teerlink T, Weitzberg E, Lundberg JO: **Dietary nitrate attenuates oxidative stress, prevents cardiac and renal injuries, and reduces blood pressure in salt-induced hypertension.** *Cardiovasc Res* 2011, **89:**574–585.

27. Derave W, Taes Y: **Beware of the pickle: health effects of nitrate intake.** *J Appl Physiol* 2009, **107:**1677. author reply 1678.

28. Lijinsky W, Epstein SS: **Nitrosamines as environmental carcinogens.** *Nature* 1970, **225:**21–23.

29. Lowery RP, Joy JM, Dudeck JE, Oliveira De Souza E, McCleary SA, Wells S, Wildman R, Wilson JM: **Effects of 8 weeks of Xpand(R) 2X pre workout supplementation on skeletal muscle hypertrophy, lean body mass, and strength in resistance trained males.** *J Int Soc Sports Nutr* 2013, **10:**44.

30. Weir JP: **Quantifying test-retest reliability using the intraclass correlation coefficient and the SEM.** *J Strength Cond Res* 2005, **19:**231–240.

31. Karagiannidis C, Hense G, Rueckert B, Mantel PY, Ichters B, Blaser K, Menz G, Schmidt-Weber CB: **High-altitude climate therapy reduces local airway inflammation and modulates lymphocyte activation.** *Scand J Immunol* 2006, **63:**304–310.

32. Delaney HD, Vargha A: *The Effect of Nonnormality on Student's Two-Sample T Test.* New Orleans: Paper presented at the Annual Meeting of the American Educational Research Association; 2000.

33. Buford TW, Kreider RB, Stout JR, Greenwood M, Campbell B, Spano M, Ziegenfuss T, Lopez H, Landis J, Antonio J: **International Society of Sports Nutrition position stand: creatine supplementation and exercise.** *J Int Soc Sports Nutr* 2007, **4:**6.

34. Hersch SM, Gevorkian S, Marder K, Moskowitz C, Feigin A, Cox M, Como P, Zimmerman C, Lin M, Zhang L, Ulug AM, Beal MF, Matson W, Bogdanov M, Ebbel E, Zaleta A, Kaneko Y, Jenkins B, Hevelone N, Zhang H, Yu H, Schoenfeld D, Ferrante R, Rosas HD: **Creatine in Huntington disease is safe, tolerable, bioavailable in brain and reduces serum 8OH2′dG.** *Neurology* 2006, **66:**250–252.

35. Bender A, Samtleben W, Elstner M, Klopstock T: **Long-term creatine supplementation is safe in aged patients with Parkinson disease.** *Nutr Res* 2008, **28:**172–178.

36. Shelmadine B, Cooke M, Buford T, Hudson G, Redd L, Leutholtz B, Willoughby DS: **Effects of 28 days of resistance exercise and consuming a commercially available pre-workout supplement, NO-Shotgun(R), on**

body composition, muscle strength and mass, markers of satellite cell activation, and clinical safety markers in males. *J Int Soc Sports Nutr* 2009, **6:**16.

37. Schmitz SM, Hofheins JE, Lemieux R: **Nine weeks of supplementation with a multi-nutrient product augments gains in lean mass, strength, and muscular performance in resistance trained men.** *J Int Soc Sports Nutr* 2010, **7:**40.

38. Kendall KL, Moon JR, Fairman CM, Spradely BD, Tai CY, Falcone PH, Carson LR, Mosman MM, Joy JJ, Kim MP, Serrano ER, Esposito EN: **Ingesting a preworkout supplement containing caffeine, creatine, β –alanine, amino acids, and B vitamins for 28 days is both safe and efficacious in recreationally active men.** *Nutr Res* 2014, **34**(5):442–449.

39. Sindelar JJ, Milkowski AL: **Human safety controversies surrounding nitrate and nitrite in the diet.** *Nitric Oxide* 2012, **26:**259–266.

40. Webb AJ, Patel N, Loukogeorgakis S, Okorie M, Aboud Z, Misra S, Rashid R, Miall P, Deanfield J, Benjamin N, Macallister R, Hobbs JA, Ahluwalia A: **Acute blood pressure lowering, vasoprotective, and antiplatelet properties of dietary nitrate via bioconversion to nitrite.** *Hypertension* 2008, **51:**784–790.

41. Hoon MW, Johnson NA, Chapman PG, Burke LM: **The effect of nitrate supplementation on exercise performance in healthy individuals: a systematic review and meta-analysis.** *Int J Sport Nutr Exerc Metab* 2013, **23:**522–532.

15

The effect of a decaffeinated green tea extract formula on fat oxidation, body composition and exercise performance

Justin D Roberts[1,2*], Michael G Roberts[2†], Michael D Tarpey[2†], Jack C Weekes[2†] and Clare H Thomas[2†]

Abstract

Background: The cardio-metabolic and antioxidant health benefits of caffeinated green tea (GT) relate to its catechin polyphenol content. Less is known about decaffeinated extracts, particularly in combination with exercise. The aim of this study was therefore to determine whether a decaffeinated green tea extract (dGTE) positively influenced fat oxidation, body composition and exercise performance in recreationally active participants.

Methods: Fourteen, recreationally active males participated in a double-blind, placebo-controlled, parallel design intervention (mean ± SE; age = 21.4 ± 0.3 yrs; weight = 76.37 ± 1.73 kg; body fat = 16.84 ± 0.97%, peak oxygen consumption [$\dot{V}O_{2peak}$] = 3.00 ± 0.10 L·min^{-1}). Participants were randomly assigned capsulated dGTE (571 mg·d^{-1}; n = 7) or placebo (PL; n = 7) for 4 weeks. Following body composition and resting cardiovascular measures, participants cycled for 1 hour at 50% $\dot{V}O_{2peak}$, followed by a 40 minute performance trial at week 0, 2 and 4. Fat and carbohydrate oxidation was assessed via indirect calorimetry. Pre-post exercise blood samples were collected for determination of total fatty acids (TFA). Distance covered (km) and average power output (W) were assessed as exercise performance criteria.

Results: Total fat oxidation rates increased by 24.9% from 0.241 ± 0.025 to 0.301 ± 0.009 g·min^{-1} with dGTE ($P = 0.05$; $\eta p^2 = 0.45$) by week 4, whereas substrate utilisation was unaltered with PL. Body fat significantly decreased with dGTE by 1.63 ± 0.16% in contrast to PL over the intervention period ($P < 0.001$; $\eta p^2 = 0.84$). No significant changes for FFA or blood pressure between groups were observed. dGTE resulted in a 10.9% improvement in performance distance covered from 20.23 ± 0.54 km to 22.43 ± 0.40 km by week 4 ($P < 0.001$; $\eta p^2 = 0.85$).

Conclusions: A 4 week dGTE intervention favourably enhanced substrate utilisation and subsequent performance indices, but did not alter TFA concentrations in comparison to PL. The results support the use of catechin polyphenols from dGTE in combination with exercise training in recreationally active volunteers.

Keywords: Green tea, Body composition, Fat oxidation, Exercise performance

Introduction

The health benefits of polyphenols found in green tea (GT), the unfermented leaves of the tea plant, *Camellia sinensis*, have been extensively investigated in the last fifteen years [1-7]. Studies have demonstrated antioxidant [8,9] and chemoprotective properties [4], as well as improvements in cardio-metabolic health from various GT strategies (including reduced circulating cholesterol and triglyerides [10], increased thermogenesis and whole body fat oxidation [1,3,11], reduced blood pressure [7,12,13] and improved body mass index ratios [5,14-17]). These health benefits, in part, relate to the bioactive catechin polyphenol content of GT, of which (−)-epigallocatechin-3-gallate (EGCG) can account for between 50–80% of the total catechin content [18].

GT catechins have been proposed to influence metabolic and thermogenic activities in the short term, via inhibition of catechol-o-methyl transferase (COMT) leading to enhanced catecholamine, cAMP and lipolytic activity

---

* Correspondence: justin.roberts@anglia.ac.uk
†Equal contributors
[1]Department of Life Sciences, Anglia Ruskin University, East Road, Cambridge, UK
[2]School of Life & Medical Sciences, University of Hertfordshire, College Lane, Hatfield, Hertfordshire, UK

[17,19,20], although this has been disputed [20]. GT catechins, particularly EGCG, may also activate endothelial nitric oxide synthase, leading to mild reductions in blood pressure [13,21].

In the longer term, GT catechins may influence specific signalling molecules, including PGC1α, leading to gene expression of fat metabolism enzymes [20]. Whilst such mechanisms are currently under debate, strategies to enhance fat oxidation, body composition and cardiovascular efficiency in conjunction with physical activity are of pertinence to the general population. Additionally the indirect sparing of glycogen stores may support improved exercise tolerance and/or performance.

Research investigating GT extracts (GTE) and exercise have produced conflicting results. Modest EGCG dosage in the short term (270 $mg \cdot d^{-1}$ EGCG for 6 days [22], and 68 $mg \cdot d^{-1}$ EGCG for 3 weeks [23,24]) did not alter metabolic or performance variables in healthy or endurance trained volunteers. However, the inclusion of 100.5 $mg \cdot d^{-1}$ EGCG over a 10 week training period enhanced whole-body metabolic efficiency elsewhere [11]. One confounding factor though is the use of caffeinated GTE in these studies. When decaffeinated GTE (dGTE) has been employed, 366 mg EGCG was found to acutely increase fat oxidation by 17% [3]. Conversely, higher dosage dGTE (624 ± 3 $mg \cdot d^{-1}$ EGCG for 28 days) did not significantly affect fat oxidation in healthy, male volunteers [25].

We were therefore invited to undertake an independent assessment of the cardio-metabolic and performance effects of a dGTE formula (571 $mg \cdot d^{-1}$ GTE providing 400 $mg \cdot d^{-1}$ EGCG) over a 4 week period in comparison to placebo in healthy, male volunteers. It was hypothesised that moderate dose dGTE would significantly improve fat oxidation and performance, supporting longer term mechanisms linking GTE catechins to enhanced metabolic enzyme gene expression.

Materials and methods

Participants

Fourteen healthy, male participants volunteered following power calculation assessment (G*Power3, Dusseldorf [26]; using α = 0.05; 1-β = 0.95; based on observed data [3,22-24] and 2 groups). Participants were required to be recreationally active non-smokers, and have no known sensitivities to tea products or be regular green tea consumers. Prior to study inclusion, all participants provided written informed consent and satisfactorily completed a general health screen. The study was approved by the University of Hertfordshire Life and Medical Sciences Ethics Committee. Participant characteristics are displayed in Table 1.

Procedures

Preliminary testing

All testing took place in the Human Physiology Laboratory, University of Hertfordshire. Participants were instructed to refrain from consuming caffeinated products for 48 hours prior to initial testing, and not be consuming other supplementation.

Peak oxygen consumption ($\dot{V}O_{2peak}$) was assessed at least one week prior to experimental trials using a standard incremental step protocol increasing by 30 W each 3 minutes until volitional exhaustion as previously reported [27]. Tests were performed on a Monark Ergomedic 874E stationary bike (Monark Exercise AB, Varberg, Sweden) using a Metalyser 3B automated gas-analyser (Cortex Biophysik, Leipzig, Germany). On a separate occasion, subjects undertook a familiarisation trial to confirm exercise intensity at 50% $\dot{V}O_{2peak}$. This intensity was selected based on pilot work in which average fat oxidation rates during sustained submaximal exercise were statistically greater at 50% $\dot{V}O_{2peak}$ compared to both 40 and 60% $\dot{V}O_{2peak}$.

Treatments

Participants were randomly assigned to an experimental or placebo group, and provided with either capsulated dGTE (571 $mg \cdot d^{-1}$ dGTE, delivering 70% or 400 $mg \cdot d^{-1}$ EGCG (equivalent to 6–7 cups of green tea per day), Changsha Active Ingredients Group Inc., Changsha, China*), or placebo (700 $mg \cdot d^{-1}$ corn flour). All participants received capsules on a weekly basis to monitor compliance, with instructions to consume one capsule daily before breakfast with 250 ml water. *Analysis of the main active ingredient (EGCG) was undertaken prior to and independently of the main study by Changsha Active Ingredients Group Inc., using high performance liquid chromatography. The certificate of analysis provided by the supplying company demonstrated that the product contained 91.21% total catechins, from which 70.74% was EGCG. The product did not appear to be assessed for other catechins, so it is likely that the remaining percentage comprised other catechins (GCG, EGC, GC, EC, ECG, etc.).

Experimental design and intervention

A randomised, double blind, placebo controlled parallel design was employed over a 4 week intervention. Participants completed three laboratory trials at week 0, 2 and 4 under controlled conditions following an overnight fast. Upon arrival, nude body mass (Seca 780, Hamburg, Germany), height (Seca 200 stadiometer, Hamburg, Germany) and body composition [28] (Tanita Body Segmental Analyser 418-BC, Tokyo, Japan) were assessed.

Participants were then fitted with a Polar FS2c telemetric monitor (Polar Electro Ltd., Kempele, Finland) and

Table 1 Baseline characteristics and resting measurements across the intervention

Variable	PL (n = 7)			dGTE (n = 7)		
Age (years)	21.4 ± 0.6			21.4 ± 0.3		
Height (m)	1.77 ± 0.03			1.78 ± 0.01		
$\dot{V}O_{2peak}$ (L·min^{-1})	3.13 ± 0.18			2.87 ± 0.08		
	Baseline	Week 2	Week 4	Baseline	Week 2	Week 4
Weight (kg)	75.46 ± 2.91	75.11 ± 2.94*	74.81 ± 2.88*	77.29 ± 2.05	76.96 ± 2.03*	76.69 ± 1.95* [B]
Bodyfat (%)	16.63 ± 1.58	16.34 ± 1.69	15.97 ± 1.69*#	17.06 ± 1.24	16.23 ± 1.39*	15.43 ± 1.33*# [A,B]
HR (bpm)	61.00 ± 2.70	62.14 ± 1.81	61.00 ± 1.83	62.00 ± 1.25	62.43 ± 2.01	62.57 ± 1.92
SBP (mm Hg)	129.29 ± 1.73	125.71 ± 3.64	127.00 ± 2.44	130.00 ± 1.18	126.57 ± 2.14	126.86 ± 3.64
DBP (mm Hg)	67.57 ± 4.35	66.14 ± 1.72	69.71 ± 2.37	69.57 ± 2.40	65.71 ± 2.55	67.71 ± 2.11

Table 1 shows the key participant characteristics for each group, including absolute changes for weight, body fat, heart rate and blood pressure over the intervention. Data are presented as mean ± SE. PL, Placebo; dGTE, decaffeinated green tea extract; $\dot{V}O_{2peak}$, peak oxygen uptake; HR, heart rate; SBP, systolic blood pressure; DBP, diastolic blood pressure. [A]denotes significant overall group x time interaction effect ($P = 0.002$). [B]denotes significant overall time interaction effect only ($P < 0.001$). *denotes significant difference ($P \leq 0.05$) to baseline only within group. #denotes significant difference to week 2 within group only ($P < 0.046$).

seated for 5 minutes prior to resting heart rate and blood pressure readings (Omron MX3 plus, Kyoto, Japan). A venous wholeblood sample was then collected into duplicate 4 ml K$_3$EDTA Vacutainers (Greiner Bio-One GmbH, Kremsmunster, Austria) by a qualified phlebotomist. Samples were centrifuged for 10 minutes at 2000 rpm, with aliquotted plasma immediately frozen at −80°C for later assessment of TFA.

Exercise trials

Exercise trials comprised a submaximal assessment and performance stage. During the submaximal assessment, participants exercised for one hour at 50% $\dot{V}O_{2peak}$ on a Monark Ergomedic 874E cycle ergometer. Gas exchange data was recorded continuously throughout exercise using a Metalyser 3B gas analyser, with average data taken over the final 45 minutes of submaximal exercise. Rating of perceived exertion (RPE) [29] and heart rate were recorded every 20 minutes.

Rates of total carbohydrate oxidation (CHO$_{TOT}$), total fat oxidation (FAT$_{TOT}$) (g·min^{-1}) and energy expenditure (EE) (kJ·min^{-1}) were calculated from $\dot{V}O_2$ and $\dot{V}CO_2$ (L·min^{-1}) using stoichiometric equations [30], with protein oxidation assumed negligible, as follows:

$$CHO_{TOT} = 4.210 \cdot (\dot{V}CO_2) - 2.962 \cdot (\dot{V}O_2) \quad (1)$$

$$FAT_{TOT} = 1.695 \cdot (\dot{V}O_2) - 1.701 \cdot (\dot{V}CO_2) \quad (2)$$

$$EE = [(0.550 \cdot \dot{V}CO_2) - (4.471 \cdot \dot{V}O_2)] \cdot 4.2 \quad (3)$$

Upon completion, seated blood pressure and post exercise venous sampling was repeated as previously described. Following this, participants were instructed to undertake a 40 minute self-paced performance trial using a Computrainer erogometer system (RaceMate

Inc., Seattle, USA). Distance covered (km) and power output (W) were recorded each 10 minutes, with only time elapsed visible to the subjects. Verbal encouragement was provided each 10 minutes. At the end of the exercise trial, subjects recovered for 5 minutes at 50 W.

Dietary intake and exercise activity

All participants recorded a 3 day dietary recall preceding each exercise trial to assess for habitual dietary compliance. Dietary analyses were undertaken using Dietplan 6.50 (Forestfield Software Ltd, West Sussex, United Kingdom), with no differences reported between groups for macronutrients and/or energy intake. Additionally, participants were requested to consume similar meals the day before the exercise trials at regular time intervals to provide increased control of oxidation variables. This was based on pilot work assessment of fat oxidation stability at 50% $\dot{V}O_{2peak}$ (assessed by calculating the amount of time (minutes) throughout the exercise that was spent within ±0.02 g·min^{-1} of the average fat oxidation rate, expressed as a percentage for each individual), which was greater when the 24 hour pre exercise period was controlled for dietary intake (68.22 ± 5.70%) compared to when only the evening meal preceding the testing session was controlled (60.78 ± 8.42%).

The standardised menu was based on typical foods consumed by participants at breakfast, lunch and dinner, and provided similar caloric intake to habitual dietary records (values as calorie totals and per kilogram mean bodyweight: energy intake: 2484.70 kcal·d^{-1} (32.68 kcal·kg^{-1}·d^{-1}); carbohydrate: 1127.7 kcal·d^{-1} (14.83 kcal·kg^{-1}·d^{-1}); fat: 565.4 kcal·d^{-1} (7.43 kcal·kg^{-1}·d^{-1}) and protein: 791.96 kcal·d^{-1} (10.42 kcal·kg^{-1}·d^{-1}). Throughout the intervention period, participants were instructed to minimise consumption of polyphenol rich foods. Participants were additionally required to cycle for one hour at 50% $\dot{V}O_{2peak}$ three times per week as part of a regulated exercise programme. All participants provided training diaries to monitor compliance.

Blood analyses

All blood analyses for TFA were independently undertaken by ABS Laboratories (Biopark, Welwyn Garden City, Hertfordshire) employing previously validated methods [31]. TFA concentrations were based on assessment of palmitic, palmitoleic, stearic, oleic and linoleic acids. Briefly, 100 µl plasma aliquots were spiked with internal standard (heptadecanoic acid), with free fatty acids being extracted using the 'Dole Extraction Solvent' (isopropanol/heptane/sulphuric acid (1 M) (40:10:1)). After drying under nitrogen, the extracts were resuspended using 200 µL of dichoromethane and the FFAs derivatised using diethylamine and Deoxo-Fluor. The diethylamide derivatives were then extracted into heptane. The heptane was then removed using nitrogen in a dry-block at 70°C. The dried extracts were reconstituted into 100 µL of heptane and quantified by gas chromatography using a mass spectrometer as the detector in the selected ion monitoring (SIM) mode.

Statistical analyses

Statistical analyses were performed using SPSS (v19, Chicago, USA). Baseline variables were assessed using an independent samples t-test. A mixed design repeated measures analysis of variance (ANOVA) was employed to assess treatment and time interactions. Where pertinent, a one way ANOVA with Bonferroni post hoc adjustments was utilised to assess within treatment effects. An alpha level of ≤0.05 was employed for statistical significance. Data are reported as means ± SE.

Results

Baseline characteristics and resting measures

Intervention groups were matched for age, height, weight, body fat and $\dot{V}O_{2peak}$ at baseline (Table 1). A significant interaction effect for bodyweight was found across time only (F = 16.98, $P < 0.001$). Net bodyweight reduction was similar between groups across the intervention (0.64 ± 0.17 kg for PL; F = 12.33, $P = 0.001$; $\eta p^2 = 0.67$), and 0.60 ± 0.21 kg for dGTE; F = 6.27, $P = 0.014$; $\eta p^2 = 0.51$ within group). There was a significant group x time interaction for percentage body fat (F = 7.81, $P = 0.002$), with an overall reduction of 1.63 ± 0.16% with dGTE ($P < 0.001$; $\eta p^2 = 0.84$ within group) compared to 0.66 ± 0.15% for PL ($P = 0.002$; $\eta p^2 = 0.66$ within group). No significant effects were reported for resting heart rate or blood pressure.

Submaximal exercise measures

Weekly contribution of substrate to total energy expenditure (EE) for PL and dGTE are reported in Figures 1 and 2 respectively. No significant differences were reported for EE either between or within groups over time ($P > 0.05$), demonstrating consistency of the submaximal exercise trials.

A significant overall group x time interaction for FAT_{TOT} was observed (F = 3.39, $P = 0.05$). FAT_{TOT} during exercise remained similar for PL across the intervention period (week 0 = 0.277 ± 0.038 g·min^{-1}; week 2 = 0.274 ± 0.031 g·min^{-1}; week 4 = 0.279 ± 0.030 g·min^{-1}, $P > 0.05$) despite a non-significant increase in percentage contribution to total EE (week 0 = 34.61 ± 3.72%; week 2 = 35.23 ± 2.99%; week 4 = 35.53 ± 2.53%, $P > 0.05$).

FAT_{TOT} for dGTE increased from 0.241 ± 0.025 g·min^{-1} at week 0 to 0.256 ± 0.023 g·min^{-1} at week 2, and to 0.301 ± 0.009 g·min^{-1} by week 4 (F = 4.10, $P = 0.05$; $\eta p^2 = 0.45$). This represented a 24.9% or 0.060 ± 0.027 g·min^{-1} increase in FAT_{TOT} with dGTE. Correspondingly, percentage contribution of total fat to exercise EE increased with dGTE from 32.61 ± 3.53% at week 0 to 34.71 ± 2.57% at week 2, and to 41.45 ± 1.31% at week 4 (F = 4.28, $P = 0.045$; $\eta p^2 = 0.46$).

A significant time interaction was observed only for CHO_{TOT} (F = 4.28, $P = 0.028$). CHO_{TOT} reduced with dGTE from 1.203 ± 0.078 g·min^{-1} at week 0, to 1.144 ± 0.044 g·min^{-1} at week 2, and finally to 1.025 ± 0.048 g·min^{-1} by week 4, representing a reduction of 14.8% or 0.178 ± 0.069 g·min^{-1} (F = 4.02, $P = 0.05$; $\eta p^2 = 0.45$).

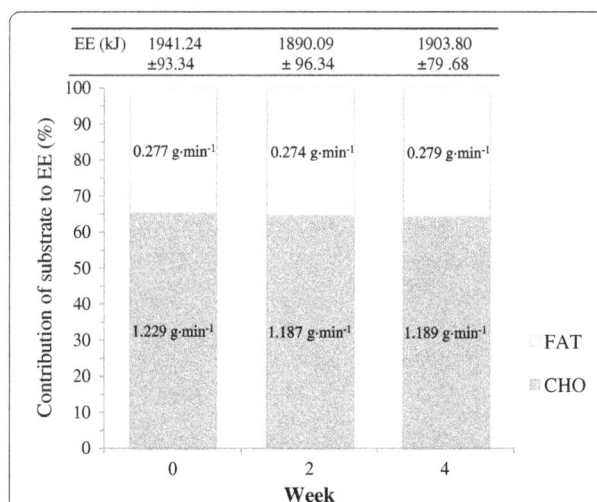

Figure 1 Weekly contribution of substrate to total energy expenditure (EE) for the PL group. Figure 1 shows the contribution of both fat and carbohydrate (based on oxidation rates) to energy expenditure during submaximal exercise for the placebo condition. Data are presented as mean ± SE. PL, Placebo; FAT, average fat oxidation rates; CHO, average carbohydrate oxidation rates. No significant differences were found with ANOVA ($P > 0.05$).

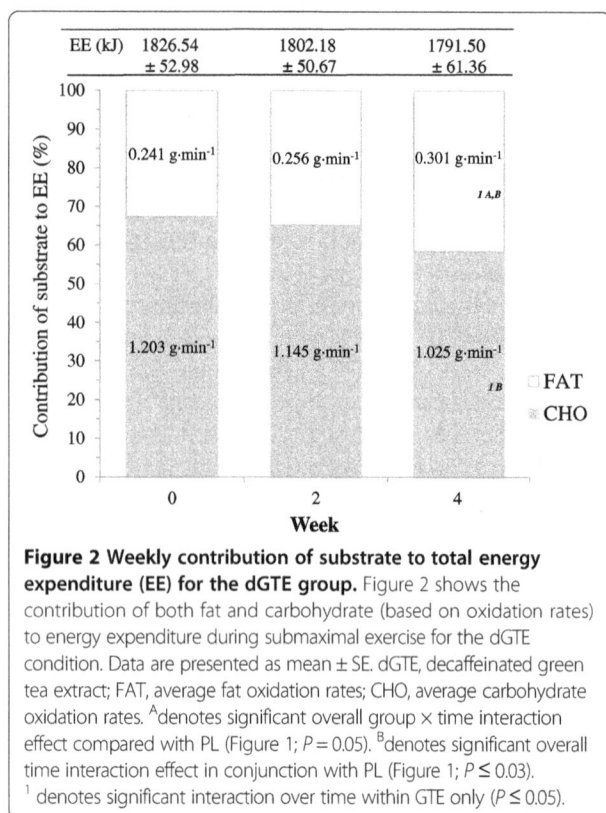

Figure 2 Weekly contribution of substrate to total energy expenditure (EE) for the dGTE group. Figure 2 shows the contribution of both fat and carbohydrate (based on oxidation rates) to energy expenditure during submaximal exercise for the dGTE condition. Data are presented as mean ± SE. dGTE, decaffeinated green tea extract; FAT, average fat oxidation rates; CHO, average carbohydrate oxidation rates. [A]denotes significant overall group × time interaction effect compared with PL (Figure 1; $P = 0.05$). [B]denotes significant overall time interaction effect in conjunction with PL (Figure 1; $P \leq 0.03$). [1] denotes significant interaction over time within GTE only ($P \leq 0.05$).

Correspondingly, percentage contribution of total CHO to exercise EE also reduced with dGTE from $67.39 \pm 3.53\%$ at week 0 to $65.28 \pm 2.57\%$ at week 2, and to $58.55 \pm 1.31\%$ at week 4 (F = 4.28, $P = 0.045$; $\eta p^2 = 0.46$). CHO_{TOT} and contribution of CHO to EE were largely unaffected with PL ($P > 0.05$).

Despite an improvement in FAT_{TOT} for dGTE, no significant differences were observed for TFA concentrations either within or between groups pre-post intervention (Figure 3, $P > 0.05$). It was however noted that TFA concentrations were elevated pre-exercise by week 4 with PL (249.3 ± 46.2 $\mu M \cdot L^{-1}$ at week 0 to 315.4 ± 98.1 $\mu M \cdot L^{-1}$ at week 4, a 26.5% increase, $P > 0.05$) and dGTE (227.9 ± 37.6 $\mu M \cdot L^{-1}$ at week 0 to 289.7 ± 54.8 $\mu M \cdot L^{-1}$ at week 4, a 27.1% increase, $P > 0.05$), with lack of significance most likely explained by individual variance.

It was also noted that whereas TFA concentrations reduced by 18.8% post exercise in the PL group from 616.5 ± 114.8 $\mu M \cdot L^{-1}$ at week 0 to 500.3 ± 141.8 $\mu M \cdot L^{-1}$ at week 4; post exercise TFA concentrations were maintained with dGTE (509.3 ± 90.0 $\mu M \cdot L^{-1}$ at week 0 to 514.3 ± 71.1 $\mu M \cdot L^{-1}$ at week 4), although no significant differences were reported within or between groups ($P > 0.05$). No significant differences were reported for any of the individual fatty acids measured.

Submaximal oxygen uptake values were not different across time either within or between groups (Table 2)

demonstrating compliance to the set intensity ($P > 0.05$). No significant interaction effects were found for expired carbon dioxide, despite a modest reduction in $\dot{V}CO_2$ during submaximal exercise with dGTE from 1.31 ± 0.05 $L \cdot min^{-1}$ at week 0, to 1.25 ± 0.05 $L \cdot min^{-1}$ at week 4 ($P > 0.05$). However, in conjunction with improved FAT_{TOT}, a significant overall group × time interaction was observed for the respiratory exchange ratio (RER; F = 3.30, $P = 0.05$), with values reducing from 0.90 ± 0.01 at week 0 to 0.87 ± 0.01 at week 4 (F = 4.36, $P = 0.044$; $\eta p^2 = 0.47$, within group) supporting reduced reliance on CHO with dGTE. No such modifications for RER were observed with PL ($P > 0.05$).

Although submaximal exercise heart rate reduced by 6.24 ± 3.85 $b \cdot min^{-1}$ (4.8% by week 4) in the PL group, significance across time was only found with dGTE where submaximal exercise heart rate reduced by 8.8% from 124.95 ± 3.69 $b \cdot min^{-1}$ at week 0 to 113.90 ± 4.03 $b \cdot min^{-1}$ at week 4 (F = 4.07, $P = 0.045$; $\eta p^2 = 0.40$). A significant overall group × time interaction was also found for RPE (F = 3.43, $P = 0.05$), with subjects perceiving exercise to be progressively easier with dGTE by week 4 (10.0 ± 0.6 relative effort rating) compared to week 0 (11.9 ± 0.4; $P = 0.015$; $\eta p^2 = 0.58$). No differences were reported for systolic or diastolic blood pressure immediately post exercise over time for either group ($P > 0.05$).

Performance measures

A significant overall group × time interaction was found for distance covered (F = 9.84, $P = 0.001$; Figure 4). The use of dGTE resulted in a progressive increase in distance covered from 20.23 ± 0.54 km at week 0, to 21.77 ± 0.49 km at week 2 and finally 22.43 ± 0.40 km by week 4, representing a 10.9% significant increase in performance (F = 28.66, $P < 0.001$; $\eta p^2 = 0.85$). A similar interaction effect was also observed for PL (F = 7.94, $P = 0.009$; $\eta p^2 = 0.61$) with distance covered significantly improving by week 2 (21.75 ± 0.40 km) compared to week 0 (20.79 ± 0.30 km; $P = 0.002$) only.

In a similar manner, a significant overall group × time interaction was found for average power output (F = 14.43, $P < 0.001$; Figure 4). Average power output increased with dGTE (F = 40.01, $P < 0.001$; $\eta p^2 = 0.89$) by 17.9% or 29.02 ± 5.53 W from week 0 (162.06 ± 10.08 W) to week 2 (191.08 ± 10.85 W; $P = 0.01$); and by 22.7% (or 36.85 ± 3.20 W) from week 0 to week 4 (198.91 ± 8.61 W; $P < 0.001$), but was not significantly different between week 2 and 4 ($P > 0.05$). No significant differences across time for average power output were observed for PL ($P > 0.05$).

Discussion

The use of a 4 week dGTE strategy significantly enhanced FAT_{TOT} by 24.9% or 0.060 ± 0.027 $g \cdot min^{-1}$ compared to

The effect of a decaffeinated green tea extract formula on fat oxidation, body composition and exercise...

127

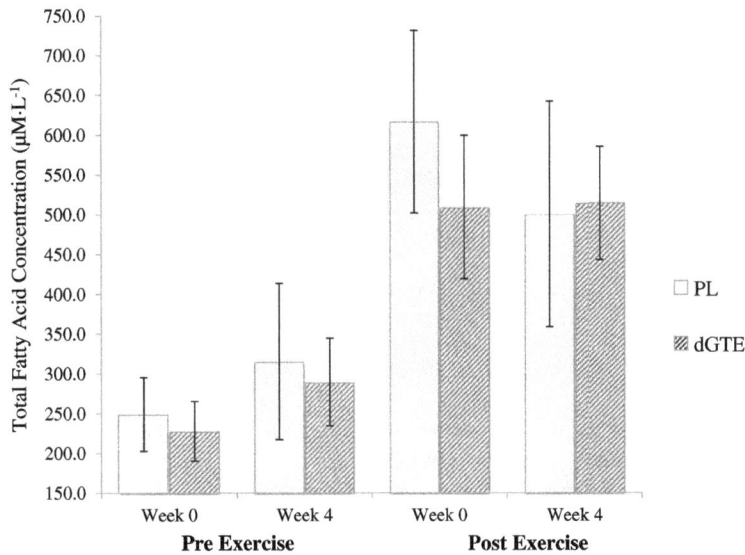

Figure 3 Total fatty acid concentrations pre and post exercise. Figure 3 shows the absolute total fatty acid concentrations at rest and post exercise for both treatment conditions at week 0 and week 4. Data are presented as mean ± SE. PL, Placebo; dGTE, decaffeinated green tea extract. No significant differences were found with ANOVA ($P > 0.05$).

PL supporting the hypothesis set. The increased contribution of total fat to EE with dGTE supports the proposal that EGCG positively influences substrate utilisation, particularly in combination with exercise training. The use of a capsulated dGTE formula in the present study potentially offers a more practical means to regularly consume a sufficient daily dosage to elicit such effects (compared to consumption of ~6-7 cups of green tea per day, especially considering the notable variability of catechin content in commercial green teas).

Improvements in FAT_{TOT} have been demonstrated elsewhere [1,11,32], with current values comparable to those reported when employing an acute dGTE strategy with similar EGCG content [3]. Conversely, higher dose

dGTE over a 28 day period did not enhance substrate metabolism in healthy, male volunteers [25] in contrast to these findings. However, in this latter study, the higher FAT_{TOT} are more typical of endurance trained athletes. It has been inferred that the combined effect of exercise training and GTE may be more relevant for untrained individuals who 'respond' to GTE intervention [25]. Participants in this study were recreationally active. It is therefore plausible that adaptations in exercise metabolism with dGTE are more pronounced with less trained individuals, as opposed to physically active or endurance trained volunteers assessed elsewhere [23-25].

Improved FAT_{TOT}, and reduced reliance on CHO_{TOT} during exercise are of clinical and performance relevance.

Table 2 Assessment of oxygen uptake, mean heart rate, perceived exertion and blood pressure related to submaximal exercise

Variable	PL (n = 7)			dGTE (n = 7)		
	Week 0	Week 2	Week 4	Week 0	Week 2	Week 4
$\dot{V}O_2$ (L·min^{-1})	1.55 ± 0.08	1.51 ± 0.08	1.52 ± 0.06	1.46 ± 0.04	1.44 ± 0.04	1.44 ± 0.05
$\dot{V}CO_2$ (L·min^{-1})	1.38 ± 0.06	1.35 ± 0.06	1.35 ± 0.05	1.31 ± 0.05	1.29 ± 0.03	1.25 ± 0.05
RER	0.89 ± 0.01	0.89 ± 0.01	0.89 ± 0.01	0.90 ± 0.01	0.89 ± 0.01	0.87 ± 0.01 [1] A,B
HR (b·min^{-1})	127.8 ± 5.5	122.7 ± 4.4	121.5 ± 3.8	124.9 ± 3.7	117.0 ± 2.5	113.9 ± 4.0 [1] B
RPE (6–20)	11.1 ± 0.8	11.7 ± 0.6	11.6 ± 0.3	11.9 ± 0.4	11.2 ± 0.4	10.0 ± 0.6* A
SBP (mm Hg)	132.7 ± 2.9	127.4 ± 3.0	127.7 ± 2.9	132.3 ± 2.4	127.6 ± 1.8	126.3 ± 2.9
DBP (mm Hg)	80.1 ± 3.3	74.7 ± 1.9	73.0 ± 2.0	74.4 ± 1.8	76.6 ± 5.1	70.1 ± 3.5

Table 2 demonstrates the influence of the dGTE on cardio-respiratory measures during submaximal steady state exercise across the intervention. Data are presented as mean ± SE. PL, Placebo; dGTE, decaffeinated green tea extract; $\dot{V}O_2$, submaximal oxygen uptake; $\dot{V}CO_2$, submaximal expired carbon dioxide; RER, respiratory exchange ratio; HR, heart rate; RPE, rating of perceived exertion; SBP, systolic blood pressure; DBP, diastolic blood pressure. [A]denotes significant overall group x time interaction effect ($P \leq 0.05$). [B]denotes significant overall time interaction effect only ($P \leq 0.02$). [1]denotes significant within group time interaction effect only ($P \leq 0.045$). [*]denotes significant difference within group to baseline ($P = 0.015$).

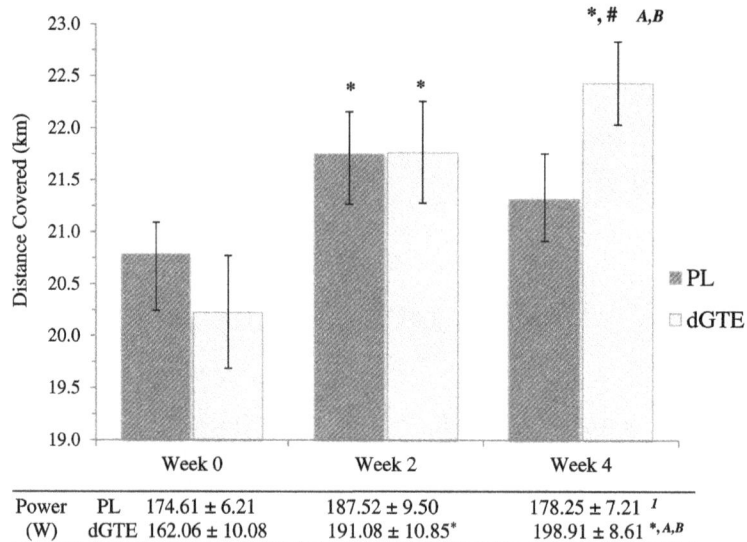

| Power | PL | 174.61 ± 6.21 | 187.52 ± 9.50 | 178.25 ± 7.21 [1] |
| (W) | dGTE | 162.06 ± 10.08 | 191.08 ± 10.85* | 198.91 ± 8.61 *,A,B |

Figure 4 Distance covered and average power output during the performance trial. Figure 4 shows the distance covered and average power output elicited during the 40 minute performance trial for both treatment conditions at week 0, 2 and 4 of the intervention. Data are presented as mean ± SE. PL, Placebo; dGTE, decaffeinated green tea extract. [A]denotes significant overall group × time interaction effect ($P \leq 0.001$). [B]denotes significant overall time interaction effect ($P < 0.001$). [1]denotes significant within group time interaction effect only ($P = 0.039$). *denotes significant difference ($P \leq 0.02$) to baseline only within group. #denotes significant difference to week 2 within group only ($P = 0.03$).

Although resting and post exercise TFAs were not significantly different between groups, the increase in FAT_{TOT} with dGTE supports the contention that the inhibition of COMT may not be a dominant mechanism.

Independently of antioxidant protective mechanisms, it has been proposed that EGCG positively modulates cell signalling via PGC1α [20], sirtuin 1 (SIRT1) and mitogen activated protein kinase (MAPK) pathways [33,34]. In the longer term (>4 weeks), it is feasible that EGCG at moderate dose facilitates up-regulation of gene expression leading to enhanced FAT_{TOT} with exercise.

Although bodyweight reductions were similar between groups, the use of dGTE combined with regulated exercise significantly reduced body fat compared to PL. These findings are similar to those reported elsewhere [10,32,35], particularly when either higher dose GTE or low dose caffeine has been employed. Alterations in body composition, coupled with increased FAT_{TOT} infer that catechin polyphenols favourably modulate cellular metabolism, possibly via a calorie restriction mimetic (CRM) action [36]. This contention is further supported via studies demonstrating enhanced glucose tolerance, insulin sensitivity and adiponectin levels with EGCG [3,37].

In the current study, resting and submaximal exercise heart rate and blood pressure decreased over the intervention period in both groups. However, results were only significant over time with dGTE for exercising heart rate and perceived exertion, possibly relating to substrate utilisation efficiency and improved exercise economy. Additionally, whilst the results could also indicate an acute training stimulus, non-significant reductions in SBP found were comparable to those observed elsewhere [10,13,37]. It is therefore suggested that any mild hypotensive effects are likely due to the short-term influence of regular aerobic activity on nitric oxide pathways than dGTE impacting on endothelial production of nitric oxide synthase.

There has been much interest in the use of GTE to enhance physical performance. In animal studies, time to exhaustion has been shown to improve with GTE by 8-24%, with corresponding evidence of increased ß-oxidation and fatty acid translocase/CD36 mRNA expression [38]. When relatively low GTE/EGCG doses have been employed in humans, improvements in time trial or performance measures have not been observed [22,24]. However, the inclusion of matched caffeine placebo or pre-exercise feeding may explain these findings. Conversely, with higher dose GTE strategies, improvements in maximal oxygen uptake and time trial performance have been observed [39,40].

To the authors' knowledge, this is the first study to demonstrate a significant impact of dGTE on subsequent exercise performance. Performance indices improved by 10.9% for distance covered, and 22.7% for average power output with dGTE. This is unlikely to be fully explained via a training effect as improvements with PL were only observed at week 2 of the trial. Reduced reliance on CHO_{TOT} may have contributed to improved performance following submaximal exercise.

Future research investigating specific effects of EGCC from dGTE on exercise tolerance, performance and recovery is warranted, particularly in light of metabolomic advances [41]. High dose GTE has been demonstrated to reduce muscle soreness following strenuous exercise [42], potentially via signalling interactions leading to reduced post exercise inflammatory cascades [43]. Results in the current study may have been augmented due to utilisation of a low polyphenol diet. Further research combining dietary polyphenols with dGTE is warranted.

Conclusions

In conclusion, dGTE in conjunction with exercise training reduced relative FAT_{TOT} and body composition in recreationally active, male volunteers. Improved metabolic efficiency during submaximal exercise may potentiate improved metabolic economy and hence adherence to longer term training programmes. Combined with the observed impact of dGTE on subsequent performance indices, this supports the contention that EGCG use may modulate cellular signalling pathways leading to more efficient substrate use, resulting in improved exercise output.

Abbreviations

CHO: Carbohydrate; CHO_{TOT}: Total carbohydrate oxidation rate (measured in $g \cdot min^{-1}$); COMT: Catechol-o-methyl transferase; dGTE: Decaffeinated green tea extract; EE: Energy expenditure (measured in $kJ \cdot min^{-1}$); EGCG: (–)-Epigallocatechin-3-gallate; FAT_{TOT}: Total fat oxidation rate (measured in $g \cdot min^{-1}$); GT: Green tea; PL: Placebo formula used in the study; RER: Respiratory exchange ratio the ratio from dividing expired carbon dioxide with oxygen uptake; RPE: Rating of perceived exertion; TFA: Total fatty acids; $\dot{V}O_2$: Volume of oxygen uptake (measured in $L \cdot min^{-1}$); $\dot{V}O_{2peak}$: Peak oxygen uptake (measured in $L \cdot min^{-1}$); $\dot{V}CO_2$: Volume of expired carbon dioxide (measured in $L \cdot min^{-1}$).

Competing interests

Research funding and product supply to support this study was received from High 5 Ltd. All data was collected, analysed and reported by the investigatory team fully independently of the company. The authors declare that they have no competing interest.

Authors' contributions

All authors were involved in the study. JDR was the principal researcher, involved with liaison with the company, project organisation, statistical analysis and manuscript generation; MGR was co-supervisor involved with project co-ordination, quality control and technical accuracy in preparation of the manuscript; MDT was involved with confirmation of statistical analyses, and manuscript editing; JCW and CHT were involved with participant recruitment, pilot data collection, experimental interventions, data analysis and manuscript editing. All authors read and approved the final manuscript.

Acknowledgements

The authors wish to acknowledge High5 Ltd. for providing the support and funding to undertake this study. dGTE was supplied by High 5 Ltd. independently of the investigatory team. The authors also wish to acknowledge the support and external collaboration with ABS Laboratories, Biopark, Welwyn Garden City, for independent assessment of blood samples.

References

1. Dulloo AG, Duret C, Rohrer D, Girardier L, Mensi N, Fathi M, et al. Efficacy of a green tea extract rich in catechin polyphenols and caffeine in increasing 24-h energy expenditure and fat oxidation in humans. Am J Clin Nutr. 1999;70:1040–50.
2. Ryu OH, Lee J, Lee KW, Kim HY, Seo JA, Kim SG, et al. Effects of green tea consumption on inflammation, insulin resistance and pulse wave velocity in type 2 diabetes patients. Diabetes Res Clin Pract. 2006;71:356–8.
3. Venables MC, Hulston CJ, Cox HR, Jeukendrup AE. Green tea extract ingestion, fat oxidation, and glucose tolerance in healthy humans. Am J Clin Nutr. 2008;87:778–84.
4. Mukhtar H, Ahmad N. Tea polyphenols: prevention of cancer and optimizing health. Am J Clin Nutr. 2000;71(6):1698S–702.
5. Maki KC, Reeves MS, Farmer M, Yasunaga K, Matsuo N, Katsuragi Y, et al. Green tea catechin consumption enhances exercise-induced abdominal fat loss in overweight and obese adults. J Nutr. 2009;139(2):264–70.
6. Moore RJ, Jackson KG, Minihane AM. Green tea (Camellia Sinensis) catechins and vascular function. Br J Nutr. 2009;102(12):1790–802.
7. Nantz MP, Rowe CA, Bukowski JF, Percival SS. Standardised capsule of Camellia sinensis lowers cardiovascular risk factors in a randomized, double-blind, placebo-controlled study. Nutr. 2009;25(2):147–54.
8. Valcic S, Burr JA, Timmermann BN, Liebler TC. Antioxidant chemistry of green tea catechins. New oxidation products of (–)-epigallocatechin gallate and (–)-epigallocatechin from their reactions with peroxyl radicals. Chem Res Toxicol. 2000;13(9):801–10.
9. Henning SM, Niu Y, Lee NH, Thames GD, Minutti RR, Wang H, et al. Bioavailability and antioxidant activity of tea flavanols after consumption of green tea, black tea, or a green tea extract supplement. Am J Clin Nutr. 2004;80:1558–64.
10. Nagao T, Hase T, Tokimitsu I. A green tea extract high in catechins reduces body fat and cardiovascular risks in humans. Obesity. 2007;15(6):1473–83.
11. Ichinose T, Nomura S, Someya Y, Akimoto S, Tachiyashiki K, Imaizumi K. Endurance training supplemented with green tea extract on substrate metabolism during exercise in humans. Scand J Med Sci Sports. 2011;21:598–605.
12. Galleano M, Pechanova O, Fraga CG. Hypertension, nitric oxide, and dietary plant polyphenols. Curr Pharm Biotech. 2010;11(8):837–48.
13. Brown AL, Lane J, Coverly J, Stocks J, Jackson S, Stephen A, et al. Effects of dietary supplementation with the green tea polyphenol epigallocatechin-3-gallate on insulin resistance and associated metabolic risk factors: a randomised control trial. Br J Nutr. 2009;101(6):886–94.
14. Rains TM, Agarwal S, Maki KC. Antiobesity effects of green tea catechins: a mechanistic review. J Nutr Biochem. 2011;22(1):1–7.
15. Phung OJ, Baker WL, Matthews LJ, Lanosa M, Thorne A, Coleman CI. Effect of green tea catechins with or without caffeine on anthropometric measures: a systematic review and meta-analysis. Am J Clin Nutr. 2010;91(1):73–81.
16. Hursel R, Viechtbauer W, Westerterp-Plantenga MS. The effects of green tea on weight loss and weight maintenance: A meta-analysis. Int J Obes. 2009;33(9):956–61.
17. Hursel R, Westerterp-Plantenga MS. Thermogenic ingredients and body weight regulation. Int J Obes. 2010;34(4):659–69.
18. Feng WY. Metabolism of green tea catechins: An overview. Curr Drug Metab. 2006;7(7):755–809.
19. Chen C, Wang CY, Lambert JD, Ali N, Welsh WJ, Yang CS. Inhibition of human liver catechol-O-methyltransferase by tea catechins and their metabolites: structure-activity relationship and molecular-modelling studies. Biochem Pharma. 2005;69(10):1523–31.
20. Hodgson AB, Randell RK, Jeukendrup AE. The effect of green tea extract on fat oxidation at rest and during exercise: Evidence of efficacy and proposed mechanisms. Adv Nutr. 2013;4:129–40.
21. Reiter CEN, Kim JA, Kwon MJ. Green tea polyphenol epigallocatechin gallate reduces endothelin-1 expression and secretion in vascular endothelial cells: Roles for AMP activated protein kinase, Akt and FOXO1. Endocrinol. 2009;151(1):103–14.
22. Dean S, Braakhuis A, Paton C. The effects of EGCG on fat oxidation and endurance performance in male cyclists. Int J Sport Nutr Exerc Metab. 2009;20(6):624–44.
23. Eichenberger P, Colombani PC, Mettler S. Effects of a 3-week consumption of green tea extracts on whole-body metabolism during cycling exercise in endurance-trained men. Int J Vitam Nutr Res. 2009;79(1):24–33.

24. Eichenberger P, Mettler S, Arnold M, Colombani PC. No effects of three-week consumption of a green tea extract on time trial performance in endurance trained men. Int J Vitam Nutr Res. 2010;80(1):54–64.

25. Randell RK, Hodgson AB, Lotito SB, Jacobs DM, Rowson M, Mela DJ. Variable duration of decaffeinated green tea extract ingestion on exercise metabolism. Med Sci Sports Exerc. 2014;46(6):1185–93.

26. Faul F, Erdfelder E, Lang A-G, Buchner A. G*power 3: a flexible statistical power analysis program for the social, behavioral, and biomedical sciences. Behav Res Meth. 2007;39(2):175–91.

27. Roberts JD, Tarpey MD, Kass LS, Tarpey RJ, Roberts MG. Assessing a commercially available sports drink on exogenous carbohydrate oxidation, fluid delivery and sustained exercise performance. J Int Soc Sports Nutr. 2014;11(8):1–14.

28. Kao M-F, Lu H-K, Jang T-R, Yang W-C, Chen C-H, Chen Y-Y, et al. Comparison of different measurement equations for body composition estimation in male athletes. Int J Sport Exerc Sci. 2010;3(1):11–6.

29. Borg G. Ratings of perceived exertion and heart rates during short term cycle exercise and their use in a new strength test. Int J Sports Med. 1982;3(3):153–8.

30. Jeukendrup AE, Wallis GA. Measurement of substrate oxidation during exercise by means of gas exchange measurements. Int J Sports Med. 2005;26(1):S28–37.

31. Kangani CO, Kelley DE, DeLany JP. New method for GC/FID and GC-C-IRMS analysis of plasma free fatty acid concentration and isotopic enrichment. J Chromatogr B Analyt Technol Biomed Life Sci. 2008;873(1):95–101.

32. Westerterp-Plantenga MS, Lejeune MPGM, Kovacs EMR. Body weight loss and weight maintenance in relation to habitual caffeine intake and green tea supplementation. Obes Res. 2005;13:1195–204.

33. Ayissi VBO, Ebrahimi A, Schluesenner H. Epigenetic effects of natural polyphenols: a focus on SIRT1-mediated mechanisms. Mol Nutr Food Res. 2014;58:22–32.

34. Kim H-S, Quon MJ, Kim J-A. New insights into the mechanisms of polyphenols beyond antioxidant properties: lessons from the green tea polyphenol, epigallocatechin 3-gallate. Redox Biol. 2014;2:187–95.

35. Wang H, Wen Y, Du Y, Yan X, Guo H, Rycroft JA, et al. Effects of catechin enriched green tea on body composition. Obesity. 2010;18:773–9.

36. Madeo F, Pietrocola F, Eisenberg T, Kroemer G. Calorie restriction mimetics: towards a molecular definition. Nat Rev: Drug Disc. 2014;13(10):727–40.

37. Potenza MA, Marasciulo FL, Tarquinio M, Tiravanti E, Colantuono G, Federici A, et al. EGCG, a green tea polyphenol, improves endothelial function and insulin sensitivity, reduces blood pressure, and protects against myocardial I/R injury in SHR. Am J Physiol Endocrinol Metab. 2007;292:E1378–87.

38. Murase T, Haramizu S, Shimotoyodome A, Tokimitsu I, Hase T. Green tea improves running endurance in mice by stimulating lipid utilization during exercise. Am J Physiol Reg Integr Comp Physiol. 2006;290(6):R1550–6.

39. MacRae HSH, Mefferd KM. Dietary antioxidant supplementation combined with quercetin improves cycling time trial performance. Int J Sport Nutr Exer Metab. 2006;16(4):405–19.

40. Richards JC, Lonac MC, Johnson TK, Schweder MM, Bell C. Epigallocatechin-3-gallate increases maximal oxygen consumption in adult humans. Med Sci Sports Exerc. 2010;42(4):739–44.

41. Nieman DC, Gillitt ND, Knab AM, Shanely RA, Pappan KL, Jin F, et al. Influence of a polyphenol-enriched protein powder on exercise-induced inflammation and oxidative stress in athletes: a randomized trial using a metabolomics approach. Plos One. 2013;8(8):1–11.

42. Moradpourian MR, Ashkavand Z, Venkatesh C, Vishwanath BS. Effect of different doses of green tea on oxidative stress and muscle soreness in downhill treadmill running. Asian J Pharm Clin Res. 2014;7(2):192–3.

43. Cunha CA, Lira FS, Neto JCR, Pimentel GD, Souza GIH, da Silva CMG, et al. Green tea extract supplementation induces the lipolytic pathway, attenuates obesity, and reduces low-grade inflammation in mice fed a high-fat diet. Mediators Inflamm. 2013;2013:1–8.

16

Undenatured type II collagen (UC-II®) for joint support: a randomized, double-blind, placebo-controlled study in healthy volunteers

James P Lugo[1], Zainulabedin M Saiyed[1], Francis C Lau[1], Jhanna Pamela L Molina[2], Michael N Pakdaman[2], Arya Nick Shamie[3] and Jay K Udani[2,4*]

Abstract

Background: UC-II contains a patented form of undenatured type II collagen derived from chicken sternum. Previous preclinical and clinical studies support the safety and efficacy of UC-II in modulating joint discomfort in osteoarthritis and rheumatoid arthritis. The purpose of this study was to assess the efficacy and tolerability of UC-II in moderating joint function and joint pain due to strenuous exercise in healthy subjects.

Methods: This randomized, double-blind, placebo-controlled study was conducted in healthy subjects who had no prior history of arthritic disease or joint pain at rest but experienced joint discomfort with physical activity. Fifty-five subjects who reported knee pain after participating in a standardized stepmill performance test were randomized to receive placebo (n = 28) or the UC-II (40 mg daily, n = 27) product for 120 days. Joint function was assessed by changes in degree of knee flexion and knee extension as well as measuring the time to experiencing and recovering from joint pain following strenuous stepmill exertion.

Results: After 120 days of supplementation, subjects in the UC-II group exhibited a statistically significant improvement in average knee extension compared to placebo ($81.0 \pm 1.3°$ vs $74.0 \pm 2.2°$; p = 0.011) and to baseline ($81.0 \pm 1.3°$ vs $73.2 \pm 1.9°$; p = 0.002). The UC-II cohort also demonstrated a statistically significant change in average knee extension at day 90 ($78.8 \pm 1.9°$ vs $73.2 \pm 1.9°$; p = 0.045) versus baseline. No significant change in knee extension was observed in the placebo group at any time. It was also noted that the UC-II group exercised longer before experiencing any initial joint discomfort at day 120 (2.8 ± 0.5 min, p = 0.019), compared to baseline (1.4 ± 0.2 min). By contrast, no significant changes were seen in the placebo group. No product related adverse events were observed during the study. At study conclusion, five individuals in the UC-II cohort reported no pain during or after the stepmill protocol (p = 0.031, within visit) as compared to one subject in the placebo group.

Conclusions: Daily supplementation with 40 mg of UC-II was well tolerated and led to improved knee joint extension in healthy subjects. UC-II also demonstrated the potential to lengthen the period of pain free strenuous exertion and alleviate the joint pain that occasionally arises from such activities.

Keywords: UC-II, Undenatured type II collagen, Joint function, Knee extension, Stepmill, Joint pain

* Correspondence: jay.udani@medicusresearch.com
[2]Medicus Research LLC, 28720 Roadside Drive, Suite 310, Agoura Hills, CA 91301, USA
[4]Northridge Hospital Integrative Medicine Program, Northridge, CA 91325, USA
Full list of author information is available at the end of the article

Introduction

The impact of strenuous exercise on knee joints may cause localized pain and stiffness, which are hallmark features of pathologic inflammatory disease [1]. It has been shown that when dogs undergo a strenuous running regimen, significant losses in articular cartilage and glycosaminoglycans occur [2]. Such studies suggest that strenuous exercise may activate some of the same physiological processes that occur in arthritic disease [2-4]. In fact, *in vitro* studies have shown that many of the cytokines implicated in the onset and progression of both rheumatoid arthritis (RA) and osteoarthritis (OA) also appear to regulate the remodeling of the normal knee extracellular matrix (ECM) following strenuous exertion [5].

When normal chondrocytes undergo strenuous mechanical stimulation under static conditions, their physiology shifts towards ECM breakdown, as indicated by the upregulation of several metalloproteinases (MMPs), such as MMP-13 as well as tumor necrosis factor (TNF)-α, interleukin (IL)-1β, IL-6, and various aggrecanases [5,6]. This *in vitro* catabolic response is mediated by changes in the phosphorylation, expression, or translocation of several transcription factors to the cell nucleus such as NF-κB, p38 MAPK, Akt, and ERK [7,8]. By contrast, normal chondrocytes produce the anti-inflammatory cytokine IL-4 when mechanically stimulated under moderate and dynamic conditions [9]. The secretion of this autocrine molecule not only helps in shifting chondrocyte metabolism towards the synthesis of aggrecan and type II collagen, it also downregulates production of nitric oxide (NO) and various MMPs and aggrecanases [10-12]. This conclusion is corroborated by the finding that pretreatment of strenuously compressed normal chondrocytes with IL-4 attenuates their catabolic response [11]. This suggests that IL-4 plays a key role in downregulating remodeling functions, restoring articular cartilage homeostasis, as well as decreasing chondrocyte apoptosis following strenuous mechanical loading [12,13].

Mechanically stressed chondrocytes also produce a number of other molecules known to participate in inflammatory responses, including prostoglandin E2, NO, and vascular endothelial growth factor [14]. These are proinflammatory molecules that, in conjunction with TNF-α, IL-6 and IL-1β, result in a localized, and transitory inflammatory-like response that is part of the normal repair process occurring in knee joints, serves to moderate remodeling events [3]. Ostrowski et al. [15] showed that healthy individuals express up to 27-fold greater concentrations of the anti-inflammatory cytokine IL-10 in blood following a marathon run when compared to IL-10 blood levels at rest. This finding is not surprising given that these same individuals also show marked increases in the proinflammatory cytokines TNF-α, IL-1β, and IL-6. It therefore appears that in healthy subjects undergoing strenuous exertion, the induction of proinflammatory cytokines is offset by the synthesis of anti-inflammatory agents as part of the recovery process. This view is supported by the observation that IL-10 reduces the catabolic impact of IL-1β and TNF-α on cartilage explants from healthy volunteers, and this effect is enhanced by combining IL-10 with IL-4 [13].

Another protein released by dynamically compressed chondrocytes is transforming growth factor (TGF)-β [16-18]. This factor is secreted by many cell types and is known to interfere with the cell cycle and arrest differentiation [19]. With regard to chondrocytes, TGF-β induces cell proliferation *in vitro* and slows terminal differentiation into hypertrophic cells [20]. Numerous studies have shown that TGF-β reverses the *in vitro* catabolic effect of various proinflammatory cytokines on normal chondrocytes as well as chondrocytes harvested from RA and OA donors [21-23].

The overall findings discussed above point to a new, unifying view of joint physiology. It suggests that many of the biological processes occurring in knee joints affected by RA and OA also participate in the maintenance of healthy knees [1,4,5]. It therefore seems appropriate to test the efficacy of natural supplements or ingredients, which have been shown to moderate joint pain in RA and OA, as possible candidates for treating the joint discomfort that occasionally results from strenuous exercise in healthy individuals.

UC-II is a natural ingredient which contains a glycosylated, undenatured type-II collagen [24]. Previous studies have shown that small doses of UC-II modulate joint health in both OA and RA [24-26]. Tong et al. [27], using an *in vivo* model of collagen induced arthritis (CIA), demonstrated that ingesting microgram quantities of undenatured type II collagen significantly reduces circulating levels of inflammatory cytokines, potentially serving to decrease both the incidence and the severity of arthritis [28]. The ability to alter immunity via the ingestion of a food, or an antigen, is called oral tolerance. This is an ongoing normal physiological process that protects the alimentary tract against untoward immunological damage [29,30]. Research into its mechanism of action has revealed that several distinct types of T regulator cells mediate this phenomenon by releasing IL-10 and TGF-β [30]. It has also been shown that this effect is transitory in nature requiring that the food, or antigen, be consumed continuously in order to maintain the tolerogenic state [30]. Given these findings, plus our current understanding of the role of various cytokines in normal joint physiology, it was hypothesized that supplementation with UC-II might relieve joint discomfort and restore joint function in healthy subjects.

The aim of this randomized, double blind, placebo-controlled study was to assess the impact of UC-II on knee function in otherwise healthy subjects with no prior history of arthritic disease who experienced knee pain upon strenuous physical exertion. The primary efficacy variable for assessing knee function included measurements of flexibility using range of motion (ROM) goniometry.

Methods

Investigational product

The investigational study product UC-II is derived from chicken sternum. It is manufactured using a patented, low-temperature process to preserve its native structure. For the clinical study, 40 mg of UC-II material (Lot 1109006), which provides 10.4 ± 1.3 mg of native type-II collagen, was encapsulated in an opaque capsule with excipients. Placebo was dispensed in an identical capsule containing only excipients (microcrystalline cellulose, magnesium stearate and silicon dioxide). Both study materials were prepared in a good manufacturing practice (GMP)-certified facility and provided by InterHealth Nutraceuticals, Inc. (Benicia, CA). Subjects were instructed to take one capsule daily with water before bedtime.

Recruitment of subjects

One hundred and six subjects were screened for eligibility using the inclusion–exclusion criteria defined in Table 1. Only healthy adults who presented with no knee joint pain at rest and no diagnosable markers indicative of active arthritic disease, as outlined by the American College of Rheumatology (ACR) guidelines [31,32], were admitted into the study. To accomplish this, all potential subjects were screened by a board certified clinician. Subjects presenting with any knee pain at rest and at least 3 of 6 clinical classification criteria, which included age greater than 50 years, morning stiffness in the joint lasting 30 minutes or less, crepitus on knee joint manipulation, body tenderness, bony enlargements, knee swelling or presence of excess fluid, and palpable warmth, were excluded. Potential subjects reporting the occasional use of NSAIDs, other pain relief medication, or anti-inflammatory supplements underwent a 2-week washout period before randomization.

Subjects were required to undergo a 10 minute period of performance testing using a standardized stepmill test developed and validated by Medicus Research (Udani JK, unpublished observation). It involved exercising at level 4 on a StepMill® model 7000PT (StairMaster® Health & Fitness Products, Inc., Kirkland, WA) until one or both knees achieved a discomfort level of 5 on an 11 point (0–10) Likert scale [33]. This pain threshold had to be achieved within a 10 minute period otherwise the subject was excluded. Once the requisite pain level was achieved the subject was asked to continue stepping for an additional two minutes in order to record the maximum pain level achieved before disembarking from the stepmill. The following knee discomfort measures were recorded from the start of the stepmill test: (1) time to onset of initial joint pain; (2) time to onset of maximum joint pain; (3) time to initial improvement in knee joint pain; (4) time to complete recovery from knee joint pain. Subjects who experienced a pain score of 5 (or greater) within one minute of starting the stress test were excluded. Out of 106 screened candidates, 55 subjects were enrolled in the study. Each subject voluntarily signed the IRB-approved informed consent form. After enrollment, the subjects were randomly assigned to either the placebo or the UC-II group.

Study design and trial site

This randomized, double blind, placebo-controlled study was conducted at the Staywell Research clinical site located in Northridge, CA. Medicus Research (Agoura Hills, CA) was the contract research organization (CRO) of record. The study protocol was approved by Copernicus Group IRB (Cary, NC) on April 25th 2012. The study followed the principles outlined in the Declaration of Helsinki (version 1996).

Randomization and blinding

Simple randomization was employed using a software algorithm based on the atmospheric noise method (www.random.org). Sequential assignment was used to determine group allocation. Once allocated, the assignment was documented and placed in individually numbered envelopes to maintain blinding. Subjects, clinical staff, plus data analysis and management staff remained blinded throughout the study.

Study schedule

The study duration was 17 weeks with a total of 7 visits that included screening, baseline, days 7, 30, 60, 90 and 120 (final visit). Table 2 summarizes the study visits and activities. Figure 1 depicts the sequence of study procedures that subjects underwent during each visit. All subjects completed a medical history questionnaire at baseline and compliance reports during follow-up evaluations at 7, 30, 60, 90 and 120 days. Subjects were assessed for anthropometric measures, vital signs, knee range of motion (flexion and extension), six-minute timed walk, as well as the onset and recovery from pain using the Udani Stepmill Procedure. A Fitbit (San Francisco, CA) device was used to measure daily distance walked, steps taken and an average step length for study participants. Subjects were also asked to complete the KOOS survey as well as the Stanford exercise scales.

Table 1 Inclusion–exclusion criteria

Inclusion

- Subject must be ≥30 and ≤65 years of age

- Body mass index (BMI) must be ≥18 and ≤35 kg/m^2

- Knee joint criteria: (1) no knee joint discomfort at rest; (2) must achieve a knee joint discomfort score of at least 5 on an 11-point Likert scale within 10 minutes of initiating the stepmill protocol

- Maintain existing food and physical activity patterns throughout the study period

- Judged by Investigator to be in general good health on the basis of medical history

- Subject understands the study procedures and provides signed informed consent to participate in the study and authorizes the release of relevant health information to the study investigator

- Females of child bearing age must agree to use approved birth control methods during the study

Exclusion

- Subjects with any indicators of arthritis, joint disorders, or history of immune system or autoimmune disorders

- Daily use of NSAIDs; however, daily use of 81 mg of aspirin for cardioprotection is allowed

- Daily use of anti-inflammatory or omega-3-fatty acid dietary supplements or using supplements to maintain joint health 30 days prior to screening

- Subjects with a history of knee or hip joint replacement surgery, or any hip or back pain which interferes with ambulation

- Use of any immunosuppressive drugs in the last 12 months (including steroids or biologics)

- Glucocorticoid injection or hyaluronic acid injection in affected knee within 3 months prior to enrollment

- History of surgery or significant injury to the target joint within 6 months prior to study enrollment, or an anticipated need for surgical or invasive procedure that will be performed during the study

- Subjects with a chronic pain syndrome and in the judgment of the Investigator is unlikely to respond to any therapy

- Participation in a clinical study with exposure to any non-registered drug product within 30 days prior

- Subjects who have any physical disability which could interfere with their ability to perform the functional performance measures included in this protocol

- Any significant GI condition that would potentially interfere with the evaluation of the study product

- Clinically significant renal, hepatic, endocrine (including diabetes mellitus), cardiac, pulmonary, pancreatic, neurologic, hematologic, or biliary disorder

- Subjects with vascular condition which interferes with ambulation

- Known allergy or sensitivity to herbal products, soy or eggs

- Vegetarian or Vegan

- History or presence of cancer in the prior two years, except for non-melanoma skin cancer.

- Individual has a condition the Investigator believes would interfere with his or her ability to provide informed consent, comply with the study protocol, which might confound the interpretation of the study results or put the person at undue risk

Table 1 Inclusion–exclusion criteria *(Continued)*

- Untreated or unstable hypothyroidism, an active eating disorder, or evidence of any neurological disorders

- Recent history of (within 12 months) or strong potential for alcohol or substance abuse

- Females who are pregnant, lactating, or unwilling to use adequate contraception during the study

Knee range of motion measurements

Knee extension was measured by goniometry. Briefly, subjects were instructed to sit in an upright position on a table edge with their backs straight (knee position defined as 90°). The axis of a goniometer was placed at the intersection of the thigh and shank at the knee joint. Subjects were asked to bring their knees to full extension without changing the position of the pelvis and lumbar spine. The extended knee joint angle was measured and recorded. For knee flexion measurement, subjects were asked to actively flex their knees while lying in a prone position with their shins off the end of the table. The range of knee flexion motion was then measured and documented.

Timed joint discomfort measurements

Briefly, a stopwatch was started when subjects began climbing the stepmill. Time to onset of pain was recorded at the first sign of pain in the target knee. The baselines at each time point were normalized to account for dropouts. Percent change in time to complete recovery from pain was measured as follows: a new stopwatch was started when the subjects disembarked from the stepmill and the time to complete recovery from pain was recorded. The baselines at each time point were normalized to account for dropouts then compared against the reference interval which was defined as the percentage change between the study baseline and day 7.

KOOS knee survey & Stanford exercise scales

The KOOS survey is a validated instrument consisting of 42 questions that are classified into sub-scales such as symptoms, stiffness, pain, daily activities, recreational activities and quality of life [34]. It measures the subjects' opinion about their knees and their ability to perform daily activities during the past week. The Stanford exercise behavior scale comprises 6 questions designed to assess exercise behaviors during the previous week [35].

Six minute timed walk

Subjects were instructed to walk up and down a hallway for 6 minutes as rapidly as possible without causing any pain. A measuring wheel (RoadRunner Wheel, Keson Industries, Aurora, IL) was used to measure distance travelled in 6 minutes.

Table 2 Protocol summary

Protocol activities	V1	V2	V3	V4	V5	V6	V7
	Day −7	Day 0	Day 7	Day 30	Day 60	Day 90	Day 120
	Screen	Baseline					End
Informed consent	X						
Inclusion/Exclusion	X						
Medical history and physical exam	X						
Vital signs/anthropometric measures	X	X	X	X	X	X	X
Urine pregnancy test	X	X					
Administer and review scales/questionnaires/diaries	X	X	X	X	X	X	X
Stressor (Udani Stepmill protocol)	X	X	X	X	X	X	X
Functional measures (6-min timed walk)	X	X	X	X	X	X	X
Goniometry (range of motion)		X	X	X	X	X	X
Review concomitant therapies	X	X	X	X	X	X	X
Intercurrent medical issues review		X	X	X	X	X	X
Compliance assessment (including phone calls)		X	X	X	X	X	X
Randomization		X					
Study supplement preparation & dispensing		X	X	X	X	X	

Rescue medication

No rescue medications were allowed during the course of the study. At all study visits, subjects were given a list of the 43 prohibited medications and supplements (Table 3). Changes in overall medication history, or the use of these substances, were then recorded by the study coordinator. Subjects found to have used any of these prohibited substances were excluded from further participation in the study as per protocol.

Statistics

Outcome variables were assessed for conformance to the normal distribution and transformed as required. Within group significance was analyzed by non-parametric Sign

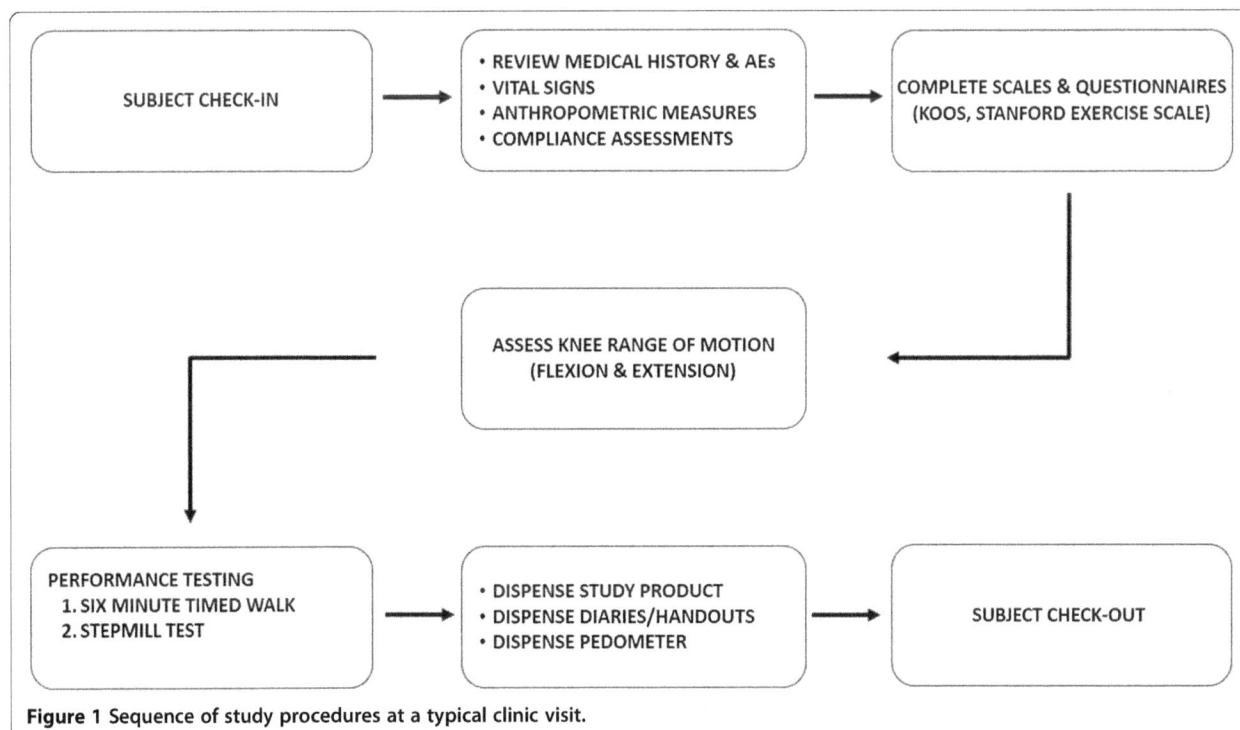

Figure 1 Sequence of study procedures at a typical clinic visit.

Table 3 Representative list of prohibited medications* by category

Category	Medications
Joint supplements (Omega-3, Omega-6 plus others)	Alpha-Linolenic acid
	Docosapentaenoic acid
	Docosahexaenoic acid
	Eicosatrienoic acid
	Eicosatetraenoic acid
	Eicosapentaenoic acid
	Hexadecatrienoic acid
	Heneicosapentaenoic acid
	Stearidonic acid
	Tetracosapentaenoic acid
	Tetracosahexaenoic acid
	Glucosamine (all forms)
	Chondroitin (all forms)
	Other herbal ingredients
NSAIDs (OTC and prescription)	Aspirin
	Diflunisal
	Diclofenac
	Celecoxib
	Etodolac
	Fenoprofen
	Flurbiprofen
	Ibuprofen
	Indomethacin
	Ketoprofen
	Meclofenamate
	Mefenamic acid
	Meloxicam
	Nabumetone
	Naproxen
	Oxaprozin
	Piroxicam
	Rofecoxib
	Sulindac
	Tolmetin
	Valdecoxib

*Selected from a list of 43 prohibited medications and supplements.

test or by non-parametric Wilcoxon Signed Rank test, while Wilcoxon Mann–Whitney test was used to analyze between groups significance. The Fisher Exact test was used to evaluate the complete loss of pain between study cohorts whereas the binomial test was used to assess the likelihood of complete loss of pain at each visit. P-values equal to or less than 0.05 were considered statistically significant. All analyses were done on a per protocol

basis using SPSS, v19 (IBM, Armonk, NY). Results were presented as mean ± SEM.

Results

Baseline demographics

A total of 55 individuals met the eligibility criteria and were randomized to the placebo (n = 28) or to the UC-II (n = 27) group. Baseline demographic characteristics for subjects in both groups were similar with respect to age, gender, height, weight and BMI (Table 4). A total of nine subjects, three in UC-II group and six in placebo group, were lost to follow-up. The results presented herein encompass 46 total subjects, 22 subjects in the placebo group plus 24 subjects in the UC-II group. It should be noted that the average age of the study participants was approximately 46 years which is about 16 years younger than the average age observed in many OA studies [36-38].

Knee extension and flexion

Figure 2 summarizes the average knee extension changes over time for subjects supplemented with either UC-II or placebo. The UC-II supplemented cohort presented with a statistically significant greater increase in the ability to extend the knee at day 120 as compared to the placebo group (81.0 ± 1.3° vs 74.0 ± 2.2°, p = 0.011) and to baseline (81.0 ± 1.3° vs 73.2 ± 1.9°, p = 0.002). The UC-II group also demonstrated a significant increase in knee extension at day 90 (78.8 ± 1.9° vs 73.2 ± 1.9°, p = 0.045) compared to baseline only. An intent to treat (ITT) analysis of these data also demonstrated a statistically significant net increase in knee extension at day 120 versus placebo (80.0 ± 1.3° vs 73.7 ± 1.8°, p = 0.006). No statistically significant changes were observed in the placebo group at any time during this study. With respect to knee flexion, no significant changes were noted in either study group (p > 0.05). The power associated with the former per protocol statistical analyses was 80%.

Time to onset of initial joint pain

Supplementation with UC-II resulted in statistically significant increases in the time to onset of initial joint pain at day 90 (2.75 ± 0.5 min, p = 0.041) and at day 120 (2.8 ± 0.5 min, p = 0.019) versus a baseline of 1.4 min for each visit. No statistically significant differences were noted for either the placebo group or between groups (Figure 3).

Five individuals in the UC-II group and one in the placebo group reported no onset of pain by the end of study (see below and Table 5). Given this unexpected finding, an additional analysis was undertaken which included these individuals in the time to onset of initial pain analysis. The 10 minute limit of the stepmill procedure was used as the lower limit to pain onset. Under

Table 4 Demographic and baseline characteristics of enrolled subjects

Characteristics	UC-II	Placebo
Total number of subjects	27	28
Number of males	11	12
Number of females	16	16
Age (years)	46.1 ± 1.5	46.6 ± 1.8
Weight (kg)	75.5 ± 2.9	77.5 ± 3.1
Height (cm)	167.1 ± 2.0	168.4 ± 2.0
BMI (kg/m^2)	26.8 ± 0.8	27.1 ± 0.7

Values are expressed as Mean ± SEM.

these conservative assumptions, supplementation with UC-II yielded statistically significant increases in time to onset of pain at day 90 (3.65 ± 0.7 min, $p = 0.011$) and day 120 (4.31 ± 0.7 min, $p = 0.002$) versus a baseline of 1.4 min for each visit. The between-group comparison at day 120 approached the statistical level of significance favoring the UC-II cohort ($p = 0.051$).

Time to onset of maximum joint pain
A statistically significant difference between groups was noted at day 60 (6.39 ± 0.5 min vs 4.78 ± 0.5 min; $p = 0.025$) favoring the UC-II cohort. This significance did not persist during the remainder of the study suggesting that this was a random occurrence.

Time to initial improvement in knee joint pain
The time to offset of joint pain was recorded immediately upon the subject stepping off the stepmill. Both groups began to recover from pain with the same rate resulting in no significant differences between groups in the time to initial offset of joint pain ($p > 0.05$).

Time to complete recovery from knee joint pain
The time to complete recovery from joint pain showed significant reductions at days 60, 90 and 120 compared to baseline for both the UC-II group as well as the placebo group (Figure 4). Percent changes in times were calculated after normalizing the baselines against the reference range of baseline to day 7. The UC-II group exhibited average reductions of $31.9 \pm 11.7\%$ ($p = 0.041$), $51.1 \pm 6.1\%$ ($p = 0.004$) and $51.9 \pm 6.0\%$ ($p = 0.011$) at days 60, 90 and 120, respectively. By contrast, the reductions for the same time points for the placebo cohort, $21.9 \pm 10.2\%$ ($p = 0.017$), $22.2 \pm 15.5\%$ ($p = 0.007$) and $30.0 \pm 11.8\%$ ($p = 0.012$), were of lower magnitude but nonetheless statistically significant versus baseline. None of these between group differences achieved statistical significance.

Time to complete loss of knee joint pain
During the course of this study it was noted that a number of subjects in both the placebo and the supplemented cohorts no longer reported any pain during the stepmill protocol. For the UC-II group, 5 subjects (21%) no longer reported pain by day 120, whereas only 1 subject (5%) in placebo group reported complete loss of pain (Table 5). This effect did not reach statistical significance between groups but there was an evident trend in the data towards a greater number of subjects losing pain in the UC-II cohort ($p = 0.126$). A binomial analysis for complete loss of pain at each visit demonstrated a statistical significance for the UC-II group by day 120 ($p = 0.031$). It is important to note that the complete loss of knee pain was not a random event. The pattern among the subjects indicates that loss of knee pain appeared to be a persistent phenomenon that spanned multiple visits (Table 5). A detailed review of the clinical report forms showed that none of these individuals consumed pain relief medication prior to their visits.

Six-minute timed walk & Daily number of steps
No significant differences were observed between the study groups for the six-minute time walk or the daily number of steps taken ($p > 0.05$). The distance walked in six-minutes by the UC-II (range = 505 to 522 meters) and the placebo (range = 461 to 502 meters) groups were within the reference range previously reported [39] for healthy adults (399 to 778 meters, males; 310 to 664 meters, females). Similarly, the average step length calculated from Fitbit data for both study groups (0.69 to 0.71 meters) also agreed with previously published results for normal adults [40].

KOOS knee survey & Stanford exercise scales
No significant differences were seen between the study groups for either the KOOS survey or the Stanford exercise scale ($p > 0.05$).

Use of analgesics and NSAIDs
Review of the clinical report forms showed that no subject in either study cohort consumed any of the 43 prohibited medicines or supplements during the study.

Safety assessments
A total of eight adverse events, equally dispersed between both groups, were noted (Table 6). None of the adverse events was considered to be associated with UC-II supplementation. All events resolved spontaneously without the need for further intervention. No subject withdrew from the study due to an adverse event. Finally, no differences were observed in vital signs after

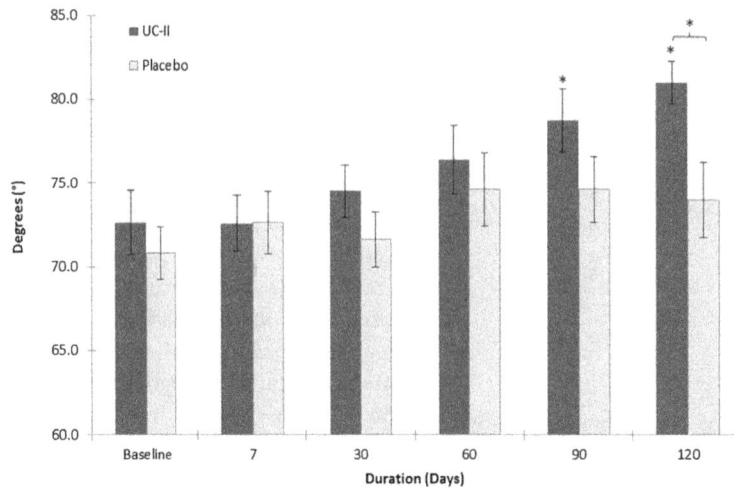

Figure 2 Knee extension as measured by goniometry. Values are presented as Mean ± SEM. *p ≤ 0.05 indicates a statistically significant difference versus baseline or placebo. Number of completers: n = 24 in UC-II group (n = 3 dropouts); n = 20 in placebo group (n = 6 dropouts; n = 2 did not participate in ROM assessment).

seventeen weeks of supplementation, and no serious adverse events were reported in this study.

Discussion

In this study, the UC-II supplement, consisting of undenatured type II collagen, was investigated for its ability to improve joint function in healthy subjects who develop joint pain while undergoing strenuous exercise. The rationale behind this approach centered on the hypothesis that strenuous exercise might uncover transient joint changes due to daily physical activities that are not attributable to a diagnosable disease. In the same way that nominally elevated blood levels of lipids, glucose plus high blood pressure and obesity can be predictive of future progression to diabetes and heart disease [41], the development of joint pain upon strenuous exercise may be indicative of possible future joint problems.

At study conclusion, we found that subjects ingesting the UC-II supplement experienced a significantly greater forward ROM in their knees versus baseline and placebo

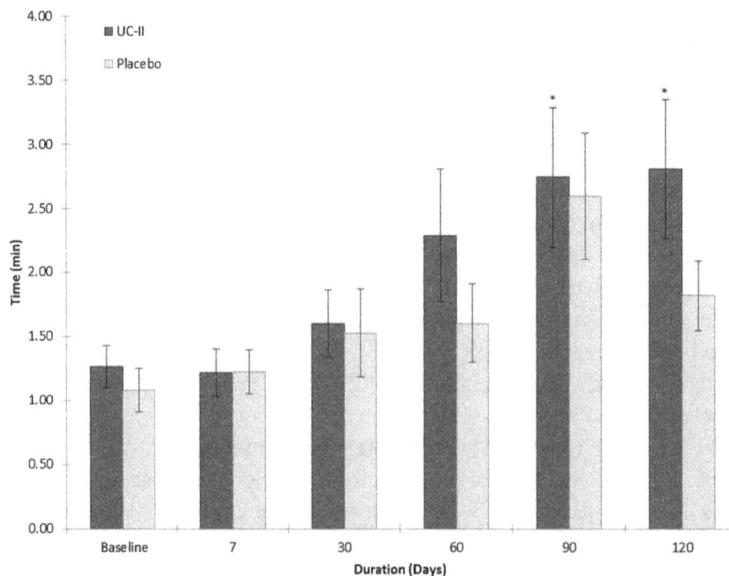

Figure 3 Impact of stepmill procedure on the onset of pain. Values are presented as Mean ± SEM. *p ≤ 0.05 indicates a statistically significant difference from baseline. Number of completers: n = 19 in UC-II group (n = 3 dropouts; n = 5 did not have pain); n = 20 in placebo group (n = 6 dropouts; n = 1 did not have pain; n = 1 did not use stepmill).

Table 5 Subjects reporting complete loss of knee pain on stepmill test

Visit	UC-II			Placebo		
	No. of pain free subjects (%)	Continuity of pain loss#	P value (Binomial test)	No. of pain free subjects (%)	Continuity of pain loss#	P value (Binomial test)
Baseline	0.0 (0)	0	NA	0.0 (0)	0	NA
Day 7	0.0 (0)	0	NA	0.0 (0)	0	NA
Day 30	1.0 (4)	1N	0.5	0.0 (0)	0	NA
Day 60	3.0 (13)	1R, 2N	0.125	0.0 (0)	0	NA
Day 90	3.0 (13)	2R, 1N	0.125	1 (5)	1N	0.5
Day 120	5.0 (21)	3R, 2N	0.031[†]	1 (5)	1R	0.5

Values denote number of subjects while parenthesis provides the percent of total subjects who did not have any pain on stepmill. Continuity indicates the number of subjects in whom the absence of pain was maintained across visits. [†]Significant at $p \leq 0.05$ based on independent binomial testing of each visit using the null hypothesis that the probability of a subject experiencing no joint pain is equal to zero. There was no statistical difference between groups. #R Repeat subject (i.e. same subject who reported no pain in previous visit), N New subject who reports no pain for the first time.

as measured by knee extension goniometry. Knee extension is necessary for daily function and sport activities. Loss of knee extension has been shown to negatively impact the function of the lower extremity [42,43]. For example, loss of knee extension can cause altered gait patterns affecting ankles and the hip which could result in difficulty with running and jumping [42,43]. Studies have further shown that a permanent loss of 3-5° of extension can significantly impact patient satisfaction and the development of early arthritis [44].

By contrast, when knee flexion, another measure of knee function, was assessed via goniometry, no differences in clinical outcomes were observed between the two study cohorts. From a structure-function perspective this outcome is not surprising. During the earliest characterized phases of OA there is an apparent preferential loss of knee extension over knee flexion, and this loss has been shown to correlate with WOMAC pain scores [45,46]. In addition, MRI imaging of the early osteoarthritic knee has shown that initial changes in knee structure appear to center on articular cartilage erosions (fibrillations) about the patella and other weight bearing regions of the knee [47]. Such changes might favor a loss in knee ROM that preferentially affects extension over flexion. The pathophysiology of the early osteoarthritic knee, we believe, provides insight regarding the effect of daily physical activities on the healthy knee insofar as it helps explain the discordance in clinical outcomes between knee extension and flexion.

Both the time to onset of initial joint pain as well as time to full recovery were measured in this study. For

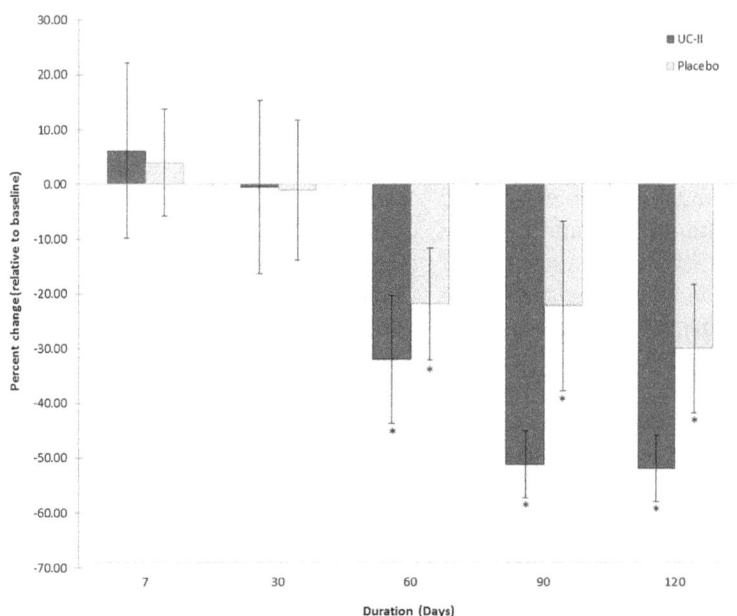

Figure 4 Percent change in time to complete recovery from pain. Values are presented as Mean ± SEM. *$p \leq 0.05$ indicates a statistically significant difference from baseline. Number of completers: n = 18 in UC-II group (n = 3 dropouts; n = 5 did not have pain; n = 1 time to complete recovery from pain was not achieved); n = 20 in placebo group (n = 6 dropouts; n = 1 did not have pain; n = 1 did not use stepmill).

Table 6 Summary of analysis of adverse events (AEs) in all subjects

Study groups	Adverse event (Body system)	Number of AEs
UC-II	Upper respiratory infection (Pulmonary)	3
	Food poisoning (Gastrointestinal)	1
Total number of AEs		**4**
Total number of subjects reporting AEs: n		**4/27**
Placebo	Bilateral ankle edema (Musculoskeletal)	1
	Right ankle fracture (Musculoskeletal)	1
	Sinusitis (Ears/Nose/Throat)	1
	Skin infection right ankle (Dermatological)	1
Total number of AEs		**4**
Total number of subjects reporting AEs: n		**2/28**

each of these measures the clinical outcomes favored the UC-II supplemented cohort versus their baseline status. The ability of UC-II to modulate knee extension may relate to its ability to moderate knee joint pain. Crowley et al. [26] and Trentham et al. [25] demonstrated that UC-II effectively enhances joint comfort and flexibility thereby improving the quality of life (QoL) in both OA and RA subjects, respectively. This effect may be attributable to the finding that microgram quantities of undenatured type II collagen moderate CIA in both the rat and the mouse via the induction of T regulator cells [27,28,48]. The induction of these T regulators takes place within gut associated lymphatic tissues (GALT), including mesenteric lymph nodes, in response to the consumption of undenatured type II collagen [27]. Studies have shown that these regulatory cells produce IL-10 and TGF-β [30,49]. A special class of CD103$^+$ dendritic cells, found almost exclusively in the GALT, facilitates this process [48,50]. Once activated, T regulator cells appear to downregulate a wide range of immunologic and proinflammatory activities resulting in the moderation of the arthritic response initiated by undenatured type II collagen [27]. The phenomenon of oral tolerance has also been demonstrated in humans, and appears to involve a similar set of T regulators [30,51-53].

The above description of how UC-II might modulate joint function is most easily understood in the context of RA given that the CIA animal model resembles this disease most closely [27,28,54]. However, the case for T regulators and immune cytokines having a moderating effect on healthy or OA knee joint function appears less apparent. This view has changed in recent years due to a growing body of evidence suggesting that both OA and normal chondrocyte biology appears to be regulated by some of the same cytokines and chemokines that regulate inflammation [5,6,55]. For example, Mannelli and coworkers [56] recently

reported that feeding microgram amounts of native type II collagen (porcine) prevents monoiodoacetate-induced articular cartilage damage in this rat model of osteoarthritis, as measured by pain thresholds and by circulating levels of cross linked c-telopeptides derived from type II collagen. This finding corroborates the efficacy of undenatured type II collagen in improving joint comfort in osteoarthritic conditions [26].

In the present study, we show for the first time that UC-II can improve joint function in healthy subjects undergoing strenuous physical exercise. This observation, when considered in context with normal chondrocyte physiology, suggests that activated T regulator cells, specific for undenatured type II collagen, home to an overstressed knee joint where their release of the anti-inflammatory cytokines, IL-10 and TGF-β reverse the catabolic changes caused by strenuous exertion [13,21,57]. In addition, the IL-10 and TGF-β produced by these T regulators may tilt the T_H balance in the knee joint towards T_H2 [30,58] responses which preferentially result in IL-4 production further fostering a shift in chondrocyte metabolism towards ECM replenishment.

Several additional tests were used in this study to assess overall joint function, QoL, and physical activity. The additional parameters and tests measured included a six minute timed walk plus the Stanford exercise scale and KOOS survey. With respect to the KOOS survey, both cohorts were statistically significant versus baseline for symptoms, pain, daily function, recreational activities and QoL but were not significant from each other. This is not an unexpected finding given that this study was carried out with healthy subjects who do not present with any joint issues at rest. It is only when the knee is stressed via the stepmill do subjects report any joint discomfort. Under these conditions, and as indicated above, the UC-II group appears to experience less joint discomfort and greater joint flexibility. No difference in clinical outcomes between groups was seen in the six minute timed walk, the daily distance walked, or the Stanford exercise scale questionnaire. Once again we are not surprised by these results given that these tests and questionnaires are designed and clinically validated to assess the severity of arthritic disease in unhealthy populations.

No clinical biomarkers associated with arthritic diseases were assessed in this study. Healthy subjects would not be expected to present with significant alterations in their inflammatory biomarker profile as they lack clinical disease [59]. In addition, it should be noted that the joint discomfort measured in this study is acute pain induced by a stressor rather than due to an ongoing inflammatory event. Therefore, any elevation in inflammation markers that might occur in these healthy subjects may simply be due to the physiological impact of strenuous exercise.

There are two study limitations to consider when reviewing these results. The first, time to onset of initial pain, was limited to a 10-minute interval. The current study design did not address the possibility that subjects might cease to experience pain on the stepmill. Future studies should allow for an extension of the exertion interval in order to gauge how much longer a subject can exercise before reporting pain. In this way better defined parameters can be placed upon the degree to which UC-II supplementation results in the cessation of joint pain due to strenuous exercise in healthy subjects.

The second limitation that merits consideration is the possibility that study subjects may have early signs of arthritis that do not meet the ACR criteria. This possible limitation was addressed by performing an extensive medical examination for signs and symptoms of OA and by excluding volunteers who experienced pain levels of 5 or greater within one minute of using the stepmill.

UC-II is a unique ingredient that supports healthy joints. Previous studies have focused on the efficacy of this ingredient in OA subjects. By including healthy subjects in this study, and using non-disease endpoints as a measure of efficacy, it is believed that the benefits that derive from UC-II usage now extends to include healthy individuals. Further, this ingredient appears to be safe for human consumption based on an extensive series of *in vivo* and *in vitro* toxicological studies as well as the absence of any adverse events in this and in previous human studies [24,26,60]. In conclusion, daily supplementation with 40 mg of UC-II supports joint function and flexibility in healthy subjects as demonstrated by greater knee extension and has the potential both to alleviate the joint pain that occasionally arises from strenuous exercise as well as to lengthen periods of pain free exertion.

Abbreviations
RA: Rheumatoid arthritis; OA: Osteoarthritis; ECM: Extracellular matrix; TNF-α: Tumor necrosis factor-alpha; IL-1β: Interleukin-1 beta; IL-6: Interleukin-6; IL-4: Interleukin 4; IL-10: Interleukin-10; MMP: Matrix metalloproteinase; NF-κB: Nuclear factor-kappa-light-chain-enhancer of activated B cells; MAPK: Mitogen activated protein kinase; ERK: Extracellular receptor kinase; NO: Nitric oxide; TGF-β: Transforming growth factor-beta; CIA: Collagen induced arthritis; KOOS: Knee injury and osteoarthritis outcome score; ROM: Range of motion; MRI: Magnetic resonance imaging; GALT: Gut associated lymphatic tissue; QoL: Quality of life; MIP-1β: Macrophage inflammatory protein-1 beta; IP-10: Interferon gamma-induced protein 10; T$_H$: T helper cell; WOMAC: Western Ontario and McMaster universities osteoarthritis index; ACR: American College of Rheumatology.

Competing interests
Medicus Research received research grants from InterHealth Nutraceuticals, Inc., Benicia, California. Dr. Udani has provided consulting services to InterHealth Nutraceuticals, Inc. Drs. JPL, ZMS, and FCL are employees of InterHealth Nutraceuticals, Inc. Medicus Research does not endorse any brand or product nor does it have any financial interests with any supplement manufacturer or distributor.

Authors' contributions
JKU was the principal investigator and together with JPL, JKU, ZMS, FCL JPM, MNP and ANS contributed to the writing, data analyses and data interpretation that are a part of this manuscript. All the authors read and approved the final draft of the manuscript.

Acknowledgements
Medicus Research thanks InterHealth Nutraceuticals, Inc., Benicia, California, for supporting this clinical trial and for providing the treatment and placebo products. We thank the entire Staywell clinical staff for their tireless efforts and dedication to the health and welfare of the subjects. The study design and the protocol preparation was the result of a collaborative effort between InterHealth Nutraceuticals, Inc., Benicia, California and Medicus Research LLC, Agoura Hills, CA, the Contract Research Organization (CRO) chosen to manage the clinical and other logistics of this study.

Funding
InterHealth Nutraceuticals, Inc., Benicia, California.

Author details
[1]InterHealth Nutraceuticals, Benicia, CA 94510, USA. [2]Medicus Research LLC, 28720 Roadside Drive, Suite 310, Agoura Hills, CA 91301, USA. [3]UCLA Medical Center, Santa Monica, CA 90401, USA. [4]Northridge Hospital Integrative Medicine Program, Northridge, CA 91325, USA.

References
1. Shek PN, Shephard RJ: Physical exercise as a human model of limited inflammatory response. *Can J Physiol Pharmacol* 1998, **76**:589–597.
2. Kiviranta I, Tammi M, Jurvelin J, et al: Articular cartilage thickness and glycosaminoglycan distribution in the canine knee joint after strenuous running exercise. *Clin Orthop Relat Res* 1992, **283**:302–308.
3. Guilak F: Biomechanical factors in osteoarthritis. *Best Pract Res Clin Rheumatol* 2011, **25**:815–823.
4. Kawamura S, Lotito K, Rodeo SA: Biomechanics and healing response of the meniscus. *Oper Tech Sports Med* 2003, **11**:68–76.
5. Ramage L, Nuki G, Salter DM: Signalling cascades in mechanotransduction: cell-matrix interactions and mechanical loading. *Scand J Med Sci Sports* 2009, **19**:457–469.
6. Honda K, Ohno S, Tanimoto K, et al: The effects of high magnitude cyclic tensile load on cartilage matrix metabolism in cultured chondrocytes. *Eur J Cell Biol* 2000, **79**:601–609.
7. Agarwal S, Deschner J, Long P, et al: Role of NF-kappaB transcription factors in antiinflammatory and proinflammatory actions of mechanical signals. *Arthritis Rheum* 2004, **50**:3541–3548.
8. Berg V, Sveinbjornsson B, Bendiksen S, et al: Human articular chondrocytes express chemR23 and chemerin; chemR23 promotes inflammatory signalling upon binding the ligand chemerin(21–157). *Arthritis Res Ther* 2010, **12**:R228.
9. Millward-Sadler SJ, Wright MO, Lee H, et al: Integrin-regulated secretion of interleukin 4: a novel pathway of mechanotransduction in human articular chondrocytes. *J Cell Biol* 1999, **145**:183–189.
10. Millward-Sadler SJ, Wright MO, Davies LW, et al: Mechanotransduction via integrins and interleukin-4 results in altered aggrecan and matrix metalloproteinase 3 gene expression in normal, but not osteoarthritic, human articular chondrocytes. *Arthritis Rheum* 2000, **43**:2091–2099.
11. Doi H, Nishida K, Yorimitsu M, et al: Interleukin-4 downregulates the cyclic tensile stress-induced matrix metalloproteinases-13 and cathepsin B expression by rat normal chondrocytes. *Acta Med Okayama* 2008, **62**:119–126.
12. Yorimitsu M, Nishida K, Shimizu A, et al: Intra-articular injection of interleukin-4 decreases nitric oxide production by chondrocytes and ameliorates subsequent destruction of cartilage in instability-induced osteoarthritis in rat knee joints. *Osteoarthritis Cartilage* 2008, **16**:764–771.
13. van Meegeren ME, Roosendaal G, Jansen NW, et al: IL-4 alone and in combination with IL-10 protects against blood-induced cartilage damage. *Osteoarthritis Cartilage* 2012, **20**:764–772.
14. Pufe T, Lemke A, Kurz B, et al: Mechanical overload induces VEGF in cartilage discs via hypoxia-inducible factor. *Am J Pathol* 2004, **164**:185–192.

15. Ostrowski K, Rohde T, Asp S, et al: Pro- and anti-inflammatory cytokine balance in strenuous exercise in humans. *J Physiol* 1999, 515(Pt 1):287–291.

16. Allen JL, Cooke ME, Alliston T: ECM stiffness primes the TGFbeta pathway to promote chondrocyte differentiation. *Mol Biol Cell* 2012, 23:3731–3742.

17. Bougault C, Aubert-Foucher E, Paumier A, et al: Dynamic compression of chondrocyte-agarose constructs reveals new candidate mechanosensitive genes. *PLoS One* 2012, 7:e36964.

18. Li TF, O'Keefe RJ, Chen D: TGF-beta signaling in chondrocytes. *Front Biosci* 2005, 10:681–688.

19. Donovan J, Slingerland J: Transforming growth factor-beta and breast cancer: cell cycle arrest by transforming growth factor-beta and its disruption in cancer. *Breast Cancer Res* 2000, 2:116–124.

20. Rosier RN, O'Keefe RJ, Crabb ID, et al: Transforming growth factor beta: an autocrine regulator of chondrocytes. *Connect Tissue Res* 1989, 20:295–301.

21. Roman-Blas JA, Stokes DG, Jimenez SA: Modulation of TGF-beta signaling by proinflammatory cytokines in articular chondrocytes. *Osteoarthritis Cartilage* 2007, 15:1367–1377.

22. Loeser RF: Aging and osteoarthritis: the role of chondrocyte senescence and aging changes in the cartilage matrix. *Osteoarthritis Cartilage* 2009, 17:971–979.

23. van Beuningen HM, van der Kraan PM, Arntz OJ, et al: Protection from interleukin 1 induced destruction of articular cartilage by transforming growth factor beta: Studies in anatomically intact cartilage in vitro and in vivo. *Ann Rheum Dis* 1993, 52:185–191.

24. Bagchi D, Misner B, Bagchi M, et al: Effects of orally administered undenatured type II collagen against arthritic inflammatory diseases: a mechanistic exploration. *Int J Clin Pharmacol Res* 2002, 22:101–110.

25. Trentham DE, Dynesius-Trentham RA, Orav EJ, et al: Effects of oral administration of type II collagen on rheumatoid arthritis. *Science* 1993, 261:1727–1730.

26. Crowley DC, Lau FC, Sharma P, et al: Safety and efficacy of undenatured type II collagen in the treatment of osteoarthritis of the knee: a clinical trial. *Int J Med Sci* 2009, 6:312–321.

27. Tong T, Zhao W, Wu YQ, et al: Chicken type II collagen induced immune balance of main subtype of helper T cells in mesenteric lymph node lymphocytes in rats with collagen-induced arthritis. *Inflamm Res* 2010, 59:369–377.

28. Nagler-Anderson C, Bober LA, Robinson ME, et al: Suppression of type II collagen-induced arthritis by intragastric administration of soluble type II collagen. *Proc Natl Acad Sci USA* 1986, 83:7443–7446.

29. Brandtzaeg P: 'ABC' of mucosal immunology. *Nestle Nutr Workshop Ser Pediatr Program* 2009, 64:23–38. discussion 38–43, 251–7.

30. Weiner HL, da Cunha AP, Quintana F, et al: Oral tolerance. *Immunol Rev* 2011, 241:241–259.

31. Aletaha D, Neogi T, Silman AJ, et al: 2010 Rheumatoid arthritis classification criteria: an american college of rheumatology/european league against rheumatism collaborative initiative. *Arthritis Rheum* 2010, 62:2569–2581.

32. Altman R, Asch E, Bloch D, et al: Development of criteria for the classification and reporting of osteoarthritis. Classification of osteoarthritis of the knee. Diagnostic and therapeutic criteria committee of the american rheumatism association. *Arthritis Rheum* 1986, 29:1039–1049.

33. Likert R: A technique for the measurement of attitudes. *Arch Psychol* 1932, 22:1–55.

34. Roos EM, Roos HP, Ekdahl C, et al: Knee injury and osteoarthritis outcome score (KOOS)–validation of a swedish version. *Scand J Med Sci Sports* 1998, 8:439–448.

35. Lorig K, Stewart A, Ritter P, et al: *Outcome measures for health education and other health care interventions. Outcome measures for health education and other health care interventions.* Thousand Oaks, CA: SAGE Publications, Inc.; 1996.

36. Hawkey C, Laine L, Simon T, et al: Comparison of the effect of rofecoxib (a cyclooxygenase 2 inhibitor), ibuprofen, and placebo on the gastroduodenal mucosa of patients with osteoarthritis: a randomized, double-blind, placebo-controlled trial. The rofecoxib osteoarthritis endoscopy multinational study group. *Arthritis Rheum* 2000, 43:370–377.

37. Pincus T, Koch GG, Sokka T, et al: A randomized, double-blind, crossover clinical trial of diclofenac plus misoprostol versus acetaminophen in patients with osteoarthritis of the hip or knee. *Arthritis Rheum* 2001, 44:1587–1598.

38. Petrella RJ, DiSilvestro MD, Hildebrand C: Effects of hyaluronate sodium on pain and physical functioning in osteoarthritis of the knee: a randomized, double-blind, placebo-controlled clinical trial. *Arch Intern Med* 2002, 162:292–298.

39. Enright PL, Sherrill DL: Reference equations for the six-minute walk in healthy adults. *Am J Respir Crit Care Med* 1998, 158:1384–1387.

40. Perry J: *Gait analysis: normal and pathological function.* Thorofare: SLACK Inc.; 1992.

41. Viera AJ: Predisease: when does it make sense? *Epidemiol Rev* 2011, 33:122–134.

42. Norkin CC, Levangie PK: *Joint structure & function: a comprehensive analysis.* Philadelphia: F.A. Davis; 1992.

43. Shah N: Increasing knee range of motion using a unique sustained method. *N Am J Sports Phys Ther* 2008, 3:110–113.

44. Shelbourne KD, Biggs A, Gray T: Deconditioned knee: the effectiveness of a rehabilitation program that restores normal knee motion to improve symptoms and function. *N Am J Sports Phys Ther* 2007, 2:81–89.

45. Serrao PR, Gramani-Say K, Lessi GC, et al: Knee extensor torque of men with early degrees of osteoarthritis is associated with pain, stiffness and function. *Rev Bras Fisioter* 2012, 16:289–294.

46. Heiden TL, Lloyd DG, Ackland TR: Knee extension and flexion weakness in people with knee osteoarthritis: Is antagonist cocontraction a factor? *J Orthop Sports Phys Ther* 2009, 39:807–815.

47. Karachalios T, Zibis A, Papanagiotou P, et al: MR imaging findings in early osteoarthritis of the knee. *Eur J Radiol* 2004, 50(3):37–40.

48. Park MJ, Park KS, Park HS, et al: A distinct tolerogenic subset of splenic IDO(+)CD11b(+) dendritic cells from orally tolerized mice is responsible for induction of systemic immune tolerance and suppression of collagen-induced arthritis. *Cell Immunol* 2012, 278:45–54.

49. Li MO, Flavell RA: TGF-beta: a master of all T cell trades. *Cell* 2008, 134:392–404.

50. Coombes JL, Siddiqui KR, Arancibia-Carcamo CV, et al: A functionally specialized population of mucosal CD103+ DCs induces Foxp3+ regulatory T cells via a TGF-beta and retinoic acid-dependent mechanism. *J Exp Med* 2007, 204:1757–1764.

51. Ilan Y, Zigmond E, Lalazar G, et al: Oral administration of OKT3 monoclonal antibody to human subjects induces a dose-dependent immunologic effect in T cells and dendritic cells. *J Clin Immunol* 2010, 30:167–177.

52. Caminiti L, Passalacqua G, Barberi S, et al: A new protocol for specific oral tolerance induction in children with IgE-mediated cow's milk allergy. *Allergy Asthma Proc* 2009, 30:443–448.

53. Ben Ahmed M, Belhadj Hmida N, Moes N, et al: IL-15 renders conventional lymphocytes resistant to suppressive functions of regulatory T cells through activation of the phosphatidylinositol 3-kinase pathway. *J Immunol* 2009, 182:6763–6770.

54. Courtenay JS, Dallman MJ, Dayan AD, et al: Immunisation against heterologous type II collagen induces arthritis in mice. *Nature* 1980, 283:666–668.

55. Pelletier JP, Martel-Pelletier J, Abramson SB: Osteoarthritis, an inflammatory disease: potential implication for the selection of new therapeutic targets. *Arthritis Rheum* 2001, 44:1237–1247.

56. Di Cesare Mannelli L, Micheli L, Zanardelli M, et al: Low dose native type II collagen prevents pain in a rat osteoarthritis model. *BMC Musculoskelet Disord* 2013, 14:228.

57. Muller RD, John T, Kohl B, et al: IL-10 overexpression differentially affects cartilage matrix gene expression in response to TNF-alpha in human articular chondrocytes in vitro. *Cytokine* 2008, 44:377–385.

58. Zouali M: *Immunological tolerance: mechanisms.* eLS: John Wiley & Sons, Ltd; 2001.

59. Chu CR, Williams AA, Coyle CH, et al: Early diagnosis to enable early treatment of pre-osteoarthritis. *Arthritis Res Ther* 2012, 14:212.

60. Marone PA, Lau FC, Gupta RC, et al: Safety and toxicological evaluation of undenatured type II collagen. *Toxicol Mech Methods* 2010, 20:175–189.

17

The effects PCSO-524®, a patented marine oil lipid and omega-3 PUFA blend derived from the New Zealand green lipped mussel (*Perna canaliculus*), on indirect markers of muscle damage and inflammation after muscle damaging exercise in untrained men: a randomized, placebo controlled trial

Timothy D Mickleborough[*], Jacob A Sinex, David Platt, Robert F Chapman and Molly Hirt

Abstract

Background: The purpose of the present study was to evaluate the effects of PCSO-524®, a marine oil lipid and *n*-3 LC PUFA blend, derived from New Zealand green- lipped mussel (*Perna canaliculus*), on markers of muscle damage and inflammation following muscle damaging exercise in untrained men.

Methods: Thirty two untrained male subjects were randomly assigned to consume 1200 mg/d of PCSO- 524® (a green-lipped mussel oil blend) or placebo for 26 d prior to muscle damaging exercise (downhill running), and continued for 96 h following the muscle damaging exercise bout. Blood markers of muscle damage (skeletal muscle slow troponin I, sTnI; myoglobin, Mb; creatine kinase, CK), and inflammation (tumor necrosis factor, TNF-α), and functional measures of muscle damage (delayed onset muscle soreness, DOMS; pressure pain threshold, PPT; knee extensor joint range of motion, ROM; isometric torque, MVC) were assessed pre- supplementation (baseline), and multiple time points post-supplementation (before and after muscle damaging exercise). At baseline and 24 h following muscle damaging exercise peripheral fatigue was assessed via changes in potentiated quadriceps twitch force ($\Delta Q_{tw,pot}$) from pre- to post-exhaustive cycling ergometer test in response to supra-maximal femoral nerve stimulation.

Results: Compared to placebo, supplementation with the green-lipped mussel oil blend significantly attenuated ($p < 0.05$) sTnI and TNF-α at 2, 24, 48, 72 and 96 h., Mb at 24, 48, 72, 96 h., and CK-MM at all-time points following muscle damaging exercise, significantly reduced ($p < 0.05$) DOMS at 72 and 96 h post-muscle damaging exercise, and resulted in significantly less strength loss (MVC) and provided a protective effect against joint ROM loss at 96 h post- muscle damaging exercise. At 24 h after muscle damaging exercise perceived pain was significantly greater ($p < 0.05$) compared to baseline in the placebo group only. Following muscle damaging exercise $\Delta Q_{tw,pot}$ was significantly less ($p < 0.05$) on the green-lipped mussel oil blend compared to placebo.

(Continued on next page)

* Correspondence: tmickleb@indiana.edu
Department of Kinesiology, Human Performance and Exercise Biochemistry Laboratory, School of Public Health-Bloomington, 1025 E. 7th St. SPH 112, Bloomington, Indiana 47401, USA

(Continued from previous page)

Conclusion: Supplementation with a marine oil lipid and *n*-3 LC PUFA blend (PCSO-524®), derived from the New Zealand green lipped mussel, may represent a useful therapeutic agent for attenuating muscle damage and inflammation following muscle damaging exercise.

Keywords: Omega-3 fatty acids, Green-lipped mussel oil blend, Muscle damage, DOMS, Eccentric

Introduction

Exercise-induced muscle damage (EIMD) can be caused by eccentric type or unaccustomed (novel) exercise, and results in decrements in muscle force production, development of delayed-onset muscle soreness (DOMS) and swelling, rise in passive tension, and an increase in blood intramuscular proteins [1]. Delayed-onset muscle soreness is generally considered a hallmark sign of EIMD [2], and it is thought that DOMS is partially related to direct muscle fiber damage, and its magnitude appears to vary with the type, duration and intensity of exercise [3]. The inflammatory response to EIMD results in the release into blood of reactive species from both neutrophils and macrophages, and an array of cytokines from the injured muscle including tumor necrosis factor (TNF)-α, interleukin (IL)-1β and IL-6, which contribute to a low-grade systemic inflammation and oxidative stress [4]. The pro- inflammatory and pro-oxidant response can provoke secondary tissue damage [5], thus prolonging the regenerative process, which is generally characterized by a restoration of muscle strength and resolution of inflammation [5].

Exercise-induced muscle damage and DOMS can potentially hinder performance in activities ranging from basic physical activity to athletic training and competition. There are a number of strategies that have been used to attenuate EIMD and DOMS such as anti-inflammatory medication, cryotherapy, massage, stretching, hyperbaric oxygen, homeopathy, ultrasound, rest, light exercise and electrotherapeutic modalities [3]. The use of non-steroidal anti- inflammatory drugs (NSAIDs) and continued exercise appear to be the most commonly used methods to treat DOMS [1]. However, while the use of NSAIDs has been shown to decrease perceived muscle soreness and pain associated with DOMS, they fail to impact the length or degree of muscle weakness [6], may be detrimental to muscle cell repair and adaptation by decreasing satellite cell activity [7], and have been shown to suppress the protein synthesis response in skeletal muscle after eccentric resistance exercise [8]. Due to the fact that there appears to be no completely effective treatment for preventing/reducing EIMD and treating DOMS [1,6], the use of complimentary therapy, in particular nutraceuticals (e.g. tart cherry juice [9], curcumin [10], and quercetin [11]) that possess anti-inflammatory properties and have the potential to attenuate EIMD-induced oxidative stress, have become of interest [1].

One class of nutrients that appears to possess both anti-inflammatory and anti-oxidant properties are the long-chain omega (*n*)-3 long chain polyunsaturated fatty acids (LC-PUFA), such as eicosapentaeoic acid (EPA; 20:5 n-3)) and docosahexaenoic acid (DHA; 22:5 n-3), found in fish oil. Numerous studies have shown that *n*-3 LC-PUFA administered at doses greater than one gram per day have beneficial actions in many inflammatory diseases, cancer, and human health in general [12], and that *n*-3 LC-PUFA may act as important energetic molecules that can modulate immune, inflammatory, and oxidative stress responses to exercise [13]. A small number of studies have sought to evaluate whether fish oil supplementation can reduce the degree of skeletal muscle injury, inflammation and oxidative stress following eccentric exercise [13]. Although more studies have demonstrated a positive effect of *n*-3 LC-PUFA in relation to ameliorating muscle damage, DOMS, inflammation, and oxidative stress following eccentric exercise [14-20], some investigations have shown no effect [14,21]. It is likely that the diversity in testing protocols, supplementation dosage and duration, subject population, timing of measurements and selection of biomarkers contribute to the discrepancies in the findings between studies. However, it is possible that different forms of marine oils may have varying effects on these responses, since these oils contain a variety of lipid mediators as well as a different amount of *n*-3 LC-PUFA.

PCSO-524® (Lyprinol®/Omega XL®) is a nutritional supplement comprising of a patented extract of a very condensed form of stabilized marine lipids from the New Zealand green lipped mussel, *Perna canaliculus*, combined with olive oil and vitamin E [22,23]. This marine oil lipid and *n*-3 PUFA blend is a multifarious mixture of sterol esters, sterols, polar lipids, triglycerides, EPA and DHA (split between the triacylglycerol and polar lipid classes), and free fatty acids [24], and has been shown to exert its anti-inflammatory effects via furan fatty acids [25], and inhibition of cyclooxygenase (COX)-2 and 5-lipoxyeganse (LOX) pathways for the metabolism of arachidonic acid, thereby leading to a subsequent reduction in pro-inflammatory leukotriene, prostaglandin, and cytokine production from inflammatory cells [22,26]. A number of human and animal studies have shown that the green-lipped mussel oil blend may have beneficial effects in treating inflammatory diseases such as osteoarthritis, rheumatoid arthritis, inflammatory bowel disease, asthma [22], and exercise- induced bronchoconstriction [27]. These preliminary findings support the potential for supplementation with the green-lipped mussel oil blend in order to attenuate muscle damage and inflammation that can occur following muscle damaging exercise.

Therefore, the primary aim of the present study was to evaluate the effects of supplementation with a green-lipped mussel oil blend on indirect markers of muscle damage, inflammation, and quadriceps fatigue following muscle damaging exercise in untrained men. We hypothesized that supplementation with a green-lipped mussel oil blend, compared to placebo, would significantly reduce blood markers of muscle damage and inflammation, and modulate quadriceps fatigue and functional measures of muscle damage following downhill running designed to induce muscle damage in untrained men.

Methods
Subjects
Forty untrained males volunteered to participate in the study, and of these thirty-two subjects (aged 22.0 ± 2 y, height 176.3 ± 7.0 cm, body mass 70.8 ± 9.8 kg, maximal oxygen consumption (VO_{2peak}) 46.0 ± 6.1 mL·kg^{-1}·min^{-1}) completed the study. Reasons for the non- inclusion of eight subject data sets in the final statistical analysis were (1) subjects failing to show up at testing sessions (incomplete data; n = 3), (2) inability of the investigators to obtain a blood sample (incomplete data; n = 3), and (3) identification of erroneous recordings of data (n = 2). Subjects were classified as 'untrained' if they exercised less than three times per wk for less than 30 min during each session. Subjects were excluded if they had a history of significant pain in hips or knees, had participated in a strength training program within 60 d prior to study participation, or regularly used nutritional supplements and over-the-counter and prescription anti-inflammatory medication. All subjects were screened for coronary artery disease risks factors as per the American College of Sports Medicine guidelines [28]. Subjects were instructed to refrain from downhill running, stair running, resistance training, plyometric or other mode of exercise that could potentially cause muscle damage, and to refrain from modifying their exercise habits during the course of the study. Adherence to these instructions was confirmed at each visit to the laboratory. The study was approved by the Indiana University Institutional Review Board for Human Subjects, and written informed consent for all subjects was obtained prior to participation in the study.

Study design
The study was conducted as a randomized, double-blind, placebo-controlled parallel group trial over 30 days. This design was chosen over a crossover design in order to avoid the repeated-bout effect acting as a confounding variable [1]. Subjects were randomly assigned to either a green-lipped mussel oil blend (PCSO-524®) supplementation group (n = 16) or a placebo group (n = 16). Supplementation with the green-lipped mussel oil blend and placebo began 26 days before an eccentric exercise bout (downhill running, designed to induce muscle damage) and continued for 4 days following the muscle damaging exercise bout. An activity diary and food frequency questionnaire was completed by each subject during the course of the study.

Pre-supplementation measures
After subjects provided written informed consent for participation and the investigators explained the study protocol, all subjects underwent an exhaustive 20-min cycle ergometer familiarization test (T1 day −21), followed one week later (T2 day −14) by an incremental treadmill load test of their maximal oxygen uptake (VO_{2max}), in order to determine the intensity (70% VO_{2peak}) the subjects will exercise at for the eccentric exercise test. One week (T3 day −7) following the VO_{2peak} test an initial (baseline) blood draw was taken in order to measure baseline blood markers of muscle damage, inflammation and DNA oxidative stress, along with baseline functional measures of muscle damage [i.e. isometric torque (MVC), knee flexion (joint range of motion), limb girth (swelling), muscle soreness, and muscle pain], which were followed one week later (T4 day 0) by measures of quadriceps muscle fatigue (quadriceps twitch force measured via femoral magnetic nerve stimulation before and after a 20-min exhaustive cycle ergometer test).

Post-supplementation measures
Following the 26 days of supplementation a venous blood draw was taken and functional measures of muscle damage conducted (T5 day 26), which was directly followed by the downhill running protocol specifically designed to induce muscle damage [29,30] (T6 day 26). Immediately (T7 day 26) and 2 h following the muscle damaging exercise a venous blood draw was taken (T8 day 26), followed by additional blood draws and functional measures of muscle damage at 24 h (T9 day 27), 48 h (T10 day 28), 72 h (T11 day 29) and 96 h (T12 day 30) post-muscle damaging exercise. Quadriceps muscle fatigue was measured 24 h following the muscle damaging exercise bout (T8 day 27). The timing of this measurement was chosen in order to correspond with expected decrements in muscle strength, range of motion and significant increases in swelling, tenderness and soreness. On testing days T3 day −7, T5 day 26, T9 day 27, T10 day 28, T11 day 29 and T12 day

30 the sequence of procedures comprised the following order: blood draws, DOMS, range of motion, pressure pain threshold, thigh girth (swelling) and isometric torque (MVC). On testing T9 day 27 only, subjects underwent the protocol for the measurement of quadriceps muscle fatigue before and after the 20-min exhaustive cycle ergometer trial.

Supplementation

Subjects ingested either 8 capsules per d of PCSO-524® (Lyprinol®/Omega XL®; Pharmalink International Ltd, Hong Kong) (n = 16), which equaled 800 mg olive oil, 400 mg lipid extract (~58 mg EPA and 44 mg DHA) and 1.8 mg vitamin E (d-alpha-tocopherol) or 8 placebo capsules containing olive oil (1200 mg olive oil) (n = 16) for 30 d. Each PCSO-524® capsule contains 50 mg lipid extract (fatty acids), 7.3 mg (14%) EPA, 5.5 mg (11%) DHA, 100 mg olive oil and 0.225 mg vitamin E, and 1 placebo capsule contains 150 mg olive oil. The active PCSO-524® capsules containing the green-lipped mussel oil blend were identical in size, color, texture and taste to their respective placebo counterpart. Product specification was provided to the investigators by the trial sponsor (Pharmalink). Cawthron Laboratories (Nelson, NZ), an independent laboratory, completed the fatty acid analysis of the raw material, and Chemisches Labor (Hannover, Germany) conducted the final fatty acid testing of the finished PCSO-524 ® capsuled product. Alpha laboratories (Auckland, NZ) conduced the fatty acid analysis on the placebo (olive oil) capsules. While Table 1 presents the fatty acid analysis conducted on the PCSO-524® (Batch No. A6530-01) and placebo (Batch No. 7820) capsules used in the present study, a detailed fatty acid analysis of the PCSO-524® and placebo capsules has been published elsewhere [31,32]. Wolyniak et al. [23] have shown that the 'lipid extract' portion of the green-lipped mussel oil blend contains up to 91 fatty acids (including EPA and DHA). Of the 91 fatty acids reported [23], 16 represented more than 1% of the total FA. In decreasing order of abundance, these were EPA, C16:0 (Palmitic acid), DHA, C14:0 (Myristic acid), C16:1n-7 (Palmitoleic acid), C18:0 (Steroic acid), C18:1n-5, C18:4n-3 (Stearidonic acid), C18:2n-6 (Linoleic acid), C20:4n-6 (Arachidonic acid), C18:3n- 3 (Alpha-linoleic acid), C16:1n-5, C20:1n-9 (Eicosenoic acid), C18:1n-9 (Oleic acid), C15:0 (Pentadecanoic acid), and C16:1n-9 (7-(hexadecenoic acid). PCSO-524® is a natural product subject to variations in the New Zealand Marlborough Sounds ecosystems. Values in the specification of this organic compound can vary according to season and climate temperatures, and therefore, during the manufacturing process a variance of +/− 10% in the saturated, monounsaturated and PUFA composition of PCSO-524® is deemed acceptable.

Table 1 Fatty acid composition (%) of PCSO-524®, a marine oil extract of the New Zealand green-lipped mussel (*Perna canaliculus*) * and placebo (olive oil) ** capsules

FA nomenclature	Fatty acid name	PCSO-524®capsules (Weight, %)	Placebo (Olive oil) capsules (Weight, %)
14:0	Myristic acid	1.7	
16:0	Palmitic acid	13.4	9.2
16:1	Palmitoleic acid	3.6	3.0
18:0	Stearic acid	3.6	3.5
18:1	Oleic acid	58.2	81.0
18:2n-6	Linoleic acid	5.7	2.6
18:3n-3	Alpha-linolenic acid	0.9	0.4
18:4n-3	Octadecatetraenoic acid	1.0	
20:0	Arachidic acid	0.4	0.3
20:1	Eicosamonoenoic acid	0.7	
20:4n-6	Arachidonic acid	0.1	
20:4n-3	Eicosatetraenoic acid	0.3	
20:5n-3	Eicosapentaenoic acid	5.8	
22:5n-3	Docosapentaenoic acid	0.3	
22:6n-3	Docosahexaenoic acid	3.0	
Others		1.3	

*Batch number: A6530-01. **Batch number: 7820. FA nomenclature: number of carbon atoms (chain length), number of double bonds, and position of the last double bond from the methyl (omega) end.

Experimental measures
Peak aerobic exercise capacity (VO$_{2peak}$)

Subjects performed a peak aerobic exercise capacity test, adapted from a previously published protocol from our laboratory [33], on a motor driven treadmill (Model 18–60, Quinton, Seattle, WA), while fitted with a heart rate monitor (Polar Electro Inc., Lake Success, NY) and breathing mask (7450 Series V2, Hans Rudolph, Shawnee, KS USA). The protocol started with a warm-up period of 5 min, in which subjects chose a comfortable running speed that they would be expected to be able to continue on a level treadmill for 15 min; selected speeds ranged from 7.2 – 13.8 km/h. After 5 min of seated rest, the exercise portion of the test began with each subject running at 0% grade at a speed of 1.6 k/h less than the selected (warm-up) speed for 2 min. Following the initial stage, the speed was increased to the predetermined speed. After 3 min, the slope of the treadmill was increased to 4% for 3 min, and then increased an additional 2% every 3 min until volitional exhaustion or valid test criteria were met. Ventilatory and metabolic data were collected using open-circuit, indirect calorimetry. Dried expired gases were sampled at a rate of 300 mL·min^{-1} for fractional concentrations of O_2 and CO_2 using an Applied Electrochemistry S-3A oxygen analyzer and a CD-3A carbon dioxide analyzer (Ametek, Thermox Instruments, Pittsburgh, PA). Inspired ventilation was measured with a pneumotachometer (Hans Rudolph 3813).

Eccentric muscle damaging exercise

All subjects performed a 20-min downhill running bout on a motorized treadmill (A.R. Young Company, Indianapolis) modified to run in reverse at a −16% grade, which is a protocol that has previously been shown to elicit a significant degree of muscle damage following downhill running [29,30]. Once the test commenced subjects were not allowed to stop, and treadmill speed was adjusted so that the subjects maintained a heart rate that corresponded to 70% VO_{2max}. It has been shown that downhill running is effective in causing skeletal muscle damage, symptoms of DOMS, and loss of muscle force [34].

Delayed onset muscle soreness and pain threshold

Lower limb soreness was assessed using a visual analog (numeric) rating pain scale with "no soreness" indicated at one end (score 0) and "unbearably painful" at the other (score 10) Subjects stood with hands on hips and feet approximately shoulder width apart. The subject was asked to squat down to 90° (internal angle), rise to the start position and then indicate on the numeric scale the soreness felt in the lower limbs.

The pressure pain threshold was measured at five specific sites on the quadriceps with a digital algometer (Force One, Wagner Instruments, Greenwich, CT.) to quantify muscle tenderness. The same investigator performed all measurements throughout the study. Specific sites for assessment were determined using established literature and landmarks [32], involving two anatomical points (anterior superior iliac spine (ASIS) and superior pole of the patella (SPP). All measurements were taken on the right side with the subject in the supine position. A longitudinal axis was created between the ASIS and the SPP from which the sites were marked with a permanent marker to ensure accuracy at each time point. The measured sites were: 15 cm distal to the ASIS, 4 cm proximal to the SPP, midpoint of the ASIS and SPP along the axis, then 2 cm lateral and 2 cm medial of this midpoint. Subjects were instructed to let the investigator know when the pressure transformed into pain at which point the amount of force was recorded in newtons (N).

Range of motion (knee flexion), swelling (thigh girth) and isometric strength (torque)

Range of motion has been shown to be an accurate method of determining the extent of muscle damage [35]. Subjects were instructed to lay prone on a massage table with both knees fully extended. Subjects flexed their left knee with no assistance from the investigator, and the angle measured with a goniometer (Prestige Medical, Northridge, CA) using universal landmarks (lateral epicondyle of the femur, lateral malleolus and greater trochanter) that were marked with a permanent marker to ensure consistency on subsequent measures. Three measurements were averaged and reported in degrees. This method for a assessing ROM has been validated previously [36].

In order to determine the presence of swelling/edema within a muscle thigh circumference was assessed at the midpoint of the ASIS and SPP of the right leg with an anthropometric tape (Idass, Glastonbury, UK). Subjects were standing fully relaxed in the anatomical position. Subjects were instructed to put all their weight on the opposite leg and 3 measurements were taken. Measurement sites were marked to ensure consistent measurements and the average was reported.

Isometric torque was assessed at a knee angle of 80° using previously described protocol [37]. Subjects were seated in a chair, secured with a belt across the legs and chest, and their left leg secured to a force transducer (Model Z Tension Load Cell, Dillon, Fairmont, MN) with a non-compliant strap. Subjects were familiarized with the equipment by performing three warm-up contractions (two submaximal, 1 maximal) separated by 10 seconds of rest, followed by a 5 min recovery. After the recovery period, subjects performed 3 maximum voluntary contractions (MVCs) of the quadriceps, interspersed with a 10 s recovery interval between contractions. The highest peak torque from the 3 contractions was recorded. Subjects were verbally encouraged during the contractions to produce a maximum effort.

Quadriceps muscle fatigue

Potentiated quadriceps twitch force was measured in the subject's left leg to quantify an index of muscle fatigue following a 20 min exhaustive cycle ergometer test. Subjects lay semirecumbent on a table with a left knee joint angle of 90 degrees. The subject's ankle was wrapped in a non-compliant strap, placed just superior to the ankle malleoli. The strap was attached to a calibrated load cell (Model Z Tension Load Cell, Dillon, Fairmont, MN) for the measurement of force connected to a custom amplifier (Hector Engineering Co. Inc., Ellettsville, IN). A magnetic stimulator (Magstim 200, Magstim, Whitland, UK) connected to a double 70 mm coil was used to stimulate the femoral nerve, causing an involuntary contraction of the quadriceps muscle. Nerve stimulation followed two protocols, which have been described previously [38].

Assessment of maximal nerve stimulation

Prior to the exhaustive 20 min cycle ergometer test, a series of single twitches were obtained at varying levels of stimulator intensity (80%, 85%, 90%, 95%, and 100% of maximal stimulator power output) to determine when supramaximal stimulation had been reached. The position of the stimulator coil was placed over the femoral triangle and adjusted to determine an acceptable location for each subject. Stimulator placement was determined to be acceptable when repeatable and measurable quadriceps contractions were obtained. Stimulator placement was marked on the subject's skin with an indelible marker to insure repeatability of the location and measurement. Typical stimulator output required to achieve supramaximal stimulation has been found to be a mean of approximately 83% of stimulator output [39].

Exhaustive 20 min cycle ergometer test

Following a 5 min warm up at a self-selected intensity, subjects completed a 20 min exercise task on a cycle ergometer (Velotron, RacerMate Inc., Seattle, Washington, USA). Subjects were allowed to change resistance freely and were asked to complete the furthest possible distance, and to achieve the highest possible power output, during the 20 min ergometer test.

Assessment of fatigue

Prior to and immediately following the exhaustive cycle ergometer test, an assessment of quadriceps twitch force ($Q_{tw,pot}$) was performed. Twitch force prior to the 20 min cycle ergometer test was used as a baseline for twitch force obtained after the time trial. The assessment of fatigue protocol consisted of six repetitions of potentiation and magnetic stimulation with 30 s of rest between repetitions. For each repetition, subjects performed a maximal voluntary isometric contraction (MVC) of the quadriceps muscle for 5 s. At the end of the 5 s MVC, the subject received a supra-maximal magnetic stimulation of the femoral nerve, and a second stimulation after 5 seconds of rest [40]. The force produced during the second twitch of each repetition was recorded as $Q_{tw,pot}$. Force values from the first two repetitions were discarded based on previous findings that the degree of potentiation is smaller after the first two measurements [38]. Force values from the final four repetitions were averaged to produce a $Q_{tw,pot}$ force value for each trial.

Blood sampling and analysis

All blood draws were taken from the antecubital vein and collected into 10 ml plain Vacutainer® clot tubes (PulmoLab, Porter Ranch, CA). The tubes were gently inverted five times after collection to mix the clot activator with blood, and then placed on ice for at least 30 minutes before centrifugation (Allegra ™ X-22R Centrifuge, Beckman Coulter, Inc., Brea, CA) at 20°C at 3000 RPM for 15 min. Serum was removed after spinning and allocated to storage tubes and stored immediately at –80°C until later analysis of muscle damage, inflammation and oxidative stress markers using enzyme immunoassay techniques [Powerwave XS™ Spectrophotometer (Bio-Tek Instruments, Winooski, VT)] according to manufacturer's instructions.

Skeletal and cardiac muscle damage

Creatine kinase, muscle (CK-MM) was assessed using a sandwich enzyme linked immunoassay test (sensitivity: 12.8 U/L; Detection range: 31.2 – 2,000 U/L. Intra-assay precision: CV < 10%; Inter-assay precision: CV < 12% as per the manufacturer's (Caltag Medsystems Ltd, Milton Keynes, UK) protocol. Skeletal muscle slow troponin I (sTnI) was assessed using a sandwich enzyme linked immunoassay test (Minimum detectable concentration typically 5.4 pg/ml; Detection range: 15.6-1,000 pg/ml; Intra-assay precision: CV < 10%; Inter-assay precision: CV < 12% as per the manufacturer's (USCN Life Science Inc., Hubei, Peoples Republic of China) protocol. Myoglobin (Mb) was assessed using an enzyme-linked immunoassay test (minimum detectable concentration: 5.0 ng/ml; sensitivity: 25 ng/ml; Detection range: 25.0-1,000 ng/ml) following the manufacturer's recommendations (Calbiotech, Spring Valley, CA, USA). Cardiac troponin I (CTnI) was analyzed a using sandwich enzyme-linked immunoassay test (minimum detectable concentration: 0.45 ng/ml; Detection range: 0.48-5.0 ng/ml; inter-assay precision: <10%) as per the manufacturer's (Abnova, Taipei, Taiwan) recommendations. Human heart fatty acid binding protein (hFABP) was assessed using a sandwich enzyme linked immunoassay test (minimum detectable concentration: 156 pg/ml; Detection range: 312 – 20,000 pg/ml. Intra-assay precision: CV < 4-6%; Inter-assay precision: CV < 8-10%) following the manufacturer's (Innovative Research, Novi, MI, USA) recommendations.

Inflammatory and DNA oxidative stress markers

Tumor necrosis factor (TNF)-α was assessed using a sandwich enzyme linked immunoassay test (sensitivity: 1.7 pg/ml; Detection range: 15.6 – 1,000 pg/ml. Intra-assay precision: CV < 4.4%; Inter-assay precision: CV < 7.5% as per the manufacturer's (Invitrogen Corp., Camarillo, CA, USA) protocol. 8-Oxo-2'-deoxyguanosine (8-OhdG) was analyzed using a competitive enzyme linked immunoassay test (Detection range: 100 pg/ml – 20 ng/ml) as per the manufacturer's (Cell Biolabs Inc., San Diego, CA, USA) recommendations.

Nutrient intake and compliance

All subjects were given an activity diary to record frequency, mode and duration of exercise. Nutrient intake was monitored to ensure that dietary factors would do not change through the course of the study, and potentially affect the dependent measures. Nutrient data was collected using the GSEL food frequency questionnaire (FFQ) developed by the Nutrition Assessment Shared Resource (NASR) of Fred Hutchinson Cancer Research Center. Subjects completed the GSEL version of the questionnaire before supplementation and at the end of the 30 day supplementation period. Analysis of GSEL for nutrient intake was conducted at the Fred Hutchinson Cancer Research Center. Nutrients of interest obtained from the GSEL analysis included macronutrient composition, antioxidants (α-tocopherol, β-carotene, lycopene, Vitamin C), certain minerals (magnesium, sodium, zinc), and types of dietary fatty acids (omega-3, total polyunsaturated fatty acids, saturated fatty acids). While the FFQ has been shown to be valid and reliable in the collection of dietary data [41], we acknowledge that diet may act as confounding factor, since it was not directly controlled for in our study. Adherence to the treatment regimen was monitored by asking the subjects to document the dose of capsules consumed daily and to return any unused capsules. For the purpose of the present study a compliance of $\geq$90% was considered acceptable.

Data analysis

The data were analyzed using a two-way (group, 2; time, 6–8) split-plot repeated measures ANOVA using SPSS version 20.0 (IBM Corporation, Chicago, IL, USA) statistical software. The data was assessed for normality using the Kolmogorov–Smirnov test, and Levene's test was used to test for homogeneity of variance between groups. Mauchly's test was conducted to determine whether sphericity is violated. If sphericity is violated, the repeated-measures ANOVA was corrected using the Greenhouse–Geiser correction factor. A fisher's protected least-square difference post-hoc test was used *a priori* to determine differences in dependent measures within and between groups. Statistical significance was set at $p \leq 0.05$. Data are expressed as mean $\pm$ SD.

To determine an appropriate sample size for present study, a post-hoc power analysis of existing literature was conducted using G*Power version 3.0.5 (Universität Kiel, Germany). Based on two studies [19,20] investigating the efficacy of *n*-3 LC-PUFA on DOMS, and blood markers of muscle damage and inflammation following eccentric exercise, achieving an experiment-wise error rate of 0.05 required 15 subjects within each treatment group. In these studies, Tartibian et al. [19,20] has shown that ingestion of *n*-3 LC-PUFA (n = 9–15) for 30 days compared to placebo/control (n = 9–15) significantly

reduced inflammatory markers, and perceived pain and symptoms, following eccentric exercise, with effect sizes ranging from 0.64-0.75 for a study power of 0.82 and 0.84 respectively.

Results

Subject characteristics

There were no significant differences ($p > 0.05$) for age, height, BMI, VO_{2max} (L) and VO_{2peak} (mL/kg/min) between the green-lipped mussel oil blend (PCSO-524™) and placebo group (Table 2). However, body mass (kg) was significantly different ($p < 0.05$) between groups.

Delayed onset muscle soreness and pain threshold

Muscle soreness significantly increased ($p < 0.05$) in both groups after the muscle damaging exercise protocol, peaking between 24 and 48 h and declining toward baseline at 72 and 96 h (Table 3). Significant effects for time were found in the green-lipped mussel oil blend group ($p < 0.001$) and placebo group ($p < 0.001$). Post-hoc pairwise comparisons between groups at each time point revealed significantly lower DOMS in the treatment group, compared to placebo, at 72 h [p = 0.027; mean difference (Δ), 1.25 $\pm$ 2.41; 95% CI (difference of means), 0.08 to 2.52] and 96 h (p = 0.037; Δ, 1.25 $\pm$ 1.95; 95% CI, 0.13 to 2.63%) following muscle damaging exercise. However, there were no significant differences ($p > 0.05$) between groups prior to supplementation (baseline) and following supplementation (before, and at 24 and 48 h following muscle damaging exercise).

The test of within-subject effects indicated that there was no significant effect ($p > 0.05$) of time on percent change from baseline in all post-supplementation time points for pressure pain threshold (PPT) values within the green-lipped mussel oil blend group. Post-hoc pairwise comparisons within the placebo group revealed a significant increase (p = 0.034; Δ, 0.12 $\pm$ 0.25%; 95% CI, 0.01 to 0.26%) in muscle tenderness at 24 h post-muscle damaging exercise only compared to before muscle damaging exercise in the placebo group (Table 3).

Table 2 Subjects' baseline characteristics

	Green-lipped mussel oil blend (n = 16)	Placebo (n = 16)	p-value
Age (years)	21.7 + 1.7	21.5 + 2.4	0.803
Height (cm)	178.1 + 5.8	174.2 + 6.7	0.091
Body mass (kg)	74.8 + 8.8	66.6 + 9.7	0.018*
BMI (kg/m²)	23.6 + 2.9	21.9 + 2.8	0.102
VO_{2peak} (L)	3.4 + 0.5	3.0 + 0.6	0.073
VO_{2peak} (ml/kg/min)	46.4 + 6.2	45.6 + 6.1	0.732

*Significantly different (p < 0.05) between groups. BMI, body mass index.
VO2peak, peak oxygen consumption. Values are expressed as mean ± SD.

Table 3 Effect of supplementation on functional measures of muscle damage and fatigue following eccentric exercise

Variables/ Groups	Pre-supplementation (Baseline)	Post-supplementation Before muscle damaging exercise	24 h after muscle damaging exercise	48 h after muscle damaging exercise	72 h after muscle damaging exercise	96 h after muscle damaging exercise
DOMS (arbitrary units)						
Green-lipped mussel oil blend	2.3 ± 1.7	2.0 ± 2.0	4.9 ± 2.7[¥,#]	4.6 ± 2.2[¥]	2.7 ± 1.7[#]	1.8 ± 1.6[#]
Placebo	1.9 ± 1.6	1.4 ± 1.5	4.4 ± 2.1[¥, #]	4.8 ± 1.8[¥]	3.9 ± 1.8[¥,#]	3.0 ± 2.2[¥,#]
p-value*	0.700	0.563	0.847	0.441	0.029*	0.037*
Pressure Pain Threshold (% Δ from baseline)						
Green-lipped mussel oil blend	-	−0.08 ± 0.32%	−0.13 ± 0.26%	−0.12 ± 0.28%	−0.07 ± 0.34%	−0.01 ± 0.34%
Placebo	-	−0.03 ± 0.35%	−0.15 ± 0.27%[#]	−0.10 ± 0.39%	−0.07 ± 0.41%	0.01 ± 0.50%
p-value*	-	0.643	0.844	0.824	0.978	0.896
Knee Flexion Range of Motion (degrees)						
Green-lipped mussel oil blend	47.5 ± 6.1	46.7 ± 5.0	47.4 ± 5.2	44.6 ± 5.9[#]	45.7 ± 5.4	46.7 ± 4.4
Placebo	45.8 ± 8.4	46.9 ± 9.8	47.3 ± 9.0	43.4 ± 7.1[#]	44.9 ± 8.5	41.8 ± 5.3[¥]
p-value*	0.476	0.939	0.980	0.628	0.760	0.007*
Thigh Girth (swelling) (% Δ from baseline)						
Green-lipped mussel oil blend	-	0.01 ± 0.02%	0.02 ± 0.02%	0.01 ± 0.02%	0.01 ± 0.02%	0.02 ± 0.04%
Placebo	-	0.00 ± 0.02%	0.02 ± 0.02%	0.01 ± 0.02%	0.02 ± 0.02%	0.02 ± 0.06%
p-value*	-	0.631	0.970	0.953	0.582	0.971
Maximum Voluntary Isometric torque (Strength) (Nm)						
Green-lipped mussel oil blend	72.8 ± 22.2	82.1 ± 19.7[#]	76.2 ± 19.8[#]	78.7 ± 21.5	79.9 ± 20.2	84.6 ± 22.4[¥,#]
Placebo	75.4 ± 19.3	82.1 ± 22.4[#]	74.9 ± 19.4[#]	74.6 ± 22.5	76.2 ± 20.8	83.9 ± 14.4
p-value*	0.721	0.843	0.987	0.569	0.608	0.872
%ΔQ$_{tw,pot}$						
Green-lipped mussel oil blend	−27.8 ± 26.2	-	−30.4 ± 14.3	-	-	-
Placebo	−23.9 ± 24.0	-	−39.5 ± 24.3[¥]	-	-	-
p-value*	0.669	-	0.039	-	-	-

*, p-value between groups at distinct time points (p < 0.05 denotes statistical significance between groups; p > 0.05 denotes no statistical significance between groups); ¥, significantly different (p < 0.05) to pre- supplementation (baseline) within group; #, significantly different (p < 0.05) from previous time point within group. Pressure pain threshold and thigh girth (swelling) are expressed as % change (Δ) from the pre- supplementation (baseline) value within group, since baseline values were significantly different (p < 0.05) between groups. DOMS, delayed onset muscle soreness; % ΔQ$_{tw,pot}$, % change in potentiated quadriceps twitch force from pre- to post-exercise (cycling time trial). Values expressed as mean ± SD.

Range of motion (knee flexion), swelling (thigh Girth) and isometric strength (torque)

The test of within-subject effects indicated that there was a significant effect (p < 0.01) of time on ROM within each group. Range of motion was significantly reduced (p < 0.05) at 48 h compared to 24 h post-muscle damaging exercise within the green-lipped mussel oil blend and placebo group. However, while no significant difference (p > 0.05) was found between groups for ROM values at baseline and post-supplementation (prior to, and at 24, 48 and 72 h post-muscle damaging exercise) a

significant reduction (p < 0.05) in ROM occurred in the placebo group compared to the green-lipped mussel oil blend group at 96 h post-muscle damaging exercise (p = 0.007; Δ, −4.94 ± 8.10 degrees; 95% CI, −1.42 to −8.45 degrees) (Table 2). No significant difference (p > 0.05) was observed for the percent change from baseline in thigh girth (swelling) within or between groups at all-time points (Table 3).

The test of within-subject effects revealed that there was a significant effect (p < 0.01) of time on MVC (torque) within the both groups (Table 3). For both groups post- supplementation MVC significantly increased immediately prior to muscle damaging exercise compared to the baseline value (Placebo: $p = 0.009$; Δ, 6.68 ± 10.1 Nm; 95% CI, 1.30 to 12.10 Nm. Green-lipped mussel oil blend: $p = 0.014$; Δ, 9.41 ± 15.48 Nm; 95% CI, 1.16 to 17.66 Nm), and was significantly reduced at 24 h post-muscle damaging exercise compared to the MVC value obtained immediately prior to muscle damaging exercise (Placebo: $p = 0.002$; Δ, 7.13 ± 8.4 Nm; 95% CI, -2.65 to -11.61 Nm. Green-lipped mussel oil blend: $p = 0.022$, Δ, $6.02 + 11.00$ Nm; 95% CI, -0.16 to -11.89 Nm). In addition, within the green-lipped mussel oil blend group only, MVC increased significantly at 96 h compared to 72 h post-muscle damaging exercise ($p = 0.014$; Δ, 4.67 ± 7.69 Nm; 95% CI, 0.57 to 8.77 Nm) and baseline ($p = 0.003$; Δ, 11.83 ± 15.24 Nm; 95% CI, 3.71 to 19.95 Nm). No significant difference ($p > 0.05$) in MVC was observed at any time point between groups.

Quadriceps muscle fatigue

There was no significant difference ($p > 0.05$) in the percent change (%Δ) in $Q_{tw, pot}$ between groups at baseline, or within the green-lipped mussel oil blend group when comparing the %$\Delta Q_{tw,pot}$ at baseline with 24 h following muscle damaging exercise. However, %$\Delta Q_{tw,pot}$ was significantly greater at 24 h following muscle damaging exercise compared to baseline within the placebo group ($p = 0.018$ Δ, $-11.4 \pm 23.3\%$, 95% CI, -2.7 to -25.4%), and %$\Delta Q_{tw,pot}$ was significantly greater for the placebo group compared with the green-lipped mussel oil blend group at 24 h following muscle damaging exercise ($p = 0.039$; Δ, $-10.1 \pm 24.7\%$; 95% CI, -4.3 to -29.1%) (Table 3), indicating greater muscle quadriceps fatigue in the placebo group.

Skeletal and cardiac muscle damage blood markers

Serum sTnI levels were not significantly different ($p > 0.05$) for baseline (pre- supplementation), immediately prior to, and immediately following (0 h) muscle damaging exercise (post-supplementation) either within or between groups (Figure 1). However, a significant increase ($p < 0.05$) in serum sTnI concentration, compared to baseline, was observed at 2, 24, 48, 72, and 96 h post- muscle damaging exercise within each group. Serum sTnI concentration peaked at 24 h following muscle damaging exercise, and compared to baseline increased by $260.2 \pm 170.6\%$ in the placebo group and by $165.1 \pm 139.1\%$ in the green-lipped mussel oil blend group. There was a significant reduction in the green-lipped mussel oil blend mean serum sTnI concentration compared to the placebo group at 2 h ($p = 0.007$; Δ, -4.5 ± 5.8 ng/ml; 95% CI, -0.9 to -8.0 ng/ml), 24 h ($p < 0.001$; Δ, -9.9 ± 10.1 ng/ml; 95% CI, -4.4 to -15.4 ng/ml), 48 hr. ($p < 0.001$, Δ, -9.4 ± 10.0 ng/ml; 95% CI, -4.7 to -14.0 ng/ml), 72 h ($p = 0.003$; Δ, -6.8 ± 9.1 ng/ml; 95% CI, -2.5 to -11.1 ng/ml), and 96 h ($p = 0.02$, Δ, -5.4 ± 10.5 ng/ml; 95% CI, -0.3 to -10.4 ng/ml) (Figure 1) following muscle damaging exercise.

Serum CK-MM levels were not significantly different ($p > 0.05$) for baseline, and immediately prior to muscle damaging exercise either within or between groups (Figure 2). However, a significant increase ($p < 0.05$) in serum CK-MM concentration, compared to baseline, was observed at 0, 2, 24, 48, 72, and 96 h post-muscle damaging exercise within each group. Serum CK-MM

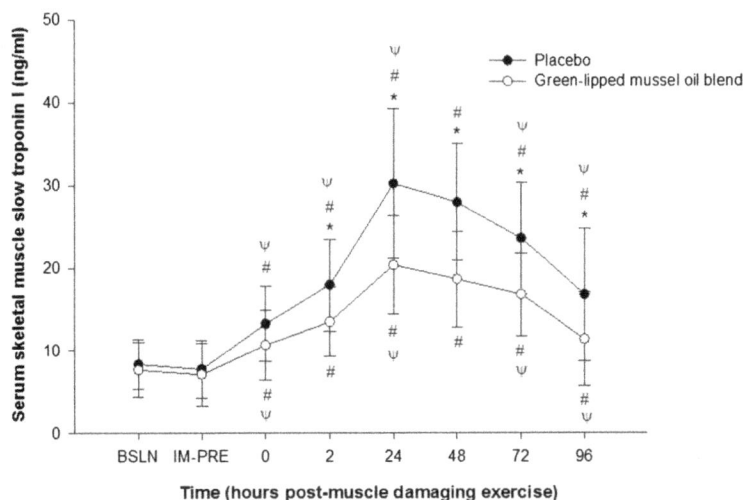

Figure 1 Effect of supplementation on mean serum skeletal muscle slow troponin I concentration (ng/ml) pre- and post-eccentric exercise. *, designates a statistical difference ($p < 0.05$) between groups at distinct time points. #, designates a significant difference ($p < 0.05$) compared to baseline (BSLN; pre-supplementation before eccentric exercise).ψ, designates a significant difference ($p < 0.05$) from previous time point within group. IM-PRE, immediately prior to eccentric exercise (post-supplementation). Data are expressed as mean ± SD.

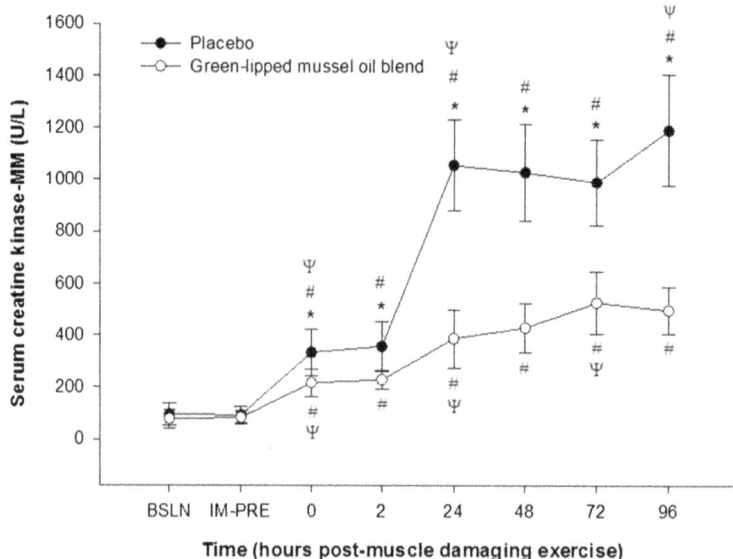

Figure 2 Effect of supplementation on mean serum creatine kinase-MM concentration (ng/ml) pre- and post-eccentric exercise. *, designates a statistical difference (p < 0.05) between groups at distinct time points. #, designates a significant difference (p < 0.05) compared to baseline (BSLN; pre-supplementation before eccentric exercise).ψ, designates a significant difference (p < 0.05) from previous time point within group. IM-PRE, immediately prior to eccentric exercise (post-supplementation). Data are expressed as mean ± SD.

concentration peaked at 24 h following muscle damaging exercise for the placebo group and 72 h for the green-lipped mussel oil blend group, and compared to baseline increased by 1006.5 ± 631.2% in the placebo group and by 579.8 ± 287.4% in the green-lipped mussel oil blend group. A significant attenuation in the green- lipped mussel oil blend mean serum CK-MM concentration, compared to the placebo group, was detected at 0 h (p < 0.001; Δ, −116.1 ± 112.0 ng/ml; 95% CI, − 63.0 to −169.2 ng/ml), 2 h (p < 0.001; Δ, −127.3 + 101.7 ng/ml; 95% CI, −76.0 to −178.6 ng/ml), 24 hr. (p < 0.001; Δ, −386.1 ± 201.0 ng/ml; 95% CI, −562.6 to −775.6 ng.ml), 48 h (p < 0.001; Δ, −600.0 ± 208.5 ng/ml; 95% CI, −493.2 to −706.7 ng/ml), 72 h (p < 0.001; Δ, −463.7 ± 221.8 ng/ml; 95% CI, −360.0 to −568.0 ng/ml) and 96 h (p < 0.001; Δ, −693.0 ± 243.0 ng/ml; 95% CI, − 564.0 to −822.4 ng/ml) following muscle damaging exercise (Figure 2).

Serum Mb levels were not significantly different (p > 0.05) when comparing baseline, and immediately prior to and at 0 h and 2 h muscle damaging eccentric exercise either within or between groups. However, a significant increase (p < 0.05) in serum Mb concentration, compared to base-line, was observed at 24, 48, 72, and 96 h post-muscle damaging exercise within each group. Serum Mb concentration peaked at 72 h following muscle damaging exercise (post-supplementation) for both groups, and compared to baseline increased by 1917.6 ± 876.3% in the placebo group and by 1109.5 ± 496.2% in the green-lipped mussel oil blend group. A significant attenuation in the green-lipped mussel oil blend mean serum Mb concentration

compared to the placebo group was observed at 24 h (p < 0.001; Δ, −43.3 ± 37.1 ng/ml; 95% CI, −22.9 to −63.7 ng. ml), 48 hr. (p < 0.001; Δ, −99.4 ± 58.7 ng/ml; 95% CI, −67.7 to −131.2 ng/ml), 72 h (p < 0.001; Δ, −192.6 ± 159.8 ng/ml; 95% CI, −119.0 to −226.3 ng/ml) and 96 h (p = 0.001; Δ, −130.7 ± 161 ng/ml; 95% CI, − 49.1 to −212.2 ng/ml) following muscle damaging exercise (post-supplementation) (Figure 3). For serum cTnI and h-FABP concentration no significant differences (p > 0.05) were observed for all time points either within or between groups.

Inflammatory and DNA oxidative stress markers

Mean serum TNF-α concentration did not significantly differ (p > 0.05) for baseline, immediately prior to, and at 0 h following muscle damaging exercise either within or between groups. However, a significant increase (p < 0.05) in serum TNF-α concentration, compared to baseline, was observed at 2, 24, 48, 72, and 96 h post-muscle damaging exercise within each group. Serum TNF-α levels peaked at 24 h following muscle damaging exercise, and compared to baseline increased by 156.2 ± 65.7% in the placebo group and by 93.3 ± 49.4% in the green-lipped mussel oil blend group. There was a significant reduction in mean serum TNF-α concentration for the green-lipped mussel oil blend group compared to the placebo group at 2 h (p = 0.042; Δ, −4.9 ± 8.1 pg/ml; 95% CI, −0.4 to −10.6 pg/ml), 24 h (p < 0.001; Δ, −19.8 ± 13.4 pg/ml; 95% CI, −11.1 to −28.5 pg/ml), 48 hr. (p < 0.001, Δ, −18.1 ± 12.7 pg/ml; 95% CI, −10.7 to −25.7 pg/ml), 72 h (p = 0.003; Δ, −19.9 ± 13.0 pg/ml; 95% CI, −11.3 to −28.5 pg/ml), and 96 h

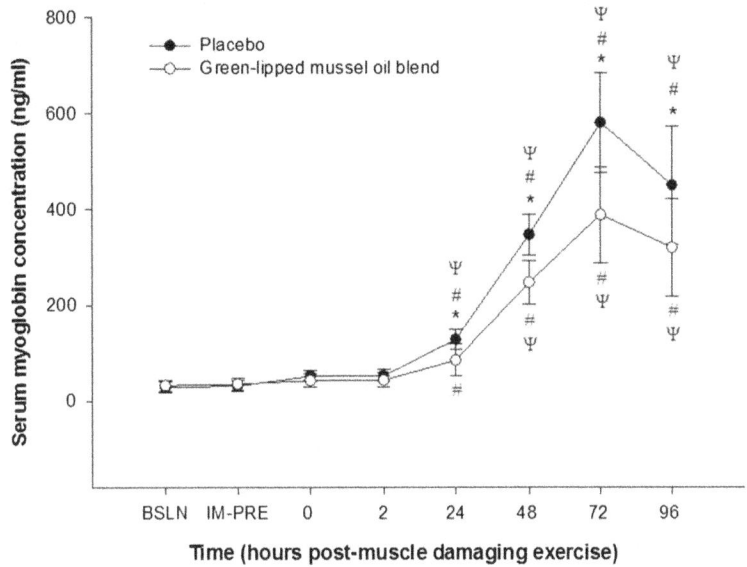

Figure 3 Effect of supplementation on mean serum myoglobin concentration (ng/ml) pre- and post-eccentric exercise. *, designates a statistical difference (p < 0.05) between groups at distinct time points. #, designates a significant difference (p < 0.05) compared to baseline (BSLN; pre-supplementation before eccentric exercise).ψ, designates a significant difference (p < 0.05) from previous time point within group. IM-PRE, immediately prior to eccentric exercise (post-supplementation). Data are expressed as mean ± SD.

(p < 0.001, Δ, −24.8 ± 15.1 pg/ml; 95% CI, −16.8 to −32.8 pg/ml) following muscle damaging exercise (Figure 4).

Mean serum 8-OHdG concentration was not significantly changed (p > 0.05) either within or between groups for all time points.

Nutrient intake and compliance

Mean daily nutrient intake, such as, for example, α-tocopherol, β-carotene, lycopene, vitamin C, magnesium, sodium, zinc, omega-3, total polyunsaturated fatty acids and saturated fatty acids did not differ

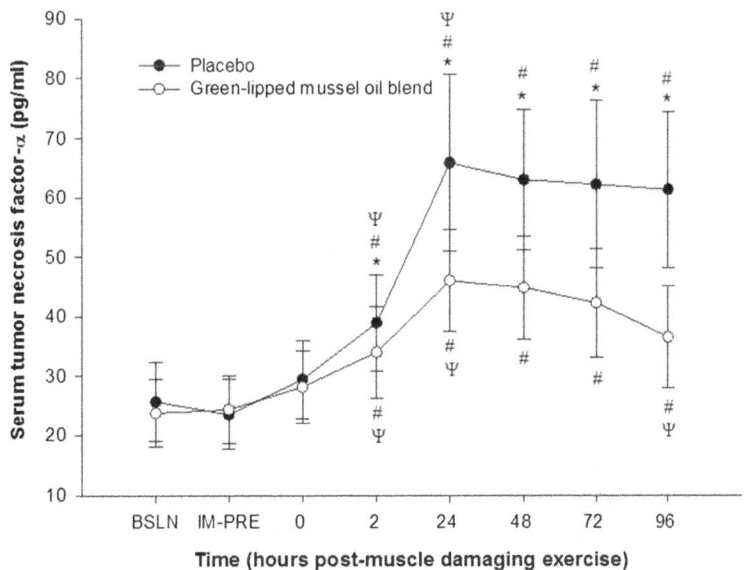

Figure 4 Effect of supplementation on mean serum tumor-necrosis factor-α concentration (pg/ml) pre- and post-eccentric exercise. *, designates a statistical difference (p < 0.05) between groups at distinct time points. #, designates a significant difference (p < 0.05) compared to baseline (BSLN; pre-supplementation before eccentric exercise).ψ, designates a significant difference (p < 0.05) from previous time point within group. IM-PRE, immediately prior to eccentric exercise (post-supplementation). Data are expressed as mean ± SD.

significantly (p > 0.05) between groups during the course of the study. Compliance as estimated from return-capsule count was high (median, 99%).

Discussion

The present study has shown that supplementing the diet of untrained men for 4 wk with a marine oil lipid and n-3 LC PUFA blend (PCSO-524®), derived from the New Zealand green lipped mussel (*P. canaliculus*), significantly reduced lower limb DOMS, quadriceps pain (tenderness), and peripheral muscle fatigue, and provided a protective effect against ROM (knee flexion) and isometric strength (torque) loss that can occur following downhill running designed to induce muscle damage. In addition, although blood markers of muscle damage and inflammation, sTnI, CK-MM, MB, and TNF-α, significantly increased following eccentric exercise in both groups, the rise in these blood markers were significantly suppressed on the green-lipped mussel oil blend supplemented diet compared to the placebo diet at most time points following muscle damaging exercise. No significant changes occurred between the green-lipped mussel oil blend and placebo group following eccentric exercise for swelling (thigh girth), and serum h-FABP, cTnI and 8-OHdG concentrations. Our findings may have implications for those who train regularly, especially since it has recently been shown that EPA and DHA levels (Omega-3 Index: percentage of EPA and DHA in total erythrocyte fatty acids) were low in a cohort of German elite winter endurance athletes [42], and importantly that n-3 LC-PUFA supplementation leads to a higher Omega-3 index level and decreased incidence of DOMS in healthy college aged individuals [43].

To date only two studies have been conducted in order to determine the efficacy of supplementation with this specific green-lipped mussel oil blend (PCSO-524®) on markers of EIMD and DOMS following muscle damaging [32] and exhaustive exercise [31]. While Baum et al. [31] found that 11 wk. of the green-lipped mussel oil blend supplemented diet reduced DOMS following an exhaustive 30 km run in male and female trained distance runners, Pumpa et al. [32] found no effect of 8 wk of supplementation with this specific green-lipped mussel oil blend on DOMS and functional and blood markers of EIMD following downhill running in trained men from a variety of sports. The divergent findings between the present study and the Pumpa et al. study [32] are difficult to reconcile, but is likely related to Pumpa and colleagues [32] using a lower dose (600 mg/day) of green-lipped mussel oil blend supplementation compared to the present study (1200 mg/day), and using a downhill running protocol of insufficient intensity to promote muscle damage and a robust inflammatory response in trained individuals.

Effect of green-lipped mussel oil blend supplementation on delayed onset muscle soreness and pain threshold

We observed a significant decrease in DOMS at 96 h following muscle damaging exercise on the green-lipped mussel oil blend supplemented diet compared to the placebo diet, which is in agreement with some studies [15,17,19], but not all [14,21,32], that have shown that supplementing the diet with n-3 LC-PUFA prior to muscle damage attenuates DOMS following eccentric exercise and a 30 km run [31]. Delayed-onset muscle soreness appears many hours after muscle damaging exercise and peaks 24–72 h post-eccentric exercise [5], as was observed in both groups in the present study. What is clear is that while DOMS is not considered a disease or a disorder, it can limit further exercise in the days following an initial training bout [3].

In the present study the quadriceps pressure pain threshold (PPT) was used as an additional measure of muscle soreness in an attempt to ameliorate the subjective nature of the visual analog scale measure of soreness. We observed no change in the PPT for all time points within the green-lipped mussel oil blend group or between groups. However, in the placebo group perceived pain increased significantly 24 h following muscle damaging exercise compared to before muscle damaging exercise. These data seem to suggest that the green-lipped mussel oil blend supplemented diet may have afforded a protective effect against perceived pain developing in the quadriceps, and may be partially explained by the attenuation in muscle damage and the inflammatory response that occurred in this group [5]. While Tartibian et al. [19] have demonstrated that n-3 LC-PUFA supplementation for 30 days reduced perceived pain 48 hr. following eccentric exercise compared to placebo, other studies [16,21,32] have found no change in perceived pain following eccentric exercise when pre-treated with n-3 LC-PUFA.

Effect of green-lipped mussel oil blend supplementation on range of motion (knee flexion), swelling (thigh Girth) and isometric strength (torque)

Among the numerous indirect markers of EIMD, muscle function measures such as muscle strength (MVC torque) and ROM are considered the best tools for quantifying muscle damage [2]. Eccentric-biased downhill running protocols typically generate 10-30% force loss after exercise, and that the reduction in MVC torque resulting from injury persists until the muscle function returns to its pre-injury condition (~24 h) [2]. Strength losses following eccentric exercise are likely due to the effects of muscle damage, and evidence suggests that excitation-contraction coupling failure plays a role [44]. In the present study there were no significant change observed for MVC torque at all-time points between groups or within the placebo group. However,

MVC torque significantly increased compared to baseline (pre- supplementation) at 96 h following muscle damaging exercise on the green-lipped mussel oil blend supplemented diet. In support of this finding of an increase in muscle strength, Rajabi et al. [17] observed a significant increase in isotonic voluntary contractile strength of the quadriceps 24, 48 and 72 h following leg press eccentric exercise on a 30 day n-3 LC-PUFA supplemented diet compared to a placebo diet. Conversely, Gray et al. [14] observed no changes in MVC torque following 200 eccentric knee contractions, while Pumpa et al. [32] and Lenn et al. [21] observed no difference in muscle strength of the right and left quadriceps and non-dominant arm respectively between a placebo and n-3 LC-PUFA supplemented diet.

Many studies have documented decreases in the voluntary ROM (~20-45 degrees) following eccentric exercise, with full recovery not achieved until 10 days after exercise [44]. The mechanism to explain this decrease has been attributed to an increase in resting cytosol calcium levels, ultrastructure damage and/or an increase in fluid accumulation (swelling), and the measurement of joint ROM in muscle damage studies has been used as an indicator of passive muscle stiffness and soreness [45]. Our data indicate that muscle damaging exercise induced no loss of ROM in the green-lipped mussel oil blend group. However, within the placebo group ROM was significantly reduced (~4 deg) at 96 h post-muscle damaging exercise compared to baseline, and was significantly less (~4.9 deg) at 96 h following muscle damaging exercise on the placebo diet compared to the green-lipped mussel oil blend supplemented diet°. The protective effect provided by the n-3 LC-PUFA rich diet against ROM loss in the present study is similar to Tartibian et al. [19] and Rajabi et al. [17] who observed that on a n-3 LC-PUFA supplemented diet, compared to a placebo diet, the loss of knee ROM was significantly less post-eccentric bench stepping exercise and leg press eccentric exercise respectively, but are in contrast to the findings of Lenn et al. [21] and Phillips et al. [21] who observed no change in joint ROM following eccentric elbow flexion exercise.

Although swelling has been shown to occur following eccentric exercise and to be associated with the mechanisms of DOMS induced by eccentric exercise [46], there are studies that have shown a dissociation between when swelling and DOMS occur following eccentric exercise. Rodenburg et al. [47] have shown that MRI changes indicating the presence of edema do not to coincide with soreness following eccentric exercise (left forearm flexors) [47], while Clarkson et al. [35] noted that peak soreness occurred 2–3 d post-eccentric exercise (forearm flexor muscles) while peak swelling occurred 5 d following maximal effort eccentric actions of the forearm flexor muscles, while Yu et al. [48] has demonstrated that eccentric exercise (downstairs running) does induce muscle fiber swelling (soleus muscle), but it emerges at 7–8 d, and not at 2–3 d post-eccentric exercise when DOMS peaked. Based on the data from these studies [35,47,48] it is possible that we missed a potential effect of treatment on limb girth (swelling) since our final measurement of limb girth was at 96 h post-muscle damaging exercise.

Effect of green-lipped mussel oil blend supplementation on quadriceps muscle fatigue

Potentiated quadriceps twitch force ($Q_{tw,pot}$) assessed via magnetic stimulation before and after a 20-min cycling time trial pre- and post-supplementation (24 h following muscle damaging exercise) was used to quantify the degree of quadriceps muscle fatigue ($\Delta Q_{tw,pot}$). The measurement of quadriceps twitch force produced by supramaximal magnetic stimulation of the femoral nerve has been shown to be a reliable method to detect quadriceps fatigue following loading [38,40,49]. This study has shown for the first time in humans that n-3 LC-PUFA supplementation provided a protective effect against the development of quadriceps muscle fatigue following a 20 min exhaustive cycling ergometer test compared to placebo supplementation. While the $\%\Delta Q_{tw,pot}$ was unaltered between pre- and post- supplementation (24 h following muscle damaging exercise) for the green-lipped mussel oil blend group, there was a significant decline (~65%) in the $\%\Delta Q_{tw,pot}$ post-supplementation compared to pre-supplementation for the placebo group. Our data are in agreement with animal studies [50,51] that have shown that rats fed fish oil, hindlimb skeletal muscle were more resistant to fatigue during continuous muscle twitch contractions, and recovered contractile force better between repeat bouts, compared to an n-6 LC-PUFA or saturated fat enriched diet.

Effect of green-lipped mussel oil blend supplementation on blood markers of muscle damage, inflammation and DNA oxidative stress

Although a few studies have shown that eccentric exercise leads to myofibrillar remodeling specifically through Z-band related proteins, rather than muscle necrosis and inflammation [48,52], we have shown that supplementing the diet with a green-lipped mussel oil blend can mitigate the rise in a number of indirect markers of skeletal muscle damage and inflammation, and this effect persists for up to 96 h following muscle damaging exercise.

Slow skeletal troponin I is considered an early marker of EIMD, since it is particularly susceptible to calpain digestion, which may contribute to the early rise in plasma sTnI levels following eccentric exercise [53]. Our data are in agreement with Sorichter et al. [29] and Willoughby et al. [54] that a significant increase in serum sTnI can be detected within 2 h following muscle damaging exercise, and peaks within 24 h after the muscle injury- inducing sessions. In addition, we have shown for the first time that n-3 LC-PUFA supplementation can mitigate the increase in serum sTnI following muscle damaging exercise.

We observed a significant attenuation in serum Mb concentration in the green-lipped mussel oil blend group, compared to the placebo group, at 24, 48, 72 and 96 h following muscle damaging exercise, which is similar to the findings from a previous study [20] that showed that 30 d of n-3 LC-PUFA supplementation can moderate the rise in serum Mb at 24 and 48 h after eccentric exercise in untrained men. Myoglobin is an oxygen-binding heme protein found in skeletal and cardiac muscle, and thus is not specific for skeletal muscle, and h- FABP, which is involved in the transport and metabolism of fatty acids, is found in higher concentrations in the heart compared to human skeletal muscle [53]. However, both myoglobin and h-FABP have been proposed as useful markers of skeletal muscle injury in the absence of cardiac damage [30]. In the present study we did not observe any significant change in serum cTnI or h-FABP following muscle damaging exercise at any time point within either group, which suggests that the increase in serum myoglobin following muscle damaging exercise was likely the result of skeletal and not cardiac muscle damage.

Myofibrillar CK-MM is a cytosolic enzyme specifically bound to the myofibrillar M-line structure located in the sarcomere, and is also found in the space of the I-band sarcomeres where it provides support for muscle energy requirements. Whist we found that serum CK- MM significantly increased immediately following muscle damaging exercise and remained elevated in both groups for a further 96 h, there was a significant attenuation in serum CK- MM in the green-lipped mussel oil blend group, compared to the placebo group, for all-time points following muscle damaging exercise. A number of studies assessing the efficacy of n-3 LC-PUFA supplementation on EIMD and DOMS have not used serum CK-MM, but rather total serum CK concentration as an indirect marker of muscle damage. Given that total serum CK has not been shown to correlate with histological evidence of skeletal muscle damage [55] it is not surprising that considerable variability is observed in this blood marker among studies assessing the impact of n-3 LC-PUFA supplementation on muscle damage and DOMS following eccentric exercise [14,16,17,20,21,32].

An important aspect associated with the initiation and amplification of acute inflammation is the production of cytokines that are synthesized de nova by lymphocyte's and monocytes at the site of muscle injury, and aid in directing inflammatory-related events [56]. At the onset of inflammation there is an upregulation of the pro-inflammatory cytokines interleukin-1β, and tumor-necrosis factor (TNF)-α. While IL-1β and TNF-α are most likely released by resident macrophages at the site of injury [56], and initiate the inflammatory response, TNF- α, in particular, has been shown to play a significant role in the muscle regeneration phase following muscle injury [57,58]. While we observed a significant increase in TNF-α for both groups following muscle damaging exercise, with serum TNF-α peaking at 24 h post-muscle damaging exercise, and remaining elevated for up to 96 h, the serum concentration of TNF-α was significantly lower in the green-lipped mussel oil blend group compared to the placebo group. At present the data are conflicting as to whether n-3 LC-PUFA can suppress the inflammatory response following eccentric exercise [16,20,21,32].

Oxidative stress-induced muscle damage has been shown to be associated with muscle soreness, and the resultant generation of free radicals causes oxidative damage to cellular DNA [59]. 8-hydroxy-2' –deoxyguanosine (8-OHdG) is a product of oxidative DNA damage induced by the action of hydroxyl radicals on the DNA base deoxyguanosine (dG) and DNA single-strand breakage, and represents the most frequently used marker to assess DNA damage. Serum 8-OHdG has been shown to increase following eccentric isokinetic exercise in humans [59], but not after downhill running in rats [60] or humans [61]. In the present study we observed no significant increase in serum 8-OHdG following muscle damaging exercise in both groups compared to baseline, and no significant difference in serum 8-OHdG between groups at any time point. The lack of change in serum 8-OHdG following muscle damaging exercise does not exclude the possibility that changes in this marker were present in the active skeletal muscle, as the serum concentration 8-OHdG may be diluted in comparison with the actual site of generation (within muscle). In addition, the intensity/duration of the stimulus may not have been sufficient to overwhelm the body's endogenous antioxidant system, and/or an upregulation of protective mechanisms against DNA damage developing [59], may have also played a role. It is surprising that serum 8- OhdG was not increased following muscle damaging exercise, especially given that structural protein within skeletal muscle was damaged (i.e. increase in serum sTnI). Changes in oxidative stress observed following muscle damaging exercise may not be the same when comparing blood and skeletal muscle, and thus we acknowledge that a limitation to our study is that we did not include additional biomarkers of oxidative stress.

While inflammation contributes to fibrosis, and causes pain and may well impair skeletal muscle function it does appear that inflammation represents a critical aspect of skeletal muscle repair and regeneration, and therefore blocking the inflammatory response with either pharmacological drugs or nutraceuticals may well hinder recovery [62]. With this in mind an important question that needs to be resolved is whether the most beneficial course of treatment should be to inhibit the inflammatory response or to let it progress naturally. Therefore, if there is a benefit in blocking inflammation, when is the appropriate time to do so and for how long post-muscle injury? While post-treatment of skeletal muscle injury is likely a more practical tactic, regardless of whether the injury is acute or slower to materialize such as with repetitive use injuries, it is not known at present whether n-3 LC-PUFA supplementation would be as effective in ameliorating EIMD and the inflammatory response if delivered post-injury only. This is an important question to answer since in some cases of skeletal muscle injury pre-treatment with anti-inflammatory agents for long periods of time is not always a realistic option for an individual.

Anti-inflammatory mechanisms of action of PCSO-524®

In the present study the attenuation of a number of indirect markers of EIMD and inflammation cannot be explained entirely by the EPA and DHA content of PCSO-524®, since the total amount of EPA and DHA content consumed daily was 58 mg and 44 mg respectively, which are considerably lower amounts than previous studies [14-20] that have demonstrated a positive effect of n-3 LC-PUFA supplementation (0.3 - 2.0 g EPA/day and 0.2 – 1.0 g DHA/day) on mitigating EIMD, DOMS and inflammation. It has been shown the green-lipped mussel oil blend used in the present study, which contains up to 91 fatty acid components [23], has more potent anti-inflammatory activity than fish oil, which contains abundant EPA, in various animal models of arthritis, and inflammatory bowel disease [22]. Therefore, it is possible that additional constituents of the green-lipped mussel oil blend, which may act synergistically with the n-3 LC-PUFA, may also be partially responsible for its anti-inflammatory effects. The green-lipped mussel oil blend contains polyphenols (oleuropein and hydroxtyrosol) and oleic acid, which are anti-inflammatory, and postulated to reduce risk factors for heart disease, lower cancer mortality, and reduce inflammation [22,63]. It has been shown that furan fatty acids, which are a minor component of the green-lipped mussel oil blend, exhibit more potent anti-inflammatory activity than EPA in a rat model of adjuvant-induced arthritis [25], and which possess potent free-radical scavenging abilities [64], may explain, at least in part, why in the present study the green-lipped mussel oil blend was effective in attenuating EIMD, DOMS and inflammation, given the very low dose of EPA and DHA.

Conclusion

In conclusion, the present study has shown that supplementing the diet of untrained men for 30 days with 1200 mg/d of a marine oil lipid and n-3 LC PUFA blend (PCSO-524®), derived from the New Zealand green lipped mussel, attenuated indirect markers of muscle damage and inflammation following downhill running designed to induce muscle damage, and may represent a useful therapeutic agent for mitigating muscle damage and inflammation following unaccustomed and/or eccentric exercise.

Competing interests
The authors declare that they have no competing interests.

Authors' contributions
JS, DP collected the study data, contributed to data interpretation and assisted in the drafting the manuscript. MH assisted in data collection. TM and RC designed the study and drafted the manuscript. All authors read and approved the final manuscript.

Acknowledgments
This work was supported by a grant from Pharmalink International Ltd, Hong Kong. The funders had no role in study design, data collection and analysis, in writing the manuscript, or decision to publish.

References
1. Howatson G, van Someren KA. The prevention and treatment of exercise-induced muscle damage. Sports Med. 2008;38(6):483–503.
2. Warren GL, Lowe DA, Armstrong RB. Measurement tools used in the study of eccentric contraction-induced injury. Sports Med. 1999;27(1):43–59.
3. Cheung K, Hume P, Maxwell L. Delayed onset muscle soreness: treatment strategies and performance factors. Sports Med. 2003;33(2):145–64.
4. Hirose L, Nosaka K, Newton M, Laveder A, Kano M, Peake JM, et al. Changes in inflammatory mediators following eccentric exercise of the elbow flexors. Exerc Immunol Rev. 2004;10:75–90.
5. Clarkson PM, Hubal MJ. Exercise-induced muscle damage in humans. Am J Phys Med Rehabil. 2002;81(11 Suppl):S52–69.
6. Lewis PB, Ruby D, Bush-Joseph CA. Muscle soreness and delayed-onset muscle soreness. Clin Sports Med. 2012;31(2):255–62.
7. Mikkelsen UR, Langberg H, Helmark IC, Skovgaard D, Andersen LL, Kjaer M, et al. Local NSAID infusion inhibits satellite cell proliferation in human skeletal muscle after eccentric exercise. J Appl Physiol. 2009;107(5):1600–11.
8. Trappe TA, White F, Lambert CP, Cesar D, Hellerstein M, Evans WJ. Effect of ibuprofen and acetaminophen on postexercise muscle protein synthesis. Am J Physiol Endocrinol Metab. 2002;282(3):E551–6.
9. Connolly DA, McHugh MP, Padilla-Zakour OI, Carlson L, Sayers SP. Efficacy of a tart cherry juice blend in preventing the symptoms of muscle damage. Br J Sports Med. 2006;40(8):679–83. discussion 683.
10. Drobnic F, Riera J, Appendino G, Togni S, Franceschi F, Valle X, et al. Reduction of delayed onset muscle soreness by a novel curcumin delivery system (Meriva(R)): a randomised, placebo-controlled trial. J Int Soc Sports Nutr. 2014;11:31.
11. O'Fallon KS, Kaushik D, Michniak-Kohn B, Dunne CP, Zambraski EJ, Clarkson PM. Effects of quercetin supplementation on markers of muscle damage and inflammation after eccentric exercise. Int J Sport Nutr Exerc Metab. 2012;22(6):430–7.
12. Serhan CN, Chiang N, Van Dyke TE. Resolving inflammation: dual anti-inflammatory and pro-resolution lipid mediators. Nat Rev Immunol. 2008;8(5):349–61.

13. Mickleborough TD. Omega-3 polyunsaturated fatty acids in physical performance optimization. Int J Sport Nutr Exerc Metabol. 2012;23(1):83–96.

14. Gray P, Chappell A, Jenkinson AM, Thies F, Gray SR. Fish oil supplementation reduces markers of oxidative stress but not muscle soreness after eccentric exercise. Int J Sport Nutr Exerc Metab. 2014;24(2):206–14.

15. Jouris KB, McDaniel JL, Weiss EP. The effect of omega-3 fatty acid supplemntation on the inflammatory response to eccentric strength exercise. J Sports Sci Med. 2011;10:432–8.

16. Phillips T, Childs AC, Dreon DM, Phinney S, Leeuwenburgh C. A dietary supplement attenuates IL-6 and CRP after eccentric exercise in untrained males. Med Sci Sports Exerc. 2003;35(12):2032–7.

17. Rajabi A, Lotfi N, Abdolmaleki A, Rashid-Amiri S. The effects of omega-3 intake on delayed onset muscle soreness in non-athletic men. Pedagogies, Psychology, Medical- Biological Problems of Physical Training and Sport. 2013;1:91–5.

18. Santos EP, Silva AS, Costa MJC, Moura Junior JS, Quirino ELO, Franca GAM, et al. Omega-3 supplementation attenuates the production of c-reactive protein in military personnel during 5 days of intense phsyical stress and nutritional restriction. Biol Sport. 2012;29:93–9.

19. Tartibian B, Maleki BH, Abbasi A. The effects of ingestion of omega-3 fatty acids on perceived pain and external symptoms of delayed onset muscle soreness in untrained men. Clin J Sport Med. 2009;19(2):115–9.

20. Tartibian B, Maleki BH, Abbasi A. Omega-3 fatty acids supplementation attenuates inflammatory markers after eccentric exercise in untrained men. Clin J Sport Med. 2011;21(2):131–7.

21. Lenn J, Uhl T, Mattacola C, Boissonneault G, Yates J, Ibrahim W, et al. The effects of fish oil and isoflavones on delayed onset muscle soreness. Med Sci Sports Exerc. 2002;34(10):1605–13.

22. Doggrell SA. Lyprinol - is It a useful anti-inflammatory agent? eCAM. 2011; Article ID 307121:1–8.

23. Wolyniak CJ, Brenna JT, Murphy KJ, Sinclair AJ. Gas chromatography-chemical ionization-mass spectrometric fatty acid analysis of a commercial supercritical carbon dioxide lipid extract from New Zealand green-lipped mussel (Perna canaliculus). Lipids. 2005;40(4):355–60.

24. Miller MR, Pearce L, Bettjeman BI. Detailed distribution of lipids in Greenshell mussel (Perna canaliculus). Nutrients. 2014;6(4):1454–74.

25. Wakimoto T, Kondo H, Nii H, Kimura K, Egami Y, Oka Y, et al. Furan fatty acid as an anti-inflammatory component from the green-lipped mussel Perna canaliculus. Proc Natl Acad Sci U S A. 2011;108(42):17533–7.

26. Whitehouse MW, Macrides TA, Kalafatis N, Betts WH, Haynes DR, Broadbent J. Anti- inflammatory activity of a lipid fraction (lyprinol) from the NZ green-lipped mussel. Inflammopharmacology. 1997;5(3):237–46.

27. Mickleborough TD, Vaughn CL, Shei R-J, Davis EM, Wilhite DP. Marine lipid fraction PCSO-524 (lyprinol/omega XL) of the New Zealand green lipped mussel attenuates hyperpnea-induced bronchoconstriction in asthma. Respir Med. 2013;197:1152–63.

28. Pescatello LS, Arena R, Riebe D, Thompson PD. ACSM's guidelines for exercise testing and prescription. 9th ed. Baltimore, MD: Wolters Kluwer - Lippincott Williams & Wilkins; 2014.

29. Sorichter S, Mair J, Koller A, Gebert W, Rama D, Calzolari C, et al. Skeletal troponin I as a marker of exercise-induced muscle damage. J Appl Physiol. 1997;83(4):1076–82.

30. Sorichter S, Mair J, Koller A, Pelsers MM, Puschendorf B, Glatz JF. Early assessment of exercise induced skeletal muscle injury using plasma fatty acid binding protein. Br J Sports Med. 1998;32(2):121–4.

31. Baum K, Telford RD, Cunningham RB. Marine oil dietary supplementation reduces delayed onest muscle soreness after a 30 km run. Open Access J Sports Med. 2013;4:109–15.

32. Pumpa KL, Fallon KE, Bensoussan A, Papalia S. The effects of Lyprinol((R)) on delayed onset muscle soreness and muscle damage in well trained athletes: a double-blind randomised controlled trial. Complement Ther Med. 2011;19(6):311–8.

33. Duke JW, Stickford JL, Weavil JC, Chapman RF, Stager JM, Mickleborough TD. Operating lung volumes are affected by exercise mode but not trunk and hip angle during maximal exercise. Eur J Appl Physiol. 2014;114(11):2387–97.

34. Eston RG, Mickleborough J, Baltzopoulos V. Eccentric activation and muscle damage: biomechanical and physiological considerations during downhill running. Br J Sports Med. 1995;29(2):89–94.

35. Clarkson PM, Nosaka K, Braun B. Muscle function after exercise-induced muscle damage and rapid adaptation. Med Sci Sports Exerc. 1992;24(5):512–20.

36. Watkins MA, Riddle DL, Lamb RL, Personius WJ. Reliability of goniometric measurements and visual estimates of knee range of motion obtained in a clinical setting. Phys Ther. 1991;71(2):90–6. discussion 96–97.

37. Nunan D, Howatson G, van Someren KA. Exercise-induced muscle damage is not attenuated by beta-hydroxy-beta-methylbutyrate and alpha-ketoisocaproic acid supplementation. J Strength Cond Res. 2010;24(2):531–7.

38. Amann M, Dempsey JA. Locomotor muscle fatigue modifies central motor drive in healthy humans and imposes a limitation to exercise performance. J Physiol. 2008;586(1):161–73.

39. Polkey MI, Kyroussis D, Hamnegard CH, Mills GH, Green M, Moxham J. Quadriceps strength and fatigue assessed by magnetic stimulation of the femoral nerve in man. Muscle Nerve. 1996;19(5):549–55.

40. Amann M, Eldridge MW, Lovering AT, Stickland MK, Pegelow DF, Dempsey JA. Arterial oxygenation influences central motor output and exercise performance via effects on peripheral locomotor muscle fatigue in humans. J Physiol. 2006;575(Pt 3):937–52.

41. Willett WC, Sampson L, Stampfer MJ, Rosner B, Bain C, Witschi J, et al. Reproducibility and validity of a semiquantitative food frequency questionnaire. Am J Epidemiol. 1985;122(1):51–65.

42. von Schacky C, Kemper M, Haslbauer R, Halle M. Low omega-3 index in 106 german elite winter endurance athletes: a pilot study. Int J Sport Nutr Exerc Metab. 2014;24(5):559–64.

43. Lembke P, Capodice J, Hebert K, Swenson T. Influence of omega-3 (n3) index on performance and wellbeing in young adults after heavy eccentric exercise. J Sports Sci Med. 2014;13(1):151–6.

44. Warren GL, Lowe DA, Hayes DA, Karwoski CJ, Prior BM, Armstrong RB. Excitation failure in eccentric contraction-induced injury of mouse soleus muscle. J Physiol. 1993;468:487–99.

45. McKune AJ, Semple SJ, Peters-Futre EM. Acute exercise-induced muscle injury. Biol Sport. 2012;29:3–10.

46. Lieber RL, Friden J. Mechanisms of muscle injury after eccentric contraction. J Sci Med Sport. 1999;2(3):253–65.

47. Rodenburg JB, de Boer RW, Schiereck P, van Echteld CJ, Bar PR. Changes in phosphorus compounds and water content in skeletal muscle due to eccentric exercise. Eur J Appl Physiol Occup Physiol. 1994;68(3):205–13.

48. Yu JG, Liu JX, Carlsson L, Thornell LE, Stal PS. Re-evaluation of sarcolemma injury and muscle swelling in human skeletal muscles after eccentric exercise. PLoS One. 2013;8(4):e62056.

49. Kufel TJ, Pineda LA, Mador MJ. Comparison of potentiated and unpotentiated twitches as an index of muscle fatigue. Muscle Nerve. 2002;25(3):438–44.

50. Peoples GE, McLennan PL. Dietary fish oil reduces skeletal muscle oxygen consumption, provides fatigue resistance and improves contractile recovery in the rat in vivo hindlimb. Br J Nutr. 2010;104(12):1771–9.

51. Peoples GE, McLennan PL. Long-chain n-3 DHA reduces the extent of skeletal muscle fatigue in the rat in vivo hindlimb model. Br J Nutr. 2014;111(6):996–1003.

52. Malm C, Yu JG. Exercise-induced muscle damage and inflammation: re-evaluation by proteomics. Histochem Cell Biol. 2012;138(1):89–99.

53. Sorichter S, Puschendorf B, Mair J. Skeletal muscle injury induced by eccentric muscle action: muscle proteins as markers of muscle fiber injury. Exerc Immunol Rev. 1999;5:5–21.

54. Willoughby DS, McFarlin B, Bois C. Interleukin-6 expression after repeated bouts of eccentric exercise. Int J Sports Med. 2003;24(1):15–21.

55. Van der Meulen JH, Kuipers H, Drukker J. Relationship between exercise-induced muscle damage and enzyme release in rats. J Appl Physiol. 1991;71(3):999–1004.

56. Dinarello CA. Role of pro- and anti-inflammatory cytokines during inflammation: experimental and clinical findings. J Biol Regul Homeost Agents. 1997;11(3):91–103.

57. Collins RA, Grounds MD. The role of tumor necrosis factor-alpha (TNF-alpha) in skeletal muscle regeneration. Studies in TNF-alpha(–/–) and TNF-alpha (–/–)/LT-alpha(–/–) mice. J Histochem Cytochem. 2001;49(8):989–1001.

58. Li YP. TNF-alpha is a mitogen in skeletal muscle. Am J Physiol Cell Physiol. 2003;285(2):C370–6.

59. Radak Z, Pucsok J, Mecseki S, Csont T, Ferdinandy P. Muscle soreness-induced reduction in force generation is accompanied by increased nitric oxide content and DNA damage in human skeletal muscle. Free Radic Biol Med. 1999;26(7–8):1059–63.

60. Umegaki K, Daohua P, Sugisawa A, Kimura M, Higuchi M. Influence of one bout of vigorous exercise on ascorbic acid in plasma and oxidative damage

to DNA in blood cells and muscle in untrained rats. J Nutr Biochem. 2000;11(7–8):401–7.

61. Sacheck JM, Milbury PE, Cannon JG, Roubenoff R, Blumberg JB. Effect of vitamin E and eccentric exercise on selected biomarkers of oxidative stress in young and elderly men. Free Radic Biol Med. 2003;34(12):1575–88.

62. Urso ML. Anti-inflammatory interventions and skeletal muscle injury: benefit or detriment? J Appl Physiol. 2013;115(6):920–8.

63. Tenikoff D, Murphy KJ, Le M, Howe PR, Howarth GS. Lyprinol (stabilised lipid extract of New Zealand green-lipped mussel): a potential preventative treatment modality for inflammatory bowel disease. J Gastroenterol. 2005;40(4):361–5.

64. Lemke RA, Peterson AC, Ziegelhoffer EC, Westphall MS, Tjellstrom H, Coon JJ, et al. Synthesis and scavenging role of furan fatty acids. Proc Natl Acad Sci U S A. 2014;111(33):E3450–7.

18

The effect of acute vs chronic magnesium supplementation on exercise and recovery on resistance exercise, blood pressure and total peripheral resistance on normotensive adults

Lindsy S Kass[*] and Filipe Poeira

Abstract

Background: Magnesium supplementation has previously shown reductions in blood pressure of up to 12 mmHg. A positive relationship between magnesium supplementation and performance gains in resistance exercise has also been seen. However, no previous studies have investigated loading strategies to optimise response. The aim of this study was to assess the effect of oral magnesium supplementation on resistance exercise and vascular response after intense exercise for an acute and chronic loading strategy on a 2-day repeat protocol.

Methods: The study was a randomised, double-blind, cross-over design, placebo controlled 2 day repeat measure protocol (n = 13). Intense exercise (40 km time trial) was followed by bench press at 80% 1RM to exhaustion, with blood pressure and total peripheral resistance (TPR) recorded. 300 mg/d elemental magnesium was supplemented for either a 1 (A) or 4 (Chr) week loading strategy. Food diaries were recorded.

Results: Dietary magnesium intake was above the Reference Nutrient Intake (RNI) for all groups. Bench press showed a significant increase of 17.7% (p = 0.031) for A on day 1. On day 2 A showed no decrease in performance whilst Chr showed a 32.1% decrease. On day 2 post-exercise systolic blood pressure (SBP) was significantly lower in both A (p = 0.0.47) and Chr (p = 0.016) groups. Diastolic blood pressure (DBP) showed significant decreases on day 2 solely for A (p = 0.047) with no changes in the Chr. TPR reduced for A on days 1 and 2 (p = 0.031) with Chr showing an increase on day 1 (p = 0.008) and no change on day 2.

Conclusion: There was no cumulative effect of Chr supplementation compared to A. A group showed improvement for bench press concurring with previous research which was not seen in Chr. On day 2 A showed a small non-significant increase but not a decrement as expected with Chr showing a decrease. DBP showed reductions in both Chr and A loading, agreeing with previous literature. This is suggestive of a different mechanism for BP reduction than for muscular strength. TPR showed greater reductions with A than Chr, which would not be expected as both interventions had reductions in BP, which is associated with TPR.

Keywords: Magnesium supplementation, Blood pressure, Bench press, Acute and chronic loading

* Correspondence: L.s.kass@herts.ac.uk
University of Hertfordshire, School of Life and Medical Science, College Lane,
Hatfield, Hertfordshire AL10 9AB, UK

Background

Magnesium (Mg^{2+}) elicits significant enzymatic cellular involvement and physical regulation such as energy metabolism/production through formation of the Mg-ATP complex [1] and physiological regulation and control of neuromuscular cardiac activity, muscular contraction, vascular tone and blood pressure [2,3]. Its effect on muscular contraction and vascular tone have been shown to reduce blood pressure and subsequently vascular resistance [4].

Nutritional supplementation is a well-established method for enhancing performance in conjunction to training. Micronutrient intake has been highlighted to have gained greater prominence with athletes in relation to the importance of an adequate nutritional status [5], However, previous research highlights nutritional inadequacies and thus an impaired nutritional status (i.e. marginal nutrient deficiency) from both an athletic [5] and general population perspective [6]. This identifies physical activity as increasing the rate at which micronutrients are utilised, promoting excessive micronutrient loss via increased catabolism and excretion (sweat and urine). Magnesium is a mineral required at rest and during exercise [7]. This increase in Mg^{2+} turnover during exercise may lead to a state of insufficiency acting as a contributory factor towards an increase in blood pressure and a state of hypertension [8]. This, together with a decline in dietary intake below the RNI may have a negative impact on both performance and blood pressure.

Magnesium supplementation in relation to exercise has differed considerably in research opinion as to the dose and type of Mg2+ salt administered. It is influenced by the specific anion attachment with Mg2+, thus influencing supplemental solubility, elemental Mg2+ bioavailability and supplemental effectiveness [9]. Research has illustrated organic forms of Mg2+ supplementation i.e. Aspartate, citrate, lactate, pidolate, fumarate, acetate, ascorbate and gluconate to exemplify a greater solubility and bioavailability in comparison to inorganic forms i.e. oxide, sulphate, chloride and carbonate [10] When considered relative to the quantity needed to be ingested to release 300 mg of elemental Mg2+ along with the fact that certain magnesiums are unavailable in the UK, magnesium citrate was considered to be the best option for this protocol.

Research to date consists of both positive [11-13] and negative [14,15] findings. The research appears to agree that Mg^{2+} supplementation has no effect on physical performance when serum concentrations are within the normal range (serum Mg^{2+} 0.8-1.2 $mmol \cdot L^{-1}$) [12,16]. However, manipulating intakes of Mg^{2+} by diet or supplementation has been shown to have performance [11,17] and blood pressure enhancements [13,18]. Limitations to many of these studies is the lack of information regarding either serum magnesium or dietary intake [19]. The general consensus appears to be that Mg^{2+} supplementation has a greater effect when habitual dietary intake or serum levels are low.

Further, to the best of the authors' knowledge research to date lacks analysis of Mg^{2+} from an acute (A) and chronic (Chr) viewpoint within the same study. Therefore, the aim of the current study was to assess the effect of oral Mg^{2+} supplementation on strength performance and vascular responses from both an A and Chr loading strategy as to establish potential differences in supplemental duration and influences of dietary status and supplemental dose on performance and vascular responses.

Methods

Subjects

A total of 13 subjects (males (m) = 7 females (f) = 6) were recruited from recreational running, cycling and triathlete clubs. Six subjects were allocated randomly to the acute intervention group (m = 3, f = 3) and 7 to the chronic intervention group (m = 4, f = 3). Subjects were recruited in accordance to meeting the inclusion/exclusion criteria, (Table 1). Informed consent and health screen were completed and ethical approval was granted by the University of Hertfordshire School of Life Sciences Ethics Committee.

Experimental design

The study was a randomised, cross-over, double-blind, placebo controlled, 2 day repeated measure protocol. Subjects were assigned to either the acute or chronic intervention and the two trials ran parallel. Within each trial subjects undertook both the magnesium intervention and a placebo intervention with a one week washout period in a randomised order. The two interventions were a chronic (Chr) (4 weeks) and acute (A) (1 week) loading strategy, sub-divided into a supplemental and a placebo control group with a 1 week washout period. A maximal graded exercise test for determination of VO_{2max} was conducted to ensure participant homogeneity with a cut off of 45 ml/kg^{-1} and 35 ml/kg^{-1} oxygen for males and females respectively. The study was tested across 2 consecutive days at each treatment time-point i.e. baseline

Table 1 Subject characteristics; including group sample size (n), age, height, weight, VO_{2max}, HR_{max}

	Chronic	Acute
N	7	6
Age (years)	40.8 ± 4.4	35.8 ± 6.2
Height (cm)	176.2 ± 11	174.6 ± 12
Weight (kg)	73.2 ± 13.2	72.1 ± 13
VO2max (ml/kg)	51.8 ± 9.1	53 ± 4.8
HRmax (bpm)	176.4 ± 3.8	180.8 ± 7.7

Values are mean ± SD.

and again after either 1 or 4 weeks intervention. A one week washout was then given and then a further intervention of the opposite treatment was given (placebo or magnesium) with the same loading phase.

Protocol

After familiarisation, subjects were tested for baseline measurements Anthropometric measures (height (cm), weight (kg)) and age (y)) were recorded. All subjects attended a familiarisation session on all equipment and testing protocols prior to testing. On both day 1 and recovery day 2 participants completed a 40 km time trial on bicycles owned by the subjects and set onto a rig. A set 40 km flat course with no wind setting was used on a Computrainer Pro ergometer (Computrainer, Seattle). All on-screen course data information was blinded, verbal encouragement was not given during the exercise testing. The time trial was carried out to elicit physiological stress as normally determined by training and competition. After a 30 minute rest participants completed the following tests to determine the effect of magnesium on strength and cardiovascular parameters.

Blood pressure, and augmentation index (Aix) were recorded at rest immediately and before the bench press. Subjects then performed a bench press corresponding to a 5 repetition maximum (5-RM) protocol [20]) for determination of their 1-RM. Upon completion, a 5-minutes rest period was given. Subsequently, a bench press at 80% 1-RM was performed to exhaustion. A measure of force (Newtons) was recorded during the bench press, with additional measures of blood pressure and Aix immediately upon completion of the bench press.

Supplementation

Magnesium citrate and placebo (cornflour) were capsulated into large vegetarian capsules. Capsules consisted of a total of 75 mg of elemental Mg^{2+} citrate, (Pioneer analytical balance. OHAUS, UK), 4 capsules per day were taken orally, equating supplemental Mg^{2+} to a total daily dose of 300 mg/d elemental Mg^{2+}. Supplements were ingested evenly throughout the day on a non-testing day, or ingested 3 hours before exercise testing. Finally, the supplementation period for both placebo and Mg^{2+} accounted for a total ingestion period of 1 week or 4 weeks within the A and Chr groups, respectively.

Diet

A 4-day weighed food and beverage diary was recorded in relation to 3 weekdays and 1 weekend day, which was used for analysis of habitual dietary magnesium intake through use of dietary analysis software (Dietplan 6.70 Forestfield Software, UK).

Statistical analysis

Data were analysed using SPSS version 20 (IBM limited, UK) and Microsoft excel 2007 for Windows. Box-whisker plots measured normality/data distribution and showed that the data were not normally distributed. Therefore non-parametric Wilcoxon 2 related samples tests were carried out on all results to look for differences. Alpha value was set at 0.05.

Results

There were no statistically significant difference found between anthropometric data, VO_{2max} and HR determining a homogeneous cohort (Table 1).

Table 2 shows averaged dietary data for both the Chr and A groups. Both the Chr and A control groups showed no significant difference between macronutrient and magnesium ingestion.

Performance

Bench press

Net strength gains as determined by 1-RM showed significant increase of 17.7% with the acute Mg^{2+} loading strategy compared to baseline (p = 0.031) (Figure 1). No significant strength gains were seen in the Chr intervention group (p = 0.281).

Furthermore, A Mg^{2+} showed no decline in recovery (day 2) performance for force (N) resulting in a small day 2 (recovery day) force increase of 2.7%, showing a trend but no significicnace (Figure 2). On the contrary Chr Mg^{2+} showed a day-to-day 32.1% performance decrement (Figure 3).

Resting SBP measures from day 1 and 2 show a significant decrease within A Mg^{2+} treatment (P = 0.031), conversely placebo showed a significant increase in SBP (P = 0.047) (Table 3). Further, significant day 2 reductions in SBP were noted between A treatments of Mg^{2+}-placebo (P = 0.016). On the contrary, Chr Mg^{2+} shows no significant reductions in resting SBP on day 1 or day 2.

In relation to post SBP responses, both Chr and A Mg^{2+} treatment resulted in significant SBP reductions; however, such reductions can be noted on day 1 (P = 0.016) and day 2 (P = 0.016) for a Chr Mg^{2+} induced SBP

Table 2 Dietary intake, values are mean ± SD

	Chronic intervention	Acute intervention	Chronic placebo control	Acute placebo control
Kcal	2513 ± 1201	2686 ± 938	3985 ± 519	3785 ± 734
CHO (g)	274 ± 170	296 ± 118	397 ± 209	343 ± 79
Fat (g)	96 ± 58	115 ± 49	114 ± 63	105 ± 48
Pro (g)	119 ± 38	114 ± 37	136 ± 66	129 ± 16
Mg^{2+} (mg)	375 ± 104	368 ± 173	551 ± 347	378 ± 79

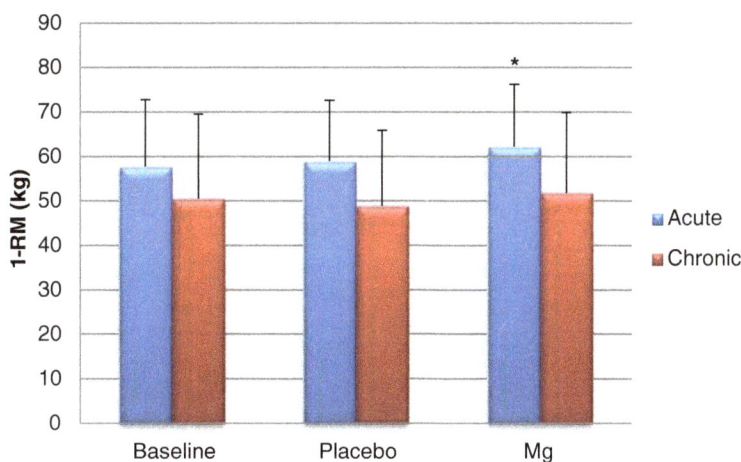

Figure 1 Acute and chronic bench press 1-RM scores on day 1 ± SD. * denotes significance.

reduction in comparison to placebo, whereas an A Mg^{2+} reduction can be accounted for on day 2 (P = 0.047) in comparison to placebo.

Resting DBP showed no difference for day 1 to day 2 between the placebo or Mg^{2+}. Post DBP showed no differences between Day 1 to Day 2 for acute supplementation group (Table 4). However, chronic intervention showed a decrease in DBP for post bench press on the recovery day 2.

Although no significance was seen for Aix at rest for both A and Chr loading strategies, a significant lowering post bench press was found as highlighted in Table 5 on day 1 for A treatment and day 2 for the Chr treatment group. Day 1 Aix reductions correspond to a significant Mg^{2+} lowering effect compared to baseline (P = 0.016) and placebo (P = 0.031), respectively. Whereas, similar Aix reductions for the Chr Mg^{2+} group is noted on day 2

post bench press resulting in significant values of P = 0.039, when compared to baseline and placebo, respectively.

Discussion

This study set out to determine whether either acute or chronic magnesium supplementation would have an effect on performance (strength and cardiovascular) and blood pressure with exercise and/or on a second bout of exercise after a 24 hr recovery period. As has been shown previously [13,21] acute magnesium supplementation has a positive effect on BP, plyometric parameters and torque, however its effect on resistance exercise has not been evident to date. Further, chronic loading strategies have not been investigated in respect to exercise as well as the effect of Mg supplementation on a second bout of exercise. It was hypothesised that as acute Mg^{2+} supplementation has been seen to have beneficial effects

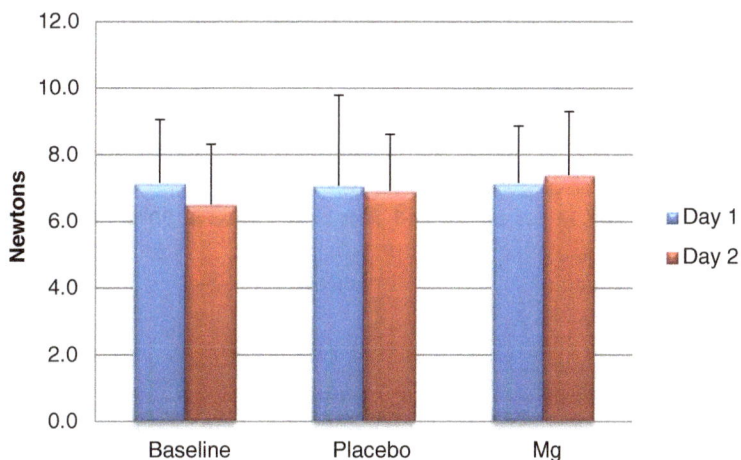

Figure 2 Acute force (newtons) output on day 1 and 2 (recovery) during repetitions to fatigue ± SD.

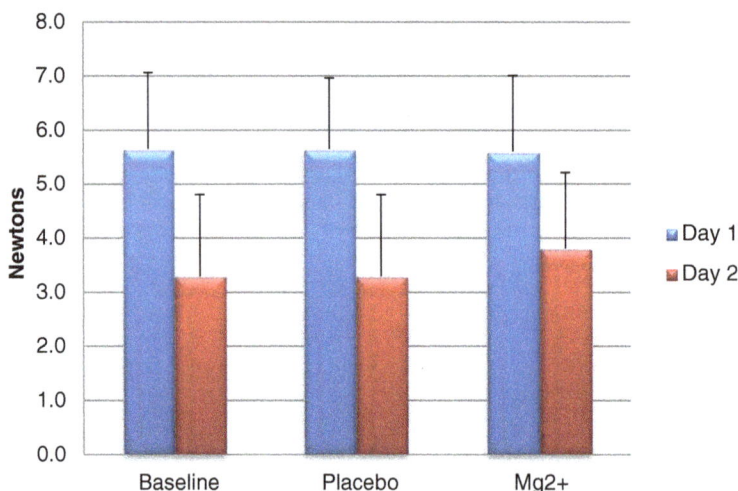

Figure 3 Chronic force (newtons) output on day 1 and 2 (recovery) during repetitions to fatigue ± SD.

on BP, CV parameters and peak torque a longer loading strategy (4 weeks) would amplify these results, giving a more beneficial and greater response. However, this study did not find that chronic loading of Mg^{2+} has a cumulative effect on the effect of supplementation, perhaps due to saturation of Mg^{2+} within the blood or limitations to transporters.

Primary findings showed variance across treatment groups on exercise (strength and recovery) and cardiovascular responses. The Chr Mg^{2+} intervention showed no significance in performance gains for bench press net strength and force output (Figures 1, 2 and 3). The A Mg^{2+} intervention showed variance in results across all variable analysed with some improvements being seen in resting HR and blood pressure for both Chr and A treatment groups regarding strength related performance (Figures 1, 2, 3 and Tables 3, 4, 5).

Strength performance

Strength related performance within the bench press showed statistical significant improvements (P = 0.031) within the A group and Chr group. Previous research has shown that Mg^{2+} significantly enhances bench press [22] and strength performance [11,23]. Acute Mg^{2+} loading

showed a significant net strength increase of 5.5 kg between baseline and supplemental Mg^{2+} trials. Other strength related measurements of force (Newtons) illustrated A Mg^{2+} induced improvements. Typically, where a decrease in force would be expected on day 2 (recovery) of training as a normal physiological response to training, an A group improvement of 0.25 Newtons (2.7%) was seen with Mg^{2+} supplementation compared to the Chr where a 2.0 Newtons (32.1%) decrement was seen.

When examining net strength of Chr compared to A groups a notable difference between baseline scores is evident implying that subjects within the A group might well be stronger due to a 7.3 kg 1-RM difference at baseline (Figure 1). Therefore, when considering the 10.5 kg difference between Chr and A group 1-RM trials after intervention of Mg^{2+}, inter-subject lifting capacity/ability could be a factor of concern for validating such a difference.

These performance enhancements for the strength associated tests are suggestive of physiological-regulatory functions of Mg^{2+} within muscle contraction and relaxation; i.e. regulating troponin expression via Ca^{2+} concentration gradients, Ca^{2+} transport, MgATP complex formation optimising energy metabolism/muscular contraction, increasing protein synthetic rate, protection against cellular

Table 3 Acute and chronic group mean SBP values at rest and post bench press at 80% 1-RM to fatigue on day 1 and 2 ±SD

Physiological variable	Treatment	Group		Physiological variable	Treatment	Group	
		C Chr	A			Chr	A
Resting SBP (mmHg) day 1	Placebo	119 ± 7	120 ± 5*[1]	Post SBP (mmHg) day 1	Placebo	143 ± 7*[3]	136 ± 5
	Mg2+	118 ± 6	122 ± 4*[2]		Mg2+	136 ± 9*[3]	137 ± 6
Resting SBP (mmHg) day 2	Placebo	121 ± 8	125 ± 2*[1, 3]	Post SBP (mmHg) day 2	Placebo	144 ± 9*[4]	144 ± 7*[5]
	Mg2+	118 ± 7	117 ± 7*[2, 3]		Mg2+	137 ± 10*[4]	134 ± 5*[5]

*Denotes significance as paired by numbers.

Table 4 Acute and chronic group mean DBP values at rest and post bench press at 80% 1-RM to fatigue on day 1 and 2 ± SD

Physiological variable	Treatment	Group		Physiological variable	Treatment	Group	
		Chr	A			Chr	A
Resting DBP (mmHg) day 1	Placebo	85 ± 7	75 ± 7	Post DBP (mmHg) day 1	Placebo	92 ± 8	85 ± 12
	Mg2+	79 ± 6	75 ± 4		Mg2+	87 ± 7	82 ± 5
Resting DBP (mmHg) day 2	Placebo	78 ± 8	79 ± 6	Post DBP (mmHg) day 2	Placebo	91 ± 5[*1, 2]	86 ± 13
	Mg2+	75 ± 7[*1]	74 ± 5[*2]		Mg2+	84 ± 8[*2]	76 ± 8[*3]

*Denotes significance as paired by numbers.

damage and, greater amount of actin-mysoin crossbridges [23-26] all of which contribute to the result of increased strength and force production. Consideration must be given as to why such a contrasting difference between Chr and A groups occur specifically when regarding strength performance measures. The A Mg^{2+} supplemented group showed day-to-day performance improvements across 3 trials, as opposed to 3 day-to-day non-performance improved trials exhibited within the Chr Mg^{2+} supplemented group which may be attributed to the different loading strategies within the current study. The Mg^{2+} supplementation within the current research was 300 mg/d, therefore equating the Chr and A group mean daily intake for Mg^{2+} to 675 mg/d and 700 mg/d, respectively, when combined with dietary Mg^{2+} intake as analysed from food diaries. This adds a sense of greater ambiguity when considering the Mg^{2+} - strength performance relationship, and comparing to research highlighting observations that intakes of 500 mg/d or greater result in further increases in strength [24,25]. It could be suggested that subjects within the Chr loading group might be more susceptible to a possible reduction threshold or cell tolerance for Mg^{2+} absorption based upon the understanding that high Mg^{2+} intakes result in a lower Mg^{2+} absorption [27]. Additionally, Mg^{2+} homeostasis may be postulated to exhibit no greater benefit from the chronic perspective due to the kidney function for Mg^{2+} excretion as to maintain a balanced concentration of Mg^{2+} [27,28]; for example, could the principle of a higher Mg^{2+} dose, longer supplemental duration and associated proportional

increase of Mg^{2+} excretion highlight the body's efficiency in maintaining a state of homeostasis? Alternatively, chronic loading through providing a regular high Mg^{2+} intake may influence extracellular Mg^{2+} concentrations which coincide with manipulation of Mg^{2+} transporter TRPM6 function, resulting in a potential decrease in TRPM6 expression in conjunction to increasing the urinary excretion of Mg^{2+} [29]. Thus, an acute ingestion rate as opposed to chronic could result in a more efficient use for Mg^{2+}.

Cardiovascular responses at rest and post bench press performance

Significant reductions in SBP and DBP are illustrated from post testing in the chronic group and rest and post testing in the acute group data across day 1 and 2 compared to baseline and placebo (Tables 3 and 4). Resting SBP was accounted for by a greater reduction in the A Mg^{2+} of 2 mmHg, in comparison to 0.7 mmHg with the Chr Mg^{2+} treatment. In addition, both resting and post DBP showed reductions with a greater day-to-day DBP reduction in the A Mg^{2+} in comparison to Chr Mg^{2+} as shown by a 69.2% and 50% (9 mmHg and 3 mmHg difference) at rest and post exercise for A and Chr groups respectively. These findings are in agreement with previous research [13,30] showing the importance of Mg^{2+} and its influence on blood pressure regulation. This is supported by findings within a recent meta-analysis [19] looking at Mg^{2+} supplementation which showed that SBP and DBP reductions of 2–3 mmHg and 3–4 mmHg, respectively. These observations oppose some previous findings which emphasise supplemental ineffectiveness of Mg^{2+} [31-33].

Such reductions in blood pressure could be speculated as being an outcome influenced by increases within the extracellular concentration of Mg^{2+}, an effect that has been associated with reductions in the arterial tension and tone. These reductions in arterial tension and tone correspond to typical Mg^{2+} induced vasodilatory actions which potentiate effects of endogenous vasodilators such as adenosine, K^+, nitric oxide and cyclo-oxygenase-dependent mechanisms via production of PGI2 [34]. In combination, Mg^{2+} acts as an antagonist to blocking Ca^{2+} channels

Table 5 Acute and chronic group mean Aix values post bench press at 80% of 1-RM to fatigue on day 1 and 2 ± SD

Physiological variable	Treatment	Group	
		Chr	A
Post Aix day 1 (%)	Baseline	7 ± 11	17 ± 5[*3]
	Placebo	9 ± 6	14 ± 6[*4]
	Mg2+	7 ± 5	10 ± 5[*3 *4]
Post Aix day 2 (%)	Baseline	14 ± 7[*1]	12 ± 6
	Placebo	14 ± 8[*2]	16 ± 4
	Mg2+	8 ± 12[*1, 2]	11 ± 6

*Denotes significance as paired by numbers.

[11,35,36] and further enzymatic mobilisation of Ca^{2+} [37]. Thus, data within the current study concur with previous research on the efficacy of Mg^{2+} supplementation in reducing blood pressure [13,38] and its capacity to suppress agonist vasoconstriction [4]. The above mechanisms may also be attributed to Mg^{2+} induced specific alterations within the vasculature, for example, Mg^{2+}'s mediatory role within the endothelium corresponds to increased nitric oxide, PGI2 and decreases platelet aggregation, in combination to stringent down-regulation of Ca^{2+} voltage operated channel activity and release from the sarcoplasmic reticulum [39].

Average dietary Mg^{2+} intakes within the A and Chr groups corresponded to 368 mg/d and 375 mg/d, respectively. However, it must be considered that the blood pressure reduction in Chr and A loading strategies, may be attributed to the Mg^{2+} supplementation. With this in mind, it could be suggested that despite average dietary intakes of Mg^{2+} meeting the UK RNI a higher requirement for Mg^{2+} may be beneficial in reducing blood pressure. Further recommendations within the U.S are 420 mg/d and 320 mg/d for males, and females, respectively, in addition to Mg^{2+} requirements within the UK being determined many years ago [40]; Research by Geleijnse et al. [41] in a comparative study between 5 European countries which included the UK, corroborates with this study suggesting a potential increase of Mg^{2+} based on supplemental blood pressure enhancements, whereby the researchers highlighted a <350 mg/d of Mg^{2+} as suboptimal, augmenting the prevalence of hypertension. The study further accounted for an 80% insufficiency corresponding to Mg^{2+} intake to be evident within the UK population analysed [41].

A principle limitation within the current study concerns lack of monitoring of the subjects' Mg^{2+} status via serum concentrations therefore this research is limited to infer indirect associations between Mg^{2+} supplementation and performance from dietary intake determined from food diaries. The study duration and the nature of a consecutive 2 day protocol both consisting of a 40 Km time trial can be seen as to limit the potential for subject recruitment and therefore final number of participants recruited. The use of males and females within groups must also be noted to account for occasional group data variance, on various parameters and a high level of standard deviation.

Conclusion

The current study showed a positive effect with A Mg^{2+} supplementation in relation to net strength and force gains with bench press, findings that support previous research [11,22,23,25]. Further, cardiovascular responses to the bench press were significantly enhanced by Mg^{2+} supplementation reducing resting SBP and DBP with the greatest effect seen with A Mg^{2+} supplementation for rest

and post exercise. Similarly, SBP, DBP and Aix showed a significantly greater and more consistent reduction in response to the A Mg^{2+} loading strategy, as opposed to the minimalistic effect induced by Chr Mg^{2+} loading strategy.

In conclusion, it can be stated that improvements seen with the A loading strategy cannot to the same extent be observed with the Chr loading of Mg^{2+}, thus potentially suggesting a regulatory effect within the body influenced by the duration of Mg^{2+} supplementation intake.

To conclude, from this study there appears to be no benefit in long term magnesium supplementation for those who have adequate dietary intake, but there are some benefits for taking an acute dose, particularly before intense exercise.

Future work may focus on the above parameters for those with low dietary Mg^{2+} intake and also for the optimum time that supplementation should be given to induce these positive findings.

Competing interests
The authors declare that they have no competing interests.

Authors' contributions
LK conceived of the study, participated in its design and coordination, statistical analysis and writing of the manuscript. FP carried out the data collection, statistical analysis and writing of the manuscript. Both authors read and approved the final manuscript.

References

1. Maguire ME. Magnesium transporters: properties, regulation and structure. Front Biosci. 2006;11:3149–63.
2. Bohl CH, Volpe SL. Magnesium and exercise. Crit Rev Food Sci Nutr. 2002;42(6):533–63.
3. Fawcett WJ, Haxby EJ, Male D a. Magnesium: physiology and pharmacology. Br J Anaesth. 1999;83:302–20.
4. Touyz RM. Role of magnesium in the pathogenesis of hypertension. Mol Aspects Med. 2003;24:107–36.
5. Lukaski HC. Micronutrients (magnesium, zinc, and copper): are mineral supplements need for athletes? Int J Sport Nutr. 1995;5suppl:S74–83.
6. Ford ES, Mokdad AH. Dietary magnesium intake in a national sample of U.S. adults. J Nutr. 2003;133:2879–82.
7. Uzun A. The acute effect of maximal strength, power endurance and interval run training on levels of some elements in elite basketball players. Life Sci J. 2013;10:2697–701.
8. Kass LS, Skinner P, Poeira F. A pilot study on the effects of magnesium supplementation with high and low habitual dietary magnesium intake on resting and recovery from aerobic and resistance exercise and systolic blood pressure. J Sports Sci Med. 2013;12:144–50.
9. Ranadel VV, Somberg JC. Bioavailability and pharmacokinetics of magnesium after administration of magnesium salts to humans. Am J Ther. 2001;8:345–57.
10. Newhouse IJ, Finstad EW. The effects of magnesium supplementation on exercise performance. Clin J Sport Med. 2000;10:195–200.
11. Santos DA, Matias CN, Monteiro CP, Silva AM, Rocha PM, Minderico CS, et al. Magnesium intake is associated with strength performance in elite basketball, handball and volleyball players. Magnes Res. 2011;24:215–9.
12. Lukaski HC, Nielsen FH. Dietary magnesium depletion affects metabolic responses during submaximal exercise in postmenopausal women. Hum Nutr Metab. 2002;132:930–5.
13. Itoh K, Kawasaka T, Nakamura M. The effects of high oral magnesium supplementation on blood pressure, serum lipids and related variables in apparently healthy Japanese subjects. Br J Nutr. 1997;78:737–50.

14. Finstad EW, Newhouse IJ. The effects of magnesium supplementation on exercise performance. Clin J Sport Med. 2001;33:493–8.

15. Terblanche S, Noakes TD, Dennis SC, Marais D, Eckert M. Failure of magnesium supplementation to influence marathon running performance or recovery in magnesium-replete subjects. Int J Sport Nutr. 1992;2:154–64.

16. Williams M. Dietary supplements and sports performance: amino acids. J Int Soc Sports Nutr. 2005;2:63–7.

17. Golf SW, Bender S, Gruttner J. On the significance of magnesium in extreme physical stress. Cardiovasc Drugs Ther. 1998;12(2):197–202.

18. Jee SH, Miller ER, Guallar E, Singh VK, Appel LJ, Klag MJ. The effect of magnesium supplementation on blood pressure: a meta-analysis of randomized clinical trials. Am J Hypertens. 2002;15:691–6.

19. Kass L, Weekes J, Carpenter L. Effect of magnesium supplementation on blood pressure: a meta-analysis. Eur J Clin Nutr. 2012;66:411–8.

20. Baechle T, Earle R. Essentials of Strength Training and Conditioning. 3rd ed. Human Kinetics: Illonois; 2008.

21. Setaro L, Santos-Silva P, Nakano E, Sales C, Nune N, Greve J, et al. Magnesium status and the physical performance of volleyball players: effects of magnesium supplemenatation. J Sport Sci. 2014;32:438–5.

22. Matias CN, Santos DA, Monteiro CP, Silva AM, Raposo MDF, Martins F, et al. Magnesium and strength in elite judo athletes according to intracellular water changes. Magnes Res. 2010;23:138–41.

23. Dominguez LJ, Barbagallo M, Lauretani F, Bandinelli S, Bos A, Corsi AM, et al. Magnesium and muscle performance in older persons: the InCHIANTI study. Am J Clin Nutr. 2006;84:419–26.

24. Lukaski HC. Vitamin and mineral status: effects on physical performance. Nutrition. 2004;20:632–44.

25. Brilla LR, Haley TF. Effect of magnesium supplementation on strength training in humans. J Am Coll Nutr. 1992;11:326–9.

26. Carvil P, Cronin J. Magnesium and implications on muscle function. Strength Cond J. 2010;32:48–54.

27. Jahnen-Dechent W, Ketteler M. Magnesium basics. Clin Kidney J. 2012;5 Suppl 1:i3–i14.

28. De Baaij JHF, Hoenderop JGJ, Bindels RJM. Regulation of magnesium balance: lessons learned from human genetic disease. Clin Kidney J. 2012;5 Suppl 1:i15–24.

29. Alexander RT, Hoenderop JG, Bindels RJ. Molecular determinants of magnesium homeostasis: insights from human disease. J Am Soc Nephrol. 2008;19:1451–8.

30. Motoyama T, Sano H, Fukuzaki H. Oral magnesium supplementation in patients with essential hypertension. Hypertension. 1989;13:227–32.

31. Dickinson HO, Mason JM, Nicolson DJ, Campbell F, Beyer FR, Cook JV, et al. Lifestyle interventions to reduce raised blood pressure: a systematic review of randomized controlled trials. J Hypertens. 2006;24:215–33.

32. Cappuccio FP. Lack of effect of oral magnesium double blind study. Br Med J. 1985;291:235–8.

33. Doyle L, Flynn a, Cashman K. The effect of magnesium supplementation on biochemical markers of bone metabolism or blood pressure in healthy young adult females. Eur J Clin Nutr. 1999;53:255–61.

34. Pokan R, Hofmann P, von Duvillard SP, Smekal G, Wonisch M, Lettner K, et al. Oral magnesium therapy, exercise heart rate, exercise tolerance, and myocardial function in coronary artery disease patients. Br J Sports Med. 2006;40:773–8.

35. Laires MJ. Biochemistry Laboratory, Faculty of Human Kinetics, Technical University of Lisbon, Portugal, 2 Genetics Laboratory, Faculty of Medicine, University of Lisbon, Portugal. Front Biosci. 2004;9:262–76.

36. O'Rourke B, Backx PH, Marban E. Phosphorylation-independent modulation of L-type calcium channels by magnesium-nucleotide complexes. Science. 1992;257:245–8.

37. Laurant P, Touyz RM. Physiological and pathophysiological role of magnesium in the cardiovascular system: implications in hypertension. J Hypertens. 2000;18:1177–91.

38. Guerrero-Romero F, Rodríguez-Morán M. Low serum magnesium levels and metabolic syndrome. Acta Diabetol. 2002;39:209–13.

39. Geiger H, Wanner C. Magnesium in disease. Clin Kidney J. 2012;5 Suppl 1:i25–38.

40. Nielsen FH, Lukaski HC. Update on the relationship between magnesium and exercise. Magnes Res. 2006;19:180–9.

41. Geleijnse JM, Grobbee DE, Kok FJ. Impact of dietary and lifestyle factors on the prevalence of hypertension in Western populations. J Hum Hypertens. 2005;19 Suppl 3:S1–4.

19

A nutrition and conditioning intervention for natural bodybuilding contest preparation: case study

Scott Lloyd Robinson[1*], Anneliese Lambeth-Mansell[2], Gavin Gillibrand[3], Abbie Smith-Ryan[4] and Laurent Bannock[1]

Abstract

Bodybuilding competitions are becoming increasingly popular. Competitors are judged on their aesthetic appearance and usually exhibit a high level of muscularity and symmetry and low levels of body fat. Commonly used techniques to improve physique during the preparation phase before competitions include dehydration, periods of prolonged fasting, severe caloric restriction, excessive cardiovascular exercise and inappropriate use of diuretics and anabolic steroids. In contrast, this case study documents a structured nutrition and conditioning intervention followed by a 21 year-old amateur bodybuilding competitor to improve body composition, resting and exercise fat oxidation, and muscular strength that does not involve use of any of the above mentioned methods. Over a 14-week period, the Athlete was provided with a scientifically designed nutrition and conditioning plan that encouraged him to (i) consume a variety of foods; (ii) not neglect any macronutrient groups; (iii) exercise regularly but not excessively and; (iv) incorporate rest days into his conditioning regime. This strategy resulted in a body mass loss of 11.7 kg's, corresponding to a 6.7 kg reduction in fat mass and a 5.0 kg reduction in fat-free mass. Resting metabolic rate decreased from 1993 kcal/d to 1814 kcal/d, whereas resting fat oxidation increased from 0.04 g/min to 0.06 g/min. His capacity to oxidize fat during exercise increased more than two-fold from 0.24 g/min to 0.59 g/min, while there was a near 3-fold increase in the corresponding exercise intensity that elicited the maximal rate of fat oxidation; 21% $\dot{V}O_{2max}$ to 60% $\dot{V}O_{2max}$. Hamstring concentric peak torque decreased (1.7 to 1.5 Nm/kg), whereas hamstring eccentric (2.0 Nm/kg to 2.9 Nm/kg), quadriceps concentric (3.4 Nm/kg to 3.7 Nm/kg) and quadriceps eccentric (4.9 Nm/kg to 5.7 Nm/kg) peak torque all increased. Psychological mood-state (BRUMS scale) was not negatively influenced by the intervention and all values relating to the Athlete's mood-state remained below average over the course of study. This intervention shows that a structured and scientifically supported nutrition strategy can be implemented to improve parameters relevant to bodybuilding competition and importantly the health of competitors, therefore questioning the conventional practices of bodybuilding preparation.

Keywords: Sports nutrition, Physique, Conditioning, Body composition, Fat oxidation, Metabolic health

Background

During bodybuilding competitions individuals are assessed on their physical or 'aesthetic' appearance and are usually required to demonstrate a high degree of muscularity and symmetry, as well as low levels of body fat. Careful attention to nutrition and exercise conditioning is undoubtedly important in facilitating the process of becoming 'competition ready'. Frequently used methods by those preparing for contest include chronic energy restriction, dehydration (water manipulation), sporadic eating and inappropriate use of diuretics and supplements of anabolic steroids and 'fat burners' [1]. These methods pose the risk of adverse health consequences that can be physiological (i.e., decreased bone mineral density [2], metabolic disruption [3], increased cardiovascular strain [4]), hormonal [5,6] and/or psychological (i.e. anger, anxiety, loss of eating control/binge eating, pre-occupation with food, short temper [1], mood disturbance [6]), in nature. Competitors may also suffer a reduction in their muscular function, strength and power during the preparation phase of competition [6,7],

* Correspondence: scott@guruperformance.co.uk
[1]Guru Performance LTD, 58 South Molton St, London W1K 5SL, UK
Full list of author information is available at the end of the article

as physique-oriented objectives are often placed above exercise performance and health goals.

A case study approach has recently been used to outline effective support strategies for the achievement of body composition and/or performance goals in professional boxing [8], professional jockeying [9], and international-standard women's football [10]. These examples highlight sports (especially boxing and horse riding) where athletes are required to repeatedly manipulate body composition to compete and perform at the highest level, similar to bodybuilding preparation. Despite insightful studies that have documented the physiological changes and dietary practices [6,11,12] that occur during prolonged bodybuilding contest preparation, there have been no case studies that provide a detailed nutrition and conditioning support strategy for the preparation phase of natural bodybuilding competition. Accordingly, we present a 14-week case study demonstrating how a scientifically designed nutrition and conditioning intervention improves body composition, resting and exercise fat oxidation, and muscular strength in an amateur bodybuilding competitor (referred to hereafter as 'The Athlete').

Case presentation
The Athlete
The Athlete was a 21-year-old male amateur bodybuilder who was aiming to compete in his first bodybuilding competition, UK Bodybuilding and Fitness Federation (UKBFF), in the Men's Physique category. He had been undertaking bodybuilding training for two years and had not previously sought any conditioning or dietary advice other than that sourced from the Internet and popular fitness magazines. Furthermore, the Athlete was not on any prescribed medication, was a non-smoker and previously supplemented his diet with whey protein only. In the 3 months prior to the intervention his diet was identical on a daily basis; comprising of four meals and two snacks that were high in carbohydrate and protein and very low in fat (Table 1). In addition to the meals he already consumed, he incorporated one 'cheat meal' approximately every two weeks, which consisted of one large take-away pizza and one serving (~200 g) of ice cream. His conditioning regime consisted of six to seven days per week of resistance training, focusing on individual muscle groups in each session (total nine hours per week).

The Athlete was fully informed of the study aims and potential risks and discomforts following which he provided written informed consent to participate in the study that received full ethical approval from the University of Worcester Ethics Committee.

Goals of the intervention
The primary goals of the support provided were to: (a) achieve the best possible aesthetic appearance in

Table 1 Example of foods consumed by the Athlete before the intervention

Item/description	Amount (g)
Meal 1	
Scrambled egg	150
Oats	40 (dry)
Meal 2	
Chicken breast	170
Broccoli	150
White rice	40 (dry)
Meal 3	
Whey protein	50
Meal 4	
Chicken breast	170
White rice	40 (dry)
Sweet potato	150
Meal 5	
Chicken breast	170
White rice	40 (dry)
Sweet potato	150
Meal 6	
Whey protein	25
Apple	100
Totals	
Energy (kcal)	2128
Carbohydrate (g)	212
Fat (g)	28
Protein (g)	257

preparation for UKBFF; (b) improve resting and exercise fat oxidation; (c) preserve muscular function and strength; (d) maintain a positive mood-state during the 14-week lead in to competition.

Metabolic assessment
Resting Metabolic Rate Assessment (RMR) was determined on six occasions (Familiarization, Baseline, Week 3, Week 8, Week 10 and Week 13) and a graded Exercise Test was completed on three occasions (Familiarization, Baseline and Week 13) to determine rates of fat oxidation during exercise and cardiorespiratory fitness ($\dot{V}O_{2max}$). For all assessments the Athlete reported to the laboratory at 07:00 h following an overnight fast from 10 pm the evening before and having abstained from strenuous physical activity, alcohol and caffeine consumption in the 24 h preceding each visit. The Athlete was asked not to perform any physical activity on the morning of testing, such as brisk walking or cycling to the laboratory, and to consume 500 ml water upon waking to encourage hydration. The

Athlete was fitted with a facemask for both the RMR and Exercise Testing (Combitox, Drager, Jaeger, Nussdorf Traunstein, Germany) and breath-by-breath measurements of oxygen consumption ($\dot{V}O_2$) and carbon dioxide production ($\dot{V}CO_2$) were measured continuously using an online gas analysis system (Oxycon Pro, Jaeger, Wuerzberg, Germany). The gas analyzer was calibrated immediately prior to testing with a known gas concentration (5% CO_2; 16% O_2; 79% N_2 [BOC Gases, Surrey, UK]) and a three-liter calibration syringe (Hans Rudolf, USA) was used to calibrate the volume transducer. Environmental conditions during testing were: humidity $51 \pm 6\%$; temperature $20 \pm 1°C$.

For the RMR Assessment the Athlete was required to lie still on a bed in the supine position for 30 minutes in a dimly lit room. There was no visual or auditory stimulation throughout this period. The Exercise Test was completed ~15 minutes after the RMR assessment. This was based on the protocol described previously by Achten and colleagues [13] with the starting speed and inclination of the treadmill (HP Cosmos, Jaeger, Nussdorf Traunstein, Germany) set at 3.5 km/h and 1%, respectively. The treadmill speed was increased by 1 km/h every three minutes until the respiratory exchange ratio (RER) reached 1.00. At this point the treadmill gradient was increased by 1% every minute until volitional exhaustion. Heart rate was measured continuously throughout testing using a heart rate monitor (Polar FT-1, Finland) and was recorded during the final 30 seconds of each exercise stage.

Calculations

Resting energy expenditure and fat oxidation were calculated during a stable measurement period i.e., a deviation in $\dot{V}O_2$ of <10% of the average $\dot{V}O_2$ between minutes 20–30 (mean ± SD recording period was 5 ± 2 minutes) using the equations of Frayn [14] and a protein correction factor of 0.11 mg/kg/min, as used previously [15,16]. During the Exercise Test $\dot{V}O_2$ and $\dot{V}CO_2$ were averaged over the last minute of each submaximal exercise stage and fat and carbohydrate oxidation were calculated according to the equations of Frayn [14], with the assumption that the urinary nitrogen excretion rate was negligible. $\dot{V}O_2$ was considered as maximal when two of the following three criteria were met; an RER >1.1, heart rate within 10 beats of predicted maximum (calculated as 220-age [17]), or an increase of <2 ml/kg/min in $\dot{V}O_2$ with a further increase in workload. $\dot{V}O_{2max}$ was calculated as the highest rolling 60 second average $\dot{V}O_2$. The results of the Exercise Test were used to create a curve of fat oxidation rate against exercise intensity, expressed as% $\dot{V}O_{2max}$. The maximal rate of fat oxidation during exercise (MFO) was determined by visual inspection i.e., by judging the peak of the curve and its corresponding rate of fat oxidation.

Fat_{max} was defined as the exercise intensity (%$\dot{V}O_{2max}$) that corresponded to MFO, as described previously [18].

Diet and activity recordings

At Baseline, the Athlete was provided with two sets of digital weighing scales (Electronic Kitchen Scale SF 400 and Swees Digital Pocket Weighing Scales); blank four-day diet log and physical activity diaries; and detailed instructions to enable the completion of these at week 3, 6, 10 and 12. The Athlete was instructed to record all consumed food and drink items accurately and in as much detail as possible. The activity diary was based on Bouchard et al. [19] and required the Athlete to record level-of-activity every 15 minutes, using a code from a 12-point scale (provided). The diary was completed over a 24-hour period on each of the four days. The scale ranged from 'sleeping' to 'vigorous exercise' and provided examples of activities at each point to assist the Athlete. To ensure the highest possible level of accuracy in estimations of energy expenditure, he was encouraged to make notes on any sport or exercise performed during the four days sampled. Diet logs were analyzed using Nutritics dietary analysis software (Nutritics v3.06, Ireland).

Daily energy expenditure was estimated using the factorial approach [20]. Here, each of the 12 codes, which had a corresponding metabolic equivalent (MET) value, was assigned a Physical Activity Level (PAL) [21] and a daily PAL was determined by multiplying each of the 12 codes by the total amount of time spent at the activity level. Where he had made notes on a specific sport and exercise activity undertaken during the 4 days, the Compendium of Physical Activities [22] was used to calculate the specific PAL value. Daily energy expenditure was then estimated by multiplying the daily PAL value by the age and sex specific resting metabolic rate (RMR; kcal/d) using height, weight and the World Health Organization (WHO) equation [23]:

$$\text{Energy Expenditure(kcal/d; men} < 30 \text{ years)}$$
$$: \text{Daily PAL value} * \text{RMR}(15.4 * \text{body mass[kg]})$$
$$-(27.0 * \text{height[m]}) + 717)$$

Anthropometric assessment

Baseline assessments are shown in Table 2. Height (Stadiometer, Seca, UK), mass (Seca, UK) and body composition using skin-folds and girths (measured by an International Standards for Anthropometric Assessment (ISAK) Certified Anthropometrist) were assessed at Baseline and at Weeks 3, 5, 7, 10, 12, 13 and 14 of the intervention at a standardized time of 07:00 h. Body fat percentage, fat-free mass (FFM) and fat mass (FM) were calculated using updated sex and race/ethnicity specific equations [24]. All skinfold measurements followed the

Table 2 Anthropometric and physiological characteristics at baseline

Characteristic	Value
Age (y)	21
Height (cm)	178.5
Body mass (kg)	86.0
BMI (kg/m^2)	27
Body fat (%)	14
Fat mass (kg)	11.7
Fat-free mass (kg)	74.3
Maximal oxygen uptake (ml/kg/min)	49.0
Maximal rate of fat oxidation (g/min)	0.24
Fatmax (%$\dot{V}O_{2max}$)	21
Resting metabolic rate (kcal/d)	1993

ISAK i.e., measurements were taken on the right hand side of the body in duplicate or in triplicate if the total error of measurement of the first and second measurement was >5%, following which a mean value was obtained.

Additional assessments

The Brunel Mood Scale (BRUMS) [25] was completed at Baseline and at Week 13. Peak torque of the hamstring (flexors) and quadriceps (extensors) of the dominant leg were determined at Baseline and Week 14 at 08:00 h following 24 hours of rest and following meal 1. This was performed on a separate day from RMR and Exercise Testing. A HUMAC NORM Isokinetic Dynamometer (Computer Sports Medicine, Inc. [CSMI], USA) was set up in the seated position, with the adjustments identical on both testing occasions. The Athlete completed three sets of five repetitions of a concentric flexion and concentric extension at 60°/second, with 60 seconds of rest between sets. After 90 seconds of recovery the Athlete completed three eccentric contraction sets of five repetitions flexion and extension at 60°/second, with 60 seconds recovery between sets. For the concentric and eccentric contractions the initial five repetitions of each set were a warm-up, the second set was a familiarization and the final set was performed to maximal exertion. Peak torque values were recorded using the CSMI computer. Prior to isokinetic testing the weight of the limb was weighed to correct for gravity using HUMAC software (CSMI, USA).

The intervention

To encourage a reduction in fat mass, we chose to obtain an energy deficit through a combination of decreased energy intake and increased energy expenditure. Adjustments in nutritional intake and the quantity of exercise performed during the intervention were made to accommodate the target energy deficit, which was set according the rate of body composition change over the period of study.

Diet

Over the 14-week period of study the Athlete followed a set-meal plan comprising of two menus. Menus 1 and 2 were followed on Conditioning and Rest days, respectively and were designed by the authors who are all certified sports nutritionists (CISSN). Table 3 shows example foods and drinks offered by the two menus and Figure 1 shows energy and macronutrient provision over the 14-week period. A set meal plan was provided for two reasons: 1) it allowed the authors to carefully control energy and macronutrient intake; 2) the Athlete favoured this approach, as opposed to receiving macronutrient and calorie targets, as used in other similar case studies [6,11]. Absolute (relative) carbohydrate, fat, and protein intake over the 14 weeks was 100 ± 56 g/d (20 ± 3% energy), 79 ± 17 g/d (37 ± 4% energy) and 212 ± 13 g/d (45 ± 8% energy), respectively. Carbohydrate recommendations focused on low or medium glycemic index (GI) sources to improve satiety [26] and enhance lipolysis [27]. To enhance muscle glycogen restoration and for purposes of improving meal enjoyment, high GI carbohydrates were also recommended [28]. To improve satiety [26] and help retain FFM and augment fat loss whilst in an energy deficit [29] the Athlete was advised to consume high biological value protein such as chicken and eggs and distribute protein intake throughout the day. This 'pulsing' strategy has been found to stimulate daily muscle protein synthesis more effectively than skewing protein intake toward the evening meal [30]. Carbohydrate intake underwent the greatest manipulation over the 14-week period to accommodate the target energy intake (Figure 1). Reducing carbohydrate intake has been suggested as a viable strategy to allow protein intake to remain high in the face of an energy deficit [31]. Fluid suggestions were water, sugar-free cordial and flavored tea that were to be consumed *ad libitum* throughout the day.

Conditioning

The 14-week conditioning programme is presented in Table 4. Briefly; the Athlete completed four resistance-training sessions (RT) during each week of the intervention; targeting each major muscle group on two occasions per week. Each RT consisted of 6–8 exercises performed for 8–10 repetitions and 4–5 sets [32]. A combination of high intensity interval training (HIIT) and low-intensity steady-state (LISS) exercise, that was performed in the overnight fasted state (07.00-08.00 h), was completed with the aim being to up-regulate oxidative enzyme adaptations to enhance fat utilization [33] and help preserve FFM whilst on a carbohydrate restricted diet [34]. Whilst two recent studies [35,36] show that fasted-state training, compared with fed-state training, does not result in greater losses in fat mass when daily caloric deficit is similar, we prescribed fasted-state training based on the Athletes

Table 3 Menus provided on rest and training days during weeks 1–5

Menu 1: Training day		Menu 2: Rest day	
Item/description	Amount (g)	Item/description	Amount (g)
Meal 1		**Meal 1**	
Venison burger	150	Poached egg	150
Poached egg	150	Oats	50 (dry)
Spinach	50	Whey protein powder	30
Meal 2		**Meal 2**	
Whey protein powder	60	Tuna (tinned)	130
Creatine	5	Asparagus	100
Brazil nuts	20	Macadamia nuts	30
Meal 3		**Meal 3**	
Mackerel	150	Chicken breast	150
Brown rice	100	Sweet potato	150
Salad leaves	50	Almonds	20
Avocado	50		
Apple cider vinegar	12		
Meal 4		**Meal 4**	
Turkey breast	155	Salmon fillet	140
White Basmati rice	100 (dry)	White Basmati rice	50
Mushrooms	100	Broccoli	100
Coconut oil	12	**Snack**	
Snack		Chocolate flavored mousse	50
Full-fat cottage cheese	225	Coconut Oil	12
Totals		**Totals**	
Energy (kcal/d)	2413	Energy (kcal/d)	2246
Carbohydrate (g)	137	Carbohydrate (g)	143
Fat (g)	119	Fat (g)	96
Protein (g)	207	Protein (g)	212

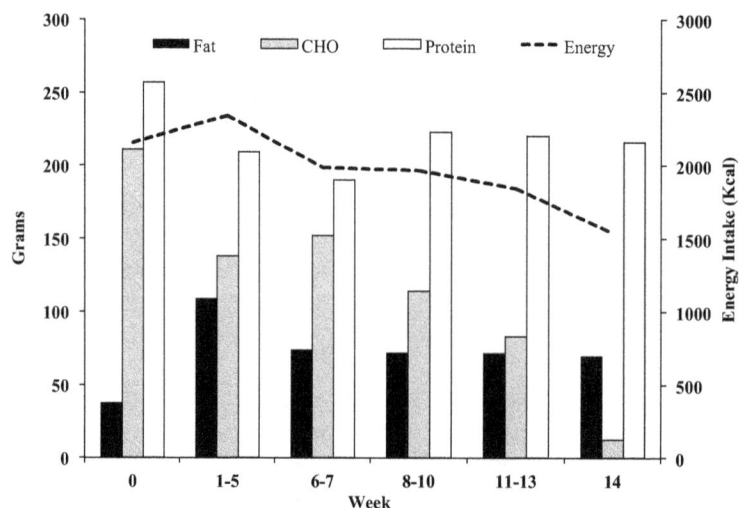

Figure 1 Energy (kcal) and macronutrient (g) intake over the 14-week period of study.

Table 4 Training program undertaken throughout the intervention period

Day (time)	Weeks 1-7	Weeks 8-10	Weeks 11-14
Monday (AM)	Rest	Sprints 10 × 10–15 sec	Sprints 10 × 10–15 sec
Monday (PM)	RT Chest and back	RT Chest and back	RT Chest and back
Tuesday (AM)	Rest	Rest	Incline walk on treadmill 40 minutes
Tuesday (PM)	RT Legs	RT Legs	RT Legs
Wednesday (AM)	Rest	Incline treadmill walk 40 minutes	Incline treadmill walk 40 minutes
Wednesday (PM)	Rest	Rest	RT Shoulders and Arms
Thursday (AM)	Rest	Rest	Incline treadmill walk 40 minutes
Thursday (PM)	RT Shoulders and arms	RT Shoulders and arms	RT Shoulders and arms
Friday (AM)	Rest	Incline treadmill walk 40 minutes	Incline treadmill walk 40 minutes
Friday (PM)	Circuit training 30 minutes	RT Legs	RT Legs
Saturday (AM)	Rest	Rest	Incline treadmill walk 40 minutes
Saturday (PM)	Rest	Rest	Rest
Sunday (AM)	Rest	Rest	Rest
Sunday (PM)	Rest	Rest	Rest

RT = Resistance Training (the mean duration of each session was 30 minutes).

preference i.e. (i) he found it difficult to perform HIIT and LISS training sessions having eaten in close-proximity (time-wise) to training and (ii) he wanted to consume his morning calories after training, as this gave him something to look forward to. The authors believe these are important practical considerations when prescribing fasted- or fed-state training to athletes.

The number of HIIT and LISS training sessions performed each week was adjusted according to the target energy deficit. In the six weeks prior to competition, "posing practice" was implemented (2–4 times per week), which involved holding isometric contraction of the major muscle groups for 30–60 seconds.

Provision of supplements

Whey protein (Optimum Nutrition, Glanbia Plc, Ireland) and one serving of a high protein (with a high whey and casein content), low carbohydrate snack in the late evening (Muscle Mousse, Genetic Supplements, Co. Durham, UK) was provided. Creatine monohydrate (Optimum

Nutrition, Glanbia Plc, Ireland) was given as 20 g per day for the first five days of the intervention, followed by 5 g per day for 93 days [37].

Evaluation of the intervention and commentary

Recorded energy intake, predicted energy expenditure and energy balance (Figure 2), and anthropometric changes (Figure 3) over the 14-week period are shown. There was a reduction in RMR over the course of the preparation period, which is consistent with previous reports that have shown a decline in RMR during periods of caloric restriction [6,38,39] (Figure 4).

Over the course of the 14-weeks total body mass loss was 11.7 kg's. This equated to an average weight loss of 0.98%/week, which is in accordance with the recommended weekly rate of 0.5-1.0% [40]. The energy deficit was 882 ± 433 kcal/d and this led to a reduction of 6.7 kg's (or 6.8% body fat or 33 mm using sum of 8 skinfolds) and 5.0 kg's, in fat mass and FFM, respectively. It is not uncommon for individuals to lose FFM whilst in a

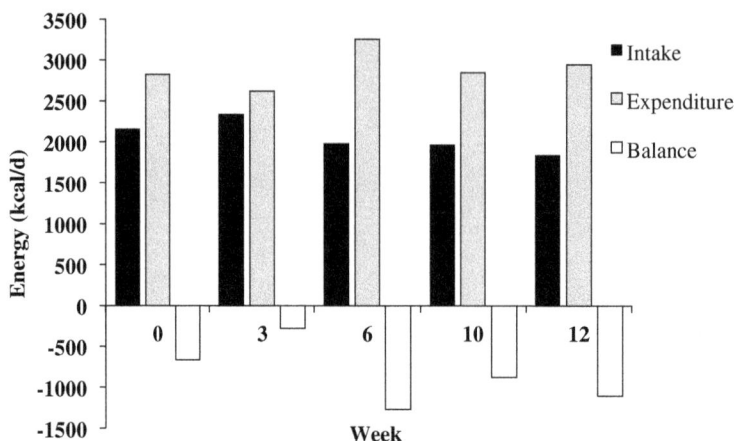

Figure 2 Recorded energy intake and predicted energy expenditure and energy balance.

negative energy balance [8,9]. Resistance training, HIIT, creatine monohydrate supplementation, and high-protein diets have all been reported to promote FFM accretion and prevent FFM loss during energy restriction (for review, see Churchward-Venne, Murphy, Longland, & Phillips [41]), however these strategies were not sufficient to prevent the decline observed in our study.

One potential reason why the Athlete lost FFM in spite of the abovementioned approaches could be because of the size of the energy deficit was larger than that applied by others. For example, one case study observed an increase (albeit only slight, 0.45 kg) in FFM during a period of less severe caloric restriction (mean ± SD energy deficit: –343 ± 156 kcal/d) [10]. A weight loss strategy that is more gradual might have induced a lesser reduction in FFM. For instance, the athlete studied in Kistler et al. [11] dieted at a rate of ~0.7% bodyweight per week and had a higher percentage of FFM loss (32% of total body mass loss) than Rossow et al. (21% of total body

mass loss) [6] where the athlete dieted at a rate of ~0.5% bodyweight per week. The Athlete in this study dieted at a rate of ~1.0% bodyweight per week and had the highest percentage of FFM loss (43% of total body mass loss). This suggests that the rate of weight loss might influence the percentage of FFM loss, even within the 0.5-1.0% bodyweight per week range as previously recommended [40]. Indeed, there is greater potential for loss of FFM as adipose tissue declines. Accordingly, an additional strategy to offset reductions in FFM whilst in energy deficit might be to reduce the size of the energy deficit as competition nears [40]. This strategy would require that the athlete allows sufficient time to reach a desirable level of body fat, such that when competition nears they do not need to place themselves in a large energy deficit to reduce body fat. Furthermore, the Athlete consumed (mean ± SD) 37 ± 4% energy from fat and 20 ± 3% energy from carbohydrate over the duration of the intervention. This is less carbohydrate and more fat (expressed as% energy) than was

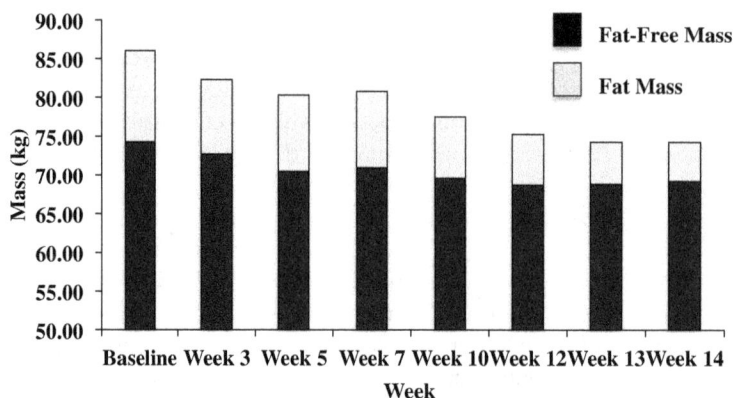

Figure 3 Anthropometrical changes over the 14-week period of study.

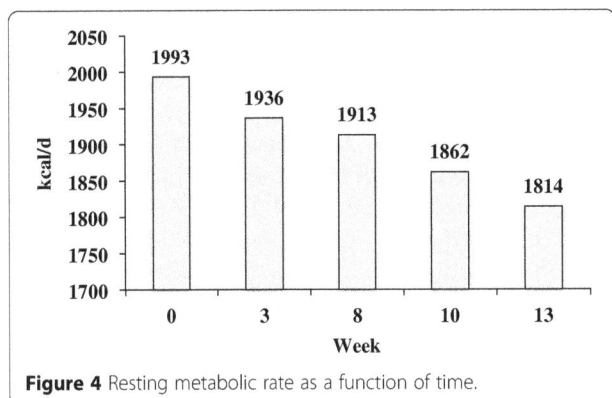

Figure 4 Resting metabolic rate as a function of time.

consumed by the athletes in Rossow et al. [6] and Kistler et al. [11] and has previously been recommended [40]. It has been shown that loss of FFM is minimal when ample carbohydrate is consumed and dietary fat reduced during a period of caloric restriction [42,43], which may offer one further reason why the Athlete lost more FFM than in other similar studies [6,11]. Finally, the Athlete undertook more endurance-based exercise than in Rossow et al. [6]. Previous work suggests that the amount of endurance exercise performed is associated with interference in muscle strength and size gains [44] and this could also provide a reason why the Athlete in our study lost a higher percentage of FFM than in Rossow et al. [6].

Maximal oxygen consumption and substrate metabolism

Absolute and relative $\dot{V}O_{2max}$ at Baseline was 4.2 L/min and 49 ml/kg/min, respectively. At Week 13, this decreased to 3.4 L/min and 46 ml/kg/min, respectively. Resting heart rate reduced from 54 beats per minute (bpm) at Baseline to 37 bpm at Week 13. Rossow and colleagues [6] and Kistler et al. [11] observed similar reductions in absolute $\dot{V}O_{2max}$ and resting heart rate during a period of competition preparation in a professional male bodybuilder. In contrast to our findings, these studies [6,11] reported an increase in relative $\dot{V}O_{2max}$ (42 ml/kg/min to 45 ml/kg/min and 42 ml/kg/min to 48 ml/kg/min, respectively).

Resting RER declined from 0.87 at Baseline to 0.82 at Week 13. Accordingly, resting fat oxidation increased from 0.04 g/min (0.53 mg/kg FFM/min) to 0.06 g/min (0.83 mg/kg FFM/min) from Baseline to Week 13, respectively, which translated to an increase in the relative contribution of fat to energy expenditure at rest by 18% from Baseline (33% of energy) to Week 13 (51% of energy). The capacity to oxidize fat during the Exercise Test also improved, as the MFO arising from the GET increased from 0.24 g/min at Baseline (3.23 mg/kg FFM/min) to 0.59 g/min (8.58 mg/kg FFM/min) at Week 13, demonstrating a greater than two-fold increase in the Athlete's capacity to oxidize fat during exercise come the

end of the intervention. The increased capacity for fat oxidation during the Exercise Test was also apparent in other ways: The number of submaximal stages completed with a RER < 1.0 increased two-fold from Baseline (5 stages) to Week 13 (10 stages). Further, Fatmax increased 39% from Baseline (21% $\dot{V}O_{2max}$) to Week 13 (60% $\dot{V}O_{2max}$). Improvements in fat oxidation could help protect towards developing an unfavourable cardiometabolic phenotype. For example, cross-sectional studies show that a reduced capacity to oxidize fat during exercise is associated with a higher clustering of metabolic syndrome risk factors [45] and unfavourable fat mass distribution (higher abdominal to lower body fat mass index, associated with metabolic disorders such as insulin resistance and dyslipidaemia [46]). Moreover, impairments in fat oxidation at the level of skeletal muscle have been associated with reduced metabolic flexibility and insulin resistance [47]. Whilst one might argue that this has little bearing on the subjective outcome of a bodybuilding competition, it is undoubtedly important for athletes and practitioners to consider the health effects of dietary and conditioning approaches. From the perspective of body composition, previous work links a high daily respiratory quotient (RQ), indicative of a low relative fat oxidation, with an increased risk of body mass gain [48] and body fat mass regain after diet-induced weight loss [49]; independent of energy expenditure. Recent research has shown that those who exhibit a higher capacity to oxidise fat during exercise (i.e. a higher MFO) also demonstrate a higher 24-hour fat oxidation and greater insulin sensitivity [50], and therefore it is not unreasonable to consider a high capacity to oxidise fat whilst physically active as beneficial for the long-term maintenance of body composition and metabolic health. Furthermore, there is some evidence that a lower use of fat as fuel during exercise [51] and on a 24-hour basis [52,53] is predictive of increased *ad libitum* energy intake, which may offer a behavioral explanation linking low fat oxidation to unfavorable body or fat mass development.

Strength and power

At Baseline, hamstring concentric and eccentric peak torque was 146 Nm (1.7 Nm/kg) and 172 Nm (2.0 Nm/kg), respectively. At Week 14, hamstring concentric strength decreased to 114 Nm (1.5 Nm/kg), whereas hamstring eccentric strength increased to 218 Nm (2.9 Nm/kg). At baseline, quadriceps concentric and eccentric peak torque was 293 Nm (3.4 Nm/kg) and 424 Nm (4.9 Nm/kg), respectively. At Week 14, absolute quadriceps concentric strength declined to (273 Nm) but increased when expressed relative to body mass (3.7 Nm/kg). Absolute quadriceps eccentric peak torque remained similar (423 Nm) but increased when considered relative to body mass (5.7 Nm/kg). Taken collectively, these findings show that the alterations in body composition observed in the present study i.e., reduced fat mass and FFM, did not compromise most measures of strength. An allied observation was made by Rossow et al. [6] who demonstrated that relative measures of strength remained similar over a six-month preparation phase, however absolute measures of strength declined (note that their method of strength testing was bench, deadlift and squat performance), which is similar to Bamman et al. [7] who observed a significant reduction (–129 N) in isometric deadlift force following a 12-week preparation period. Whilst it could be argued that strength is not essential to bodybuilding competition performance, the ability to maintain an appropriate level of strength is important for the achievement of physique-oriented goals. Indeed, Rossow et al. [6] reported that the decrements in strength observed in their study required four to six months to return to baseline and suggested that it is preferable to maintain strength during the preparation phase of competition to facilitate a quick return of training competency post-competition.

Subjective ratings of health and performance

Over the 14-week period of study, the Athlete reported no severe feelings of hunger or thirst. Previous work suggests that rigid dietary regimes, as opposed to ones that are more flexible, are associated with a higher prevalence of overeating and binging [54,55], however the Athlete in this study reported no such desires. It could be that there are large inter-individual differences in the response to particular dietary and training regimes, which might offer one explanation for the apparent discrepancy. Compared with Baseline, the Athlete described more stable energy levels, concentration and focus throughout the day as well as during conditioning sessions. These positive outcomes were reflected in the BRUMS assessment, which showed anger, confusion, depression, fatigue and tension all remained below average at the end of the intervention, whilst fatigue increased slightly from Baseline to Week 13 but remained below average (Figure 5). These favorable findings are in contrast to Rossow and colleagues [6] who reported that total mood disturbance increased in the six months leading up to competition and did not return to baseline until four months after competition. Compared with Rossow et al. [6], the Athlete in our study followed a strict meal plan, which induced a faster rate of weight loss and required a higher volume of cardiovascular training, all of which would suggest that contest preparation in the present study may also have had detrimental effects on mood, however no such decrements were reported.

Conclusions

There is a wide range of speculation regarding optimal nutrition and conditioning strategies to facilitate the achievement of an optimal figure for physique-orientated competitions such as bodybuilding. Furthermore, it has previously been suggested that some of the unfavourable physiological alterations that accompany the achievement of an optimal physique during the preparation phase i.e., a reduction in mood-state, muscular strength and power and physical performance, are a prerequisite [6]. This case study shows that a structured and scientifically supported nutrition and conditioning strategy can be effectively implemented to reduce body fat whilst

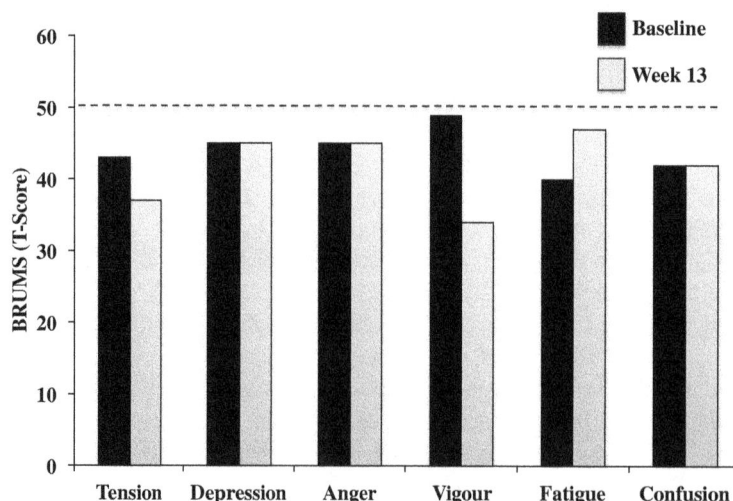

Figure 5 BRUMS scale pre- and post-intervention.

improving physiological parameters of health, maintaining a favourable mood state and positively influencing strength. Here, the Athlete consumed four meals and one snack on each day of preparation. The majority of the Athlete's nutrition came from whole foods and there was minimal reliance on dietary supplements, with the exception of those that have only strong scientific evidence in support of their ergogenic effects. Taken collectively, and in contrast to popular myth, our case study shows that it is not necessary to skip meals, neglect specific macronutrient groups, dehydrate or consume a large variety of supplements to adequately prepare for bodybuilding competition. Nevertheless, we acknowledge that 43% of the total body mass lost was FFM, which is not a favourable response. Accordingly, we propose a variety of practical strategies to assist in counteracting this. Whilst the authors appreciate that a limitation of the present study is its sample size of 1, this approach enabled us to accurately document a variety of measures that may not have been possible to acquire using a randomized control trial in a laboratory. As such, we offer this case study as a real-world applied example for other male bodybuilding competitors and coaches seeking to deploy nutrition and training strategies. Finally, the Athlete placed 7th out of 19 competitors, which he and the support team acknowledged as a successful performance given that this was his first time competing as a physique competitor.

Consent

Written informed consent was obtained from the patient for publication of this Case report and any accompanying images. A copy of the written consent is available for review by the Editor-in-Chief of this journal.

Competing interests

The authors declare that they have no competing interests.

Author's contributions

Conception of design and research: SLR, ALM, GG, LB. Implementation of exercise trials and sample collection: ALM. Data analysis: SLR, ALM. Interpretation of results: SLR, ALM, ASR, LB. Drafted manuscript: SLR, ALM. Edited and revised the manuscript: SLR, ALM, GG, ASR, LB. Approved the final version of the manuscript: SLR, ALM, GG, ASR, LB.

Acknowledgements

The authors would like to acknowledge Colin Hill and Mark Corbett (Institute of Sport & Exercise Science, University of Worcester, UK) for assistance during data collection and Dr David Hughes (University California Davis, USA) for his intellectual critique during manuscript preparation.

Author details

[1]Guru Performance LTD, 58 South Molton St, London W1K 5SL, UK. [2]Institute of Sport & Exercise Science, University of Worcester, Henwick Grove, Worcester WR2 6AJ, UK. [3]Ultimate City Fitness, 1-3 Cobb Street, London E1 7LB, UK. [4]Department of Exercise and Sport Science, University of North Carolina Chapel Hill, Office: 303A Woolen, 209 Fetzer Hall, Chapel Hill, NC, USA.

References

1. Andersen RE, Barlett SJ, Morgan GD, Brownell KD. Weight loss, psychological, and nutritional patterns in competitive male body builders. Int J Eat Disord. 1994;18:49–57.
2. Villareal DT, Fontana L, Weiss EP, Racette SB, Steger-May K, Schechtman KB, et al. Bone mineral density response to caloric restriction–induced weight loss or exercise-induced weight loss. A Randomized controlled trial. Arch Intern Med. 2006;166:2502–10.
3. Camps S, Verhoef S, Westerterp K. Weight loss, weight maintenance, and adaptive thermogenesis. Am J Clin Nutr. 2013;97:990–4.
4. Ebert TR, Martin DT, Bullock N, Mujika I, Quod MJ, Farthing LA, et al. Influence of hydration status on thermoregulation and cycling hill climbing. Med Sci Sports Exerc. 2007;39:323–9.
5. Maetsu J, Eliakim A, Jurimae J, Valter I, Jurimae T. Anabolic and catabolic hormones and energy balance of the male bodybuilders during the preparation for competition. J Strength Cond Res. 2010;24:1074–81.
6. Rossow LM, Fukuda DH, Fahs CA, Loenneke JP, Stout JR. Natural bodybuilding competition preparation and recovery: a 12-month case study. Int J Sports Physiol Perform. 2013;8:582–92.
7. Bamman MM, Hunter GR, Newton LE, Roney RK, Khaled MA. Changes in body composition, diet, and strength of bodybuilders during the 12 weeks prior to competition. J Sports Med Phys Fitness. 1993;33:383–91.
8. Morton JP, Robertson C, Sutton L, MacLaren DPM. Making the weight: a case study from professional boxing. Int J Sport Nutr Exerc Metab. 2010;20:80–5.
9. Wilson G, Chester N, Eubank M, Crighton B, Drust B, Morton JP, et al. An alternative dietary strategy to make weight while improving mood, decreasing body fat, and not dehydrating: a case study of a professional jockey. Int J Sports Nutr Exerc Metab. 2012;22:225–31.
10. Robinson SL, Morton JP, Close GL, Flower D, Bannock L. Nutrition intervention for an international-standard female football player. JACSSES. 2014;1:17–28.
11. Kistler BM, Fitschen PJ, Ranadive SM, Fernhall B, Wilund KR. Case study: natural bodybuilding contest preparation. IJSNEM. 2014;24:694–700.
12. Guardia LD, Cavallaro M, Cena H. The risks of self-made diets: the case of an amateur bodybuilder. JISSN. 2015;12:16.
13. Achten J, Venables MC, Jeukendrup AE. Fat oxidation rates are higher during running compared with cycling over a wide range of intensities. Metabolism. 2003;52:747–52.
14. Frayn KN. Calculation of substrate oxidation rates in vivo from gaseous exchange. J Appl Physiol. 1983;55:628–34.
15. Flatt JP, Ravussin E, Acheson KJ, Jequier E. Effects of dietary fat on postprandial substrate oxidation and on carbohydrate and fat balances. J Clin Invest. 1985;76:1019–24.
16. Hall LML, Moran CN, Milne GR, Wilson J, MacFarlane NG, Forouhi NG, et al. Fat oxidation, fitness and skeletal muscle expression of oxidative/lipid metabolism genes in South Asians: implications for insulin resistance? PLoS One. 2010;5:e14197.
17. Fox SMI, Naughton JP, Haskell WL. Physical activity and the prevention of coronary heart disease. Ann Clin Res. 1971;3:404–32.
18. Achten J, Gleeson M, Jeukendrup AE. Determination of the exercise intensity that elicits maximal fat oxidation. Med Sci Sports Exerc. 2002;34:92–7.
19. Bouchard C, Tremblay A, Leblanc C, Lortie G, Savard R, Theriault G. A method to assess energy expenditure in children and adults. Am J Clin Nutr. 1983;37:461–7.
20. Manore M, Meyer NL, Thompson J. Sport nutrition for health and performance. 2nd ed. Champaign, IL: Human Kinetics; 2009.
21. Subcommittee on the Tenth Edition of the Recommended Dietary Allowances, Food and Nutrition Board, Commission on Life Sciences, National Research Council. Recommended dietary allowances. 10th ed. Washington DC, USA: The National Academies Press; 1989.
22. Ainsworth BE, Haskell WL, Whitt MC, Irwin ML, Swartz AM, Strath SJ, et al. Compendium of physical activities: A second update of codes and MET values. Med Sci Sports Exerc. 2011;43:1575–81.
23. Food and Agricultural Organization, World Health Organization, United Nations University. Energy and protein requirements. Report of a joint FAO/

WHO/UNU expert consultation, World Health Organization Technical Report Series. Geneva, Switzerland: WHO; 1985. p. 724.

24. Davidson LE, Wang J, Thornton JC, Kaleem Z, Silva-Palacios F, Pierson RN, et al. Predicting fat percent by skinfolds in racial groups: Durnin and Womersley revisited. Med Sci Sports Exerc. 2011;43:542–9.

25. Terry PC, Lane AM, Lane HJ, Keohane L. Development and validation of a mood measure for adolescents. J Sports Sci. 1999;17:861–72.

26. Halton TL, Hu FB. The effects of high protein diets on thermogenesis, satiety and weight loss: a critical review. J Am Coll Nutr. 2004;23:373–85.

27. Wee SL, Williams C, Tsintzas K, Boobis L. Ingestion of a high-glycemic index meal increases muscle glycogen storage at rest but augments its utilization during subsequent exercise. J Appl Physiol. 2005;99:707–14.

28. Burke LM, Collier GR, Hargreaves M. Muscle glycogen storage after prolonged exercise: effect of the glycemic index of carbohydrate feedings. J Appl Physiol. 1993;75:1019–23.

29. Mettler S, Mitchell N, Tipton KD. Increased protein intake reduces lean body mass loss during weight loss in athletes. Med Sci Sports Exerc. 2010;42:326–37.

30. Areta JL, Burke LM, Ross ML, Camera DM, West DW, Broad EM, et al. Timing and distribution of protein ingestion during prolonged recovery from resistance exercise alters myofibrillar protein synthesis. J Physiol. 2013;591:2319–31.

31. Phillips SM, Van Loon LJC. Dietary protein for athletes: from requirements to optimum adaptation. J Sports Sci. 2011;29:29–38.

32. Helms ER, Fitschen PJ, Aragon AA, Schoenfeld BJ CJ. Recommendations for natural bodybuilding contest preparation: resistance and cardiovascular training. J Sports Med Phys Fitness. 2015;55:164–78.

33. Morton JP, Croft L, Bartlett JD, MacLaren DPM, Reilly T, Evans L, et al. Reduced carbohydrate availability does not modulate training-induced heat shock protein adaptations but does up-regulate oxidative enzyme activity in human skeletal muscle. J Appl Physiol. 2009;106:1513–21.

34. Sartor F, de Morree HM, Matschke V, Marcora SM, Milousis A, Thom JM, et al. High-intensity exercise and carbohydrate-reduced energy-restricted diet in obese individuals. Eur J Appl Physiol. 2010;110:893–903.

35. Schoenfeld BJ, Aragon AA, Wilborn CD, Krieger J, Sonmez GT. Body composition changes associated with fasted versus non-fasted aerobic exercise. JISSN. 2014;11:54.

36. Gillen GB, Percival ME, Ludzki A, Tarnopolsky MA, Gibala MJ. Interval training in the fed or fasted state improves body composition and muscle oxidative capacity in overweight women. Obesity. 2013;21:2249–55.

37. Harris RC, Söderlund K, Hultman E. Elevation of creatine in resting and exercised muscle of normal subjects by creatine supplementation. Clin Sci. 1992;83:367–74.

38. Ravussin E, Burnand B, Schutz Y, Jequier E. Energy expenditure before and during energy restriction in obese patients. Am J Clin Nutr. 1985;41:753–9.

39. Leibel RL, Rosenbaum M, Hirsch J. Changes in energy expenditure resulting from altered body weight. N Engl J Med. 1995;332:621–8.

40. Helms ER, Aragon A, Fitschen PJ. Evidence-based recommendations for natural bodybuilding contest preparation: nutrition and supplementation. JISSN. 2014;11:20.

41. Churchward-Venne TA, Murphy CH, Longland TM, Phillips SM. Role of protein and amino acids in promoting lean mass accretion with resistance exercise and attenuating lean mass loss during energy deficit in humans. Amino Acids. 2013;45:231–40.

42. Garthe I, Raastad T, Refsnes PE, Koivisto A, Sundgot-Borgen J. Effect of two different weight-loss rates on body composition and strength and power-related performance in elite athletes. Int J Sport Nutr Exerc Metab. 2011;21:97–104.

43. Murphy CH, Hector AJ, Phillips SM. Considerations for protein intake in managing weight loss in athletes. Eur J Sports Sci. 2014;1:21–8.

44. Wilson JM, Marin PJ, Rhea MR, Wilson SM, Loenneke JP, Anderson JC. Concurrent training: a meta-analysis examining interference of aerobic and resistance exercise. J Strength Cond Research. 2012;26:2293–307.

45. Rosenkilde M, Nordby P, Nielsen LB, Stallknecht BM, Helge JW. Fat oxidation at rest predicts peak fat oxidation during exercise and metabolic phenotype in overweight men. Int J Obesity. 2010;34:871–7.

46. Isacco L, Thivel D, Duclos M, Aucouturier J, Boisseau N. Effects of adipose tissue distribution on maximum lipid oxidation rate during exercise in normal weight-women. Diabetes Metab. 2014;40:215–9.

47. Kelley DE, Simoneau JA. Impaired free fatty acid utilization by skeletal muscle in non-insulin-dependent diabetes mellitus. J Clin Invest. 1994;94:2349–56.

48. Zurlo F, Lillioja S, Puente EA, Nyomba BL, Raz I, Saad MF, et al. Low ratio of fat to carbohydrate metabolism as predictor of weight gain: study of 24-h RQ. Am J Physiol Endocrinol Metab. 1990;259:650–7.

49. Ellis AC, Hyatt TC, Gower BA, Hunter GR. Respiratory quotient predicts fat mass gain in premenopausal women. Obesity. 2010;18:2255–9.

50. Robinson SL, Hattersley J, Frost GS, Chambers ES, Wallis GA. Maximal fat oxidation during exercise is positively associated with 24-hour fat oxidation and insulin sensitivity in young, healthy men. J Appl Physiol (in press)

51. Almeras N, Lavallee N, Despres JP, Bouchard C, Tremblay A. Exercise and energy intake: effect of substrate oxidation. Physiol Behav. 1995;57:995–1000.

52. Eckel RH, Hernandez TL, Bell ML, Weil KM, Shepard TY, Grunwald GK, et al. Carbohydrate balance predicts weight and fat gain in adults. Am J Clin Nutr. 2006;83:803–8.

53. Pannacciulli N, Salbe AD, Ortega E, Venti CA, Bogardus C, Krakoff J. The 24-h carbohydrate oxidation rate in a human respiratory chamber predicts ad libitum food intake. Am J Clin Nutr. 2007;86:625–32.

54. Smith CF, Williamson DA, Bray GA, Ryan DH. Flexible vs. rigid dieting strategies: relationship with adverse behavioral outcomes. Appetite. 1999;32:295–305.

55. Steen SN. Precontest strategies of a male bodybuilder. Int J Sport Nutr. 1991;1:69–78.

20

Effects of protein type and composition on postprandial markers of skeletal muscle anabolism, adipose tissue lipolysis, and hypothalamic gene expression

Christopher Brooks Mobley[1], Carlton D Fox[1], Brian S Ferguson[1], Corrie A Pascoe[1], James C Healy[1], Jeremy S McAdam[1], Christopher M Lockwood[2] and Michael D Roberts[1*]

Abstract

Background: We examined the acute effects of different dietary protein sources (0.19 g, dissolved in 1 ml of water) on skeletal muscle, adipose tissue and hypothalamic satiety-related markers in fasted, male Wistar rats (~250 g).

Methods: Oral gavage treatments included: a) whey protein concentrate (WPC, n = 15); b) 70:30 hydrolyzed whey-to-hydrolyzed egg albumin (70 W/30E, n = 15); c) 50 W/50E (n = 15); d) 30 W/70E (n = 15); and e) 1 ml of water with no protein as a fasting control (CTL, n = 14).

Results: Skeletal muscle analyses revealed that compared to CTL: a) phosphorylated (p) markers of mTOR signaling [p-mTOR (Ser2481) and p-rps6 (Ser235/236)] were elevated 2–4-fold in all protein groups 90 min post-treatment ($p < 0.05$); b) WPC and 70 W/30E increased muscle protein synthesis (MPS) 104% and 74% 180 min post-treatment, respectively ($p < 0.05$); and c) 70 W/30E increased p-AMPKα (Thr172) 90 and 180-min post-treatment as well as PGC-1α mRNA 90 min post-treatment. Subcutaneous (SQ) and omental fat (OMAT) analyses revealed: a) 70 W/30 W increased SQ fat phosphorylated hormone-sensitive lipase [p-HSL (Ser563)] 3.1-fold versus CTL and a 1.9–4.4-fold change versus all other test proteins 180 min post-treatment ($p < 0.05$); and b) WPC, 70 W/30E and 50 W/50E increased OMAT p-HSL 3.8–6.5-fold 180 min post-treatment versus CTL ($p < 0.05$). 70 W/30E and 30 W/70E increased hypothalamic POMC mRNA 90 min post-treatment versus CTL rats suggesting a satiety-related response may have occurred in the former groups. However, there was a compensatory increase in orexigenic AGRP mRNA in the 70 W/30E group 90 min post-treatment versus CTL rats, and there was a compensatory increase in orexigenic NPY mRNA in the 30 W/70E group 90 min post-treatment versus CTL rats.

Conclusions: Higher amounts of whey versus egg protein stimulate the greatest post-treatment anabolic skeletal muscle response, though test proteins with higher amounts of WPH more favorably affected post-treatment markers related to adipose tissue lipolysis.

Keywords: Whey protein, Egg protein, Hydrolyzed protein, Muscle protein synthesis, Lipolysis

* Correspondence: mdr0024@auburn.edu
[1]School of Kinesiology, Molecular and Applied Sciences Laboratory, Auburn University, 301 Wire Road, Office 286, Auburn, AL 36849, USA
Full list of author information is available at the end of the article

Background

Dietary whey protein has numerous well-known health benefits. For instance, whey protein feeding has been shown to acutely increase postprandial muscle protein synthesis (MPS) in rodents [1,2] and humans [3,4], whereas chronic whey protein supplementation has been shown to consistently increase muscle mass with exercise training [5-7]. Acute whey protein feeding has also been shown to reduce appetite 90–180 min following low-dose ingestion [8-10] by potentially affecting anorectic hormone and hypothalamic mRNA expression patterns [11,8,9]. Chronic whey protein supplementation has also been shown to reduce adiposity in rodents and humans [12-14,5]; an effect which may be explained by an increased expression of adipose tissue lipolysis-related gene expression patterns following chronic supplementation [12], an increase in protein-induced thermogenesis (reviewed in [15]), and/or a consistent reduction in food intake given its satiety-stimulatory effects as discussed above.

More recent data has focused on the potential health benefits of hydrolyzed dietary proteins. In short, commercial hydrolysis of different dietary protein sources is thought to [16-18]: a) expedite the digestion of amino acids via 'pre-digestion' thus increasing their postprandial bioavailability; and b) liberate bioactive peptides that are able to exhibit physiological responses that otherwise would be diminished from consuming intact protein sources. Indeed, *in vivo* [19,20] and *in vitro* [21] evidence suggests that hydrolyzed whey or native whey protein increases the activation of postprandial intramuscular insulin signaling markers. Putative bioactive peptides from whey protein hydrolysates (WPH) have also been shown to exhibit insulin secretagogue properties versus intact whey protein [22,23]. Likewise, we have recently demonstrated that acute WPH feeding in rats increases the appearance of di- and oligopeptides as well as numerous lipolysis-related serum markers (i.e., epinephrine, glycerol and numerous free fatty acids) compared to an isonitrogenous WPC feeding condition [18]. Thus, it is of interest to further examine how WPH versus WPC ingestion differentially affects various physiological systems.

Widespread interest has also surrounded the positive health benefits of dietary egg protein due to its high essential amino acid (EAA) content and high digestibility [24]. Similar to whey protein, egg protein feeding in rats has been found to significantly increase postprandial MPS [1]. Likewise, one report suggests that bioactives isolated from egg protein down-regulate serum myostatin (MSTN) [25]; an effect which may enhance skeletal muscle hypertrophy with chronic supplementation. However, unlike the aforementioned whey protein research, there is a paucity of data regarding the physiological effects of dietary egg protein on other tissues (i.e., adipose tissue and the hypothalamus), though there is

some evidence to suggest that egg-based breakfast meals can increase satiety post-ingestion [26] and cause weight loss in overweight individuals over the long-term [27].

Given the widespread interest regarding the physiological effects of dietary whey and egg proteins, as well as hydrolyzed versus intact protein forms, the purpose of this study was to examine how different solutions of extensively hydrolyzed whey and egg albumin protein (EPH) blends, in combination with a standardized blend of cow colostrum and egg yolk extract acutely affect post-prandial markers of skeletal muscle anabolism, adipose tissue lipolysis and thermogenesis, and hypothalamic mRNA expression patterns in rodents. Treatments included: 300 human equivalent mg of bovine colostrum and egg yolk extract (0.0057 g protein rat dose) in addition to 10 human equivalent g protein dose (0.19 g protein rat dose) of, a) high-dose WPH + low-dose EPH (70 W/30E); b) equal doses of both WPH and EPH (50 W/50E); and c) low-dose WPH + high-dose EPH (30 W/70E). An isonitrogenous amount of intact whey protein concentrate (WPC) was also fed to a fourth group of rats as a positive feeding control, and 1 ml of water with no protein was fed to a fifth group of rats as a fasting control (CTL). Based upon the aforementioned literature, we hypothesized that all protein treatments would similarly increase postprandial markers of skeletal muscle anabolism as well as satiety-related hypothalamic markers relative to CTL. We also hypothesized that higher proportions of whey protein (i.e., WPC and 70 W/30E) would induce larger increases in adipose tissue lipolysis markers relative to other feeding groups; though we also hypothesized that the hydrolysates would outperform the WPC on markers of muscle anabolism, adipose tissue lipolysis and satiety.

Experimental methods

Animals and feeding protocols

All experimental procedures described herein were approved by Auburn University's Institutional Animal Care and Use Committee. Male Wistar rats (~250 g) approximately 8–9 weeks old were purchased from Harlan Laboratories and were allowed to acclimate in the animal quarters for 5 days prior to experimentation. Briefly, animal quarters were maintained on a 12 h light: 12 h dark cycle, at ambient room temperature, with water and standard rodent chow (18.6% protein, 44.2% carbohydrate, 6.2% fat; Teklad Global #2018 Diet, Harlan Laboratories) provided to animals *ad libitum*.

The day prior to acute protein feeding experiments, food was removed from home cages resulting in an 18 h overnight fast. The morning of experimentation, animals were removed from their quarters between 0800–0900, transported to the Molecular and Applied Sciences Laboratory and were allowed to acclimate for approximately 3–5 h. Thereafter, rats were administered either WPC, 70 W/30E,

Effects of protein type and composition on postprandial markers of skeletal muscle anabolism...

181

50 W/50E, 30 W/70E at a human equivalent (eq.) dose of 10 g protein (0.19 g protein rat dose) dissolved in 1 ml of tap water via gavage feeding. Doses were calculated per the species conversion calculations of Reagan-Shaw et al. [28], whereby the human body mass for an average male was assumed to be 80 kg. The group of non-fed CTL rats was gavage-fed 1 ml of tap water. Dietary components of each test protein solution are presented in Table 1.

Of note, We examined how graded doses of WPC in solution (0.19, 0.37, and 0.93 g protein) stimulated MPS and Akt-mTOR markers 90 min post-gavage in order to

Table 1 Contents of each protein per the 0.19 g protein dose of each respective protein

Amino Acid	70 W/30E (mg)	50 W/50E (mg)	30 W/70E (mg)	WPC (mg)
Alanine	10	10	10	9
Arginine	8	8	9	6
Aspartic Acid	21	20	19	22
Cysteine	5	5	5	4
Glutamic Acid	31	29	26	34
Glycine	4	5	5	4
Histidine*	4	4	4	4
Isoleucine*†	11	11	10	12
Leucine*†	20	19	17	23
Lysine*	17	15	14	19
Methionine*	5	5	6	4
Phenylalanine*	8	9	9	7
Proline	12	11	9	17
Serine	12	12	11	12
Threonine*	11	10	9	12
Tryptophan*	3	3	3	3
Tyrosine	7	7	7	6
Valine*†	12	12	12	11
Total EAAs*	92	87	83	95
Total BCAAs*†	43	41	38	46
M.W.	70 W/30E	50 W/50E	30 W/70E	WPC
(kDa)	(%)	(%)	(%)	(%)
<1.0	40	39	40	0
1.0 - 5.0	23	22	23	7
5.0 - 10.0	6	6	6	11
>10.0	30	32	32	82

As stated in the methods, rats were administered either WPC, 70 W/30E, 50 W/50E, or 30 W/70E at a human equivalent (eq.) dose of 10 g protein (equaled a true dose of 0.191 g of protein) dissolved in 1 ml of water via gavage feeding. While not stated in the methods, total protein was determined using the Dumas (N x 6.38) test method. Furthermore, amino acid concentrations (g/100 g) were determined using liquid chromatography. Finally, molecular weight (M.W.) distribution was determined by high-performance liquid chromatography size exclusion (HPLC-SEC), on an Agilent 1290 Infinity Quaternary LC System w/ TOSOH TSKgel G2000SW 7.5 mm ID x 30 cm (10 μm) column at a wavelength of 205 nm. Symbols: * indicates an essential amino acid; † indicates a branched chain amino acid (BCAA).

determine an optimal dose that adequately elicited a postprandial physiological response. These preliminary results demonstrated that 10 human eq. g of WPC (0.19 g protein) increased markers of mTOR activation and MPS 90 min post-gavage, and this generally was equal to the 19 human eq. g (0.37 g protein) and 48 human eq. g (0.93 g protein) doses (Additional file 1: Figure S1). Thus, given that the 10 human eq. g of WPC (0.19 g protein) elicited similar anabolic responses compared to higher doses, we opted to use the 10 human eq. g (0.19 g) dose for each test protein. While this dose is not typically associated with the optimal human MPS response to protein ingestion (i.e., 20–40 g), it should be noted that the species conversion calculations of Reagan-Shaw et al. is a basis to dose rats relative to humans and, alternatively, these human eq. dosages should not be viewed in absolute terms when comparing species (i.e., 10 human eq. g appears to elicit an anabolic response in rats whereas 20–40 g in humans is needed).

The gavage feeding procedure involved placing the animals under light isoflurane anesthesia for approximately 1 min while gavage feeding occurred. Following gavage feeding, rats were allowed to recover 90 or 180 min prior to being euthanized under CO_2 gas in a 2 L induction chamber (VetEquip, Inc., Pleasanton, CA, USA). Animals that were sacrificed 180 min post-treatment were injected intraperitoneally with puromycin dihydrochloride (5.44 mg in 1 ml of diluted in phosphate buffered saline; Ameresco, Solon, OH, USA) 30 min prior to euthanasia in order to determine skeletal muscle protein synthesis via the surface sensing of translation (SUnSET) method described in detail elsewhere [29]. Of note, with the SUnSET method MPS is determined through the incorporation of puromycin into actively synthesized proteins given that it is a structural analogue of aminoacyl-transfer RNA; specifically tyrosyl-tRNA. It should also be noted that the SUnSET method is an alternative method for measuring MPS compared to radioactive isotope (e.g. ^{3}H-phenyalanine or ^{35}S-methionine), or stable isotope (e.g. ^{15}N-lysine, ^{13}C-leucine or [ring-^{13}C6]-phenyalanine) tracers. Goodman et al. [29] compared the SUnSET method to a ^{3}H-phenyalanine flooding method in *ex vivo* plantaris muscle preparations isolated from animals that had undergone synergist ablation. Remarkably, these authors determined that MPS rates increased 3.6-fold as determined by the SUnSET method and 3.4-fold as determined by the tracer method; a finding which proves the reliability of this method in detecting sensitive changes in MPS.

Immediately following euthanasia, whole blood was removed via heart sticks using a 21-gauge needle and syringe, placed in a serum separator tubes, and processed for serum extraction via centrifugation at 3,500 × *g* for 5 min. Serum was aliquoted into multiple 1.7 ml microcentrifuge tubes for subsequent biochemical assays and then frozen for later analysis. Approximately two 50 mg pieces of mixed gastrocnemius muscle was harvested using standard dissection techniques and placed in homogenizing buffer [Tris base; pH 8.0, NaCl, NP-40, sodium deoxycholate, SDS with added protease and phosphatase inhibitors (G Biosciences, St. Louis, MO, USA)] and Ribozol (Ameresco) for immunoblotting and mRNA analyses, respectively. Approximately two 50 mg pieces of subcutaneous adipose tissue (SQ) from the inguinal crease was harvested and placed in the aforementioned Tris base homogenizing buffer and Ribozol for immunoblotting and mRNA analyses, respectively. Due to tissue limitations, only one 50 mg piece of omental adipose tissue (OMAT) was harvested and placed in the aforementioned Tris base homogenizing buffer for immunoblotting. Finally, removal of the hypothalamus was performed per the methods similar to those previously employed [30]. Briefly, brains were removed and rinsed in 1x phosphate buffered saline. Brains were then placed posterior side up in a 1.0 mm acrylic sectioning apparatus (Braintree Scientific, Braintree, MA, USA) and a 2.0-mm coronal slice of each brain was made between Bregma-1.6 and-1.8 mm. Coronal slices were immediately placed on an ice-cooled stage and two bilateral punches (2.0 mm diameter) were made to capture the hypothalamus. Tissue was immediately placed in Ribozol and stored at-80°C until RNA isolation.

Gastrocnemius muscle, SQ and OMAT samples placed in Tris base homogenizing buffer were homogenized using a 1.7 ml tube using a tight-fitting micropestle, insoluble proteins were removed with centrifugation at $500 \times g$ for 5 min at 4°C, and supernatants were assayed for total protein content using a BCA Protein Assay Kit (Thermo Scientific, Waltham, MA, USA) prior to immunoblotting sample preparation. Muscle, SQ, and hypothalamus samples placed in Ribozol were subjected to total RNA isolation according to manufacturer's instructions, and concentrations were performed using a NanoDrop Lite (Thermo Scientific) prior to cDNA synthesis for mRNA analyses. Extra gastrocnemius muscle and SQ fat not processed during dissections were flash-frozen in liquid nitrogen and stored at-80°C for later potential analyses.

Directed Akt-mTOR phosphoproteomics

The PathScan® Akt Signaling Antibody Array Kit (Chemiluminescent Readout; Cell Signaling, Danvers, MA, USA) containing glass slides spotted with antibodies was utilized to detect phosphorylated proteins predominantly belonging to the Akt-mTOR signaling network.

The kit assays p-Akt (Thr308), p-Akt (Ser473), p-rps6 (Ser235/236), p-AMPKα (Thr172), p-Pras40 (Thr246), p-mTOR (Ser2481), p-GSK-3α (Ser21), p-GSK-3β (Ser9), p-p70s6k (Thr389), p-p70s6k (Thr421/Ser424), p-BAD (Ser112), p-PTEN (Ser380), p-PDK1 (Ser241), p-ERK1/2 (Thr202/Tyr204), p-4E-BP1 (Thr37/46). However,

we specifically analyzed p-Akt (Ser473), p-rps6 (Ser235/236), p-AMPKα (Thr172), p-mTOR (Ser2481), p- p-p70s6k (Thr389), and p-4E-BP1 (Thr37/46) in order follow a 'linear' analysis in Akt-mTOR signaling. Briefly, gastrocnemius homogenates were diluted to 0.5 μg/μl using cell lysis buffer provided by the kit and assayed according to manufacturer's instructions. Slides were developed using an enhanced chemiluminescent reagent provided by the kit, and spot densitometry was performed through the use of a UVP Imager and associated densitometry software (UVP, LLC, Upland, CA, USA). The calculation of each phosphorylated target was as follows:

(Density value of the target – negative control)/summation of all density values for the sample.

It should be noted that this high throughput antibody chip array for muscle phosphorylation markers was used rather than single antibodies due to resource constraints. Notwithstanding, and as discussed in the results section, the results presented herein are in agreement with past literature showing that protein feeding affects numerous targets on the aforementioned antibody array chip. Furthermore, our preliminary WPC graded-dose feedings show an increase in Akt-mTOR markers across multiple doses relative to fasting rats (Additional file 1: Figure S1). We have also internally tested this array on exercised rat muscle as well as C2C12 cell culture lysates deprived of or treated with L-leucine, and have produced reproducible results commensurate with prior literature examining these markers (i.e., increased activation of mTOR markers which parallel increases in MPS; *unpublished observations*).

Western blotting

As mentioned prior, the SUnSET method was employed in order to examine if different dietary protein blends differentially affected MPS. Briefly, 2 μg/μl gastrocnemius Western blotting preps were made using 4x Laemmli buffer. Thereafter, 20 μl of prepped samples were loaded onto pre-casted 4–20% SDS-polyacrylamide gels (C.B.S. Scientific Company, San Diego, CA, USA) and subjected to electrophoresis (200 V @ 75 min) using pre-made 1x SDS-PAGE running buffer (C.B.S. Scientific Company). Proteins were then transferred to polyvinylidene difluoride membranes, and membranes were blocked for 1 h at room temperature with 5% nonfat milk powder. For muscle samples, mouse anti-puromycin IgG (1:5,000; Millipore) was incubated with membranes overnight at 4°C in 5% bovine serum albumin (BSA), and the following day membranes were incubated with anti-mouse IgG secondary antibodies (1:2,000, Cell Signaling) at room temperature for 1 h prior to membrane development described below. Thereafter, membranes were stripped of antibodies via commercial stripping buffer (Restore Western Blot Stripping Buffer, Thermo Scientific), membranes were incubated with rabbit anti-beta-actin

(1:5,000; GeneTex, Inc., Irvine, CA, USA) as a normalizer protein overnight at 4°C in 5% BSA, and the following day membranes were incubated with anti-rabbit IgG secondary antibodies (1:2,000, Cell Signaling) at room temperature for 1 h prior to membrane development.

SQ and OMAT samples were assayed with rabbit anti-phospho-hormone sensitive lipase [p-HSL (Ser563) IgG (1:1000; Cell Signaling)] overnight at 4°C in 5% BSA. The following day membranes were incubated with anti-rabbit IgG secondary antibodies (1:2,000, Cell Signaling) at room temperature for 1 h prior to membrane development. Membranes were stripped, incubated with rabbit glyceraldehyde 3-phosphate dehydrogenase (GAPDH; 1:5,000; GeneTex) overnight at 4°C in 5% BSA, and the following day were incubated with anti-rabbit IgG secondary antibodies (1:2,000, Cell Signaling) at room temperature for 1 h prior to membrane development.

Membrane development was performed using an enhanced chemiluminescent reagent (Amersham, Pittsburgh, PA, USA), and band densitometry was performed through the use of a UVP Imager and associated densitometry software (UVP, LLC, Upland, CA, USA).

Real-time RT-PCR

RNA from each tissue (500 ng of hypothalamus RNA and 1 μg of gastrocnemius and SQ RNA) were reverse transcribed into cDNA for real time PCR analyses using a commercial cDNA synthesis kit (Quanta Biosciences, Gaithersburg, MD, USA). Real-time PCR was performed using SYBR-green-based methods with gene-specific primers [MSTN, Mighty/Akirin-1, Myosin Heavy Chain 4 (Myhc4), p21Cip1, Atrogin-1, MuRF-1, GLUT-4, Insulin-like growth factor-1ea (IGF-1Ea), proopiomelanocortin (POMC), neuropeptide Y (NPY), agouti-related protein (AGRP), leptin receptor (LEPR), peroxisome proliferator-activated receptor gamma co-activator 1-alpha (PGC-1α), uncoupling protein 3 (UCP3), carnitine palmitoyltransferase 1b (CPT1B), beta-2 microglobulin (B2M), and beta-actin] designed using primer designer software (Primer3Plus, Cambridge, MA, USA). The forward and reverse primer sequences are as follows: [MSTN: forward primer 5'-ACGCTACCACG-GAAACAATC-3', reverse primer 5'-CCGTCTTTCATG GGTTTGAT-3'; Mighty/Akirin-1: forward primer 5'-TTTGATCTTGGGGATTCTGG-3', reverse primer 5'-GCCTGGAAACAGTCCCTGTA-3'; p21Cip1: forward primer 5'-AGCAAAGTATGCCGTCGTCT-3', reverse primer 5'-ACACGCTCCCAGACGTAGTT-3'; Atrogin-1: forward primer 5'-CTACGATGTTGCAGCCAAGA –3', reverse primer 5'- GGCAGTCGAGAAGTCCAGTC-3'; MuRF-1: forward primer 5'-AGTCGCAGTTTCGAAG-CAAT-3', reverse primer 5'-AACGACCTCCAGACATG-GAC-3'; GLUT-4: forward primer 5'-GCTTCTGTTGCC CTTCTGTC-3', reverse primer 5'-TGGACGCTCTCTTT

CCAACT-3'; IGF-1Ea: forward primer 5'-TGGTGGACG CTCTTCAGTTC-3', reverse primer 5'-TCCGGAAGCA ACACTCATCC-3'; POMC: forward primer 5'-GAAG GTGTACCCCAATGTCG-3', reverse primer 5'-CTTCT CGGAGGTCATGAAGC-3'; NPY: forward primer 5'-AG AGATCCAGCCCTGAGACA-3', reverse primer 5'-AAC-GACAACAAGGGAAATGG-3'; AGRP: forward primer 5'-CGTGTGGGCCCTTTATTAGA-3', reverse primer 5'-CAGACCTTCTGATGCCCTTC-3'; LEPR: forward primer 5'-CTGGGTTTGCGTATGGAAGT-3', reverse primer 5'-CCAGTCTCTTGCTCCTCACC-3'; PGC-1α: forward primer 5'-ATGTGTCGCCTTCTTGCTCT-3', reverse primer 5'-ATCTACTGCCTGGGGACCTT-3'; UCP3: forward primer 5'-GAGTCAGGGGACTGTGGAAA-3', reverse primer 5'-GCGTTCATGTATCGGGTCTT-3'; CPT1B: forward primer 5'-CCCAGTTCTGAGACCAGCTC-3', reverse primer 5'-TAGGCACCTAAGGGCTGAGA-3'; B2M: forward primer 5'-CCCAAAGAGACAGTGGGTGT-3', reverse primer 5'-CCCTACTCCCCTCAGTTTCC-3'; beta-actin: forward primer 5'-GTGGATCAGCAAGCAGGAG T-3', reverse primer 5'-ACGCAGCTCAGTAACAGTCC-3'] and SYBR green chemistry (Quanta). Primer efficiency curves for all genes were generated and efficiencies ranged between 90% and 110%, and melt curve analyses demonstrated that one PCR product was amplified per reaction.

SQ cAMP determination

Frozen SQ samples were subjected to 3'–5'-cyclic adenosine monophosphate (cAMP) assays using a rat-specific spectrophotometric commercial assay (R&D Systems, Inc., Minneapolis, MN, USA). Briefly, approximately 50–100 mg of tissue was homogenized in 500 μl of 0.1 N HCl. Samples were subjected to 10 min of centrifugation at $10,000 \times g$ at 4°C, and neutralized with 50 μl of 1 N NaOH. Samples were then diluted 2-fold with the assay diluent provided, and cAMP concentrations were determined according to the manufacturer's recommendations.

Serum analyses

Serum samples were assayed for lipolysis markers including free fatty acids (FFAs) as well as epinephrine (EPI) and norepinephrine (NorEPI) using rat-specific spectrophotometric commercial assays according to the manufacturer's recommendations (FFAs: Abcam, Cambridge, MA, USA; EPI/NorEPI: Abnova, Taipei City, Taiwan). Serum samples were also analyzed for triiodothyronine (T3) using a rat-specific spectrophotometric commercial assay according to the manufacturer's recommendations (Abnova).

Statistics

All data are presented in figures and tables as means ± standard error values. Given that each post-treatment time point were comprised of independent groups of rats, statistical comparisons were performed using one-way ANOVAs, and statistical significance was set at $p < 0.05$ (SPSS v 22.0, IBM, Armonk, NY, USA). When between-group significance was obtained, a Fisher's LSD *post hoc* test was performed in order to determine specific between-group comparisons.

Results

A higher proportion of whey protein versus egg protein elicits the most favorable postprandial anabolic response

mTOR pathway targets were assayed in order to determine how each protein source affect post-prandial Akt-mTOR signaling substrates which, when activated, lead to increases in MPS. p-mTOR (Ser2481) was approximately 2-to-3-fold greater for protein-fed versus CTL rats 90 min post-gavage (WPC vs. CTL $p = 0.006$, 70 W/30E vs. CTL $p = 0.005$, 50 W/50E vs. CTL $p < 0.001$, 30 W/70E $p = 0.022$; Figure 1a), though it only remained significantly elevated in the 70 W/30E group 180 min post-gavage compared to CTL rats ($p = 0.010$; Figure 1a). p-p70s6k (Thr389) was significantly elevated approximately 2-fold in 70 W/30E and 50 W/50E versus CTL rats 90 min post-feeding (70 W/30E vs. CTL $p = 0.011$, 50 W/50E vs. CTL $p = 0.007$; Figure 1b), and this marker remained significantly elevated in 70 W/30E versus CTL rats 180 min post-feeding ($\sim$1.9-fold, $p = 0.020$; Figure 1b). p-rps6 (Ser235/236) was approximately 2.8-to-4-fold greater for protein-fed versus CTL rats 90 min post-gavage (WPC vs. CTL $p < 0.001$, 70 W/30E vs. CTL $p < 0.001$, 50 W/50E vs. CTL $p < 0.001$, 30 W/70E $p = 0.003$; Figure 1c), and this marker remained 2.7-to-2.9-fold elevated 70 W/30E and 50 W/50E versus CTL rats 180 min post-feeding (70 W/30E vs. CTL $p = 0.002$, 50 W/50E vs. CTL $p = 0.007$; Figure 1c). Interestingly, except for the 30 W/70E group, all protein-fed groups presented statistically 30–50% lower p-4E-BP1 (Thr37/47) values 90 min (WPC vs. CTL $p < 0.001$, 70 W/30E vs. CTL $p = 0.003$, 50 W/50E vs. CTL $p < 0.001$, 30 W/70E $p = 0.064$; Figure 1d) and 180 min (WPC vs. CTL $p = 0.036$, 70 W/30E vs. CTL $p = 0.009$, 50 W/50E vs. CTL $p < 0.011$, 30 W/70E $p = 0.107$; Figure 1d) post-feeding versus CTL rats. MPS levels were higher in WPC and 70 W/30E versus CTL rats 180 min post-feeding (WPC vs. CTL $p = 0.007$, 70 W/30E vs. CTL $p = 0.032$; Figure 1e), though there was no statistical differences between protein feeding groups.

Select gastrocnemius mRNAs related to skeletal muscle hypertrophy are differentially affected by protein type

While transient gene expression patterns in response to feeding provide limited information, mRNA expression

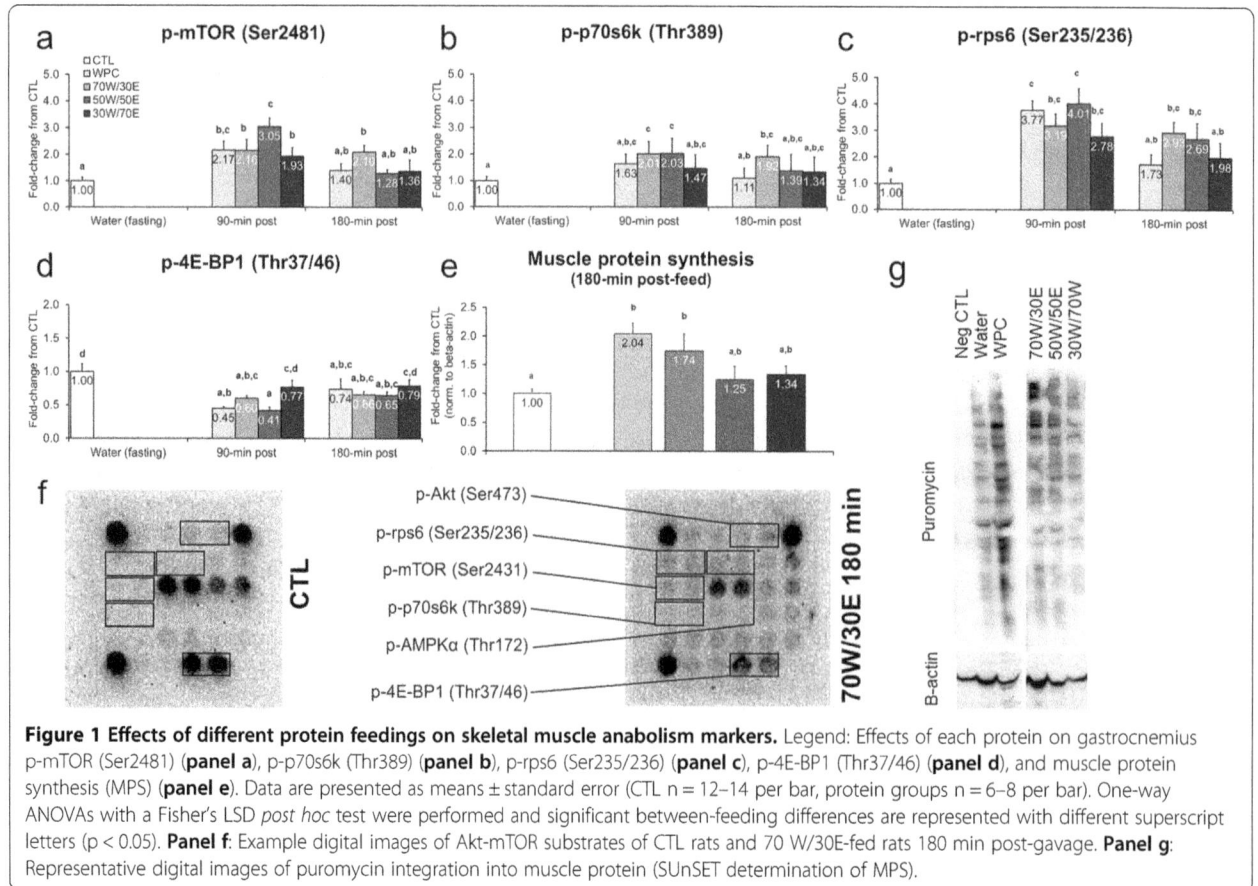

Figure 1 Effects of different protein feedings on skeletal muscle anabolism markers. Legend: Effects of each protein on gastrocnemius p-mTOR (Ser2481) (**panel a**), p-p70s6k (Thr389) (**panel b**), p-rps6 (Ser235/236) (**panel c**), p-4E-BP1 (Thr37/46) (**panel d**), and muscle protein synthesis (MPS) (**panel e**). Data are presented as means ± standard error (CTL n = 12–14 per bar, protein groups n = 6–8 per bar). One-way ANOVAs with a Fisher's LSD *post hoc* test were performed and significant between-feeding differences are represented with different superscript letters (p < 0.05). **Panel f:** Example digital images of Akt-mTOR substrates of CTL rats and 70 W/30E-fed rats 180 min post-gavage. **Panel g:** Representative digital images of puromycin integration into muscle protein (SUnSET determination of MPS).

patterns of anabolic genes are a putative index regarding whether or not a particular protein source may have a potential impact on long-term anabolism. MSTN mRNA increased in the 30 W/70E group versus fasting rats 90 min post-feeding (p < 0.001; Figure 2a), and 30 W/70E and 50 W/50E increased MSTN mRNA 180 min post-feeding versus CTL rats (30 W/70E p = 0.003, 50 W/50E p < 0.001; Figure 2a). Mighty/Akirin-1 mRNA, which is transcriptionally down-regulated by MSTN [31] and is related to muscle hypertrophy [32], was similar between groups 90 min post-treatment but: a) was greater in the WPC and 70 W/30E groups 180 min post-treatment compared to 50 W/50E rats (WPC vs. 50 W/50E p = 0.001, 70 W/30E vs. 50 W/50E p = 0.001; Figure 2b); and b) was greater in the WPC, 70 W/30E and 30 W/70E groups 180 min post-treatment compared to CTL rats (WPC vs. CTL p < 0.001, 70 W/30E vs. CTL p < 0.001, 30 W/70E vs. CTL p = 0.046; Figure 2b). p21Cip mRNA, which is a gene potentially related to skeletal muscle hypertrophy [33], remained similar between CTL and all protein-fed groups 90 min post-feeding (Figure 2c). However, p21Cip mRNA generally increased 3–4-fold in all protein groups 180 min post-treatment versus CTL rats and 90 min post-treatment values (WPC vs. CTL p = 0.005, 70 W/30E vs. CTL p = 0.001, 50 W/50E p < 0.001, 30 W/70E vs. CTL p = 0.004; Figure 2c). Atrogin-1 mRNA remained unaltered 90 min post-feeding in all protein groups compared to CTL rats, but increased in the 70 W/30E 180 min post-feeding versus CTL rats (p = 0.049; Figure 2d). MuRF-1 mRNA remained unaltered 90 min post-feeding in all protein groups compared to CTL rats, but was greater 180 min post-feeding in the WPC and 70 W/30E groups versus CTL rats at this time point (WPC vs. CTL p = 0.020, 70 W/30E vs. CTL p = 0.032;

Figure 2e). No between-group differences existed for IGF-1Ea expression patterns (Figure 2f).

Select gastrocnemius metabolic-related phosphoprotein and mRNAs are differentially affected by protein type

While markers of metabolic-related signaling and gene expression in response to feeding provide limited information, these markers also provide putative index regarding whether or not a particular protein source may have a potential impact on long-term metabolic alterations within skeletal muscle. At 90 min post-feeding, WPC and 70 W/30E increased p-Akt (Ser473) compared to CTL rats (WPC vs. CTL p = 0.012, 70 W/30E vs. CTL p = 0.031; Figure 3a), though this increase returned to CTL levels 180 min post-feeding. At 90 min post-treatment, 70 W/30E and 50 W/50E increased p-AMPKα (Thr172) versus CTL rats (70 W/30E vs. CTL p = 0.033, 50 W/50E vs. CTL p = 0.013; Figure 3b), and at 180 min post-treatment 70 W/30E induced a persistent elevation in p-AMPKα (Thr172) versus CTL rats (p = 0.040; Figure 3b). 70 W/30E increased PGC-1α mRNA versus CTL rats 90 min post-treatment (p = 0.002; Figure 3c) and all other protein groups at 90 min post-treatment (70 W/30E vs. WPC p = 0.038, 70 W/30E vs. 50 W/50E p = 0.001, 70 W/30E vs. 30 W/70E p = 0.039; Figure 3c). Though statistical differences existed between treatments for GLUT-4 mRNA, fold-changes between groups were modest (~30%) and there were no clear treatment effects (Figure 3d). Finally, 70 W/30E caused a 1.7-to-2.2-fold increase in CPT1B mRNA versus CTL rats 90 min (p = 0.012; Figure 3e) and 180 min post-treatment (p < 0.001; Figure 3e) as well as other protein groups at 90 min (70 W/30E vs. WPC p = 0.025, 70 W/30E vs. 50 W/50E p = 0.001, 70 W/30E vs. 30 W/70E p = 0.047; Figure 3e) and 180 min post-treatment (70 W/30E vs. WPC p = 0.001, 70 W/30E vs.

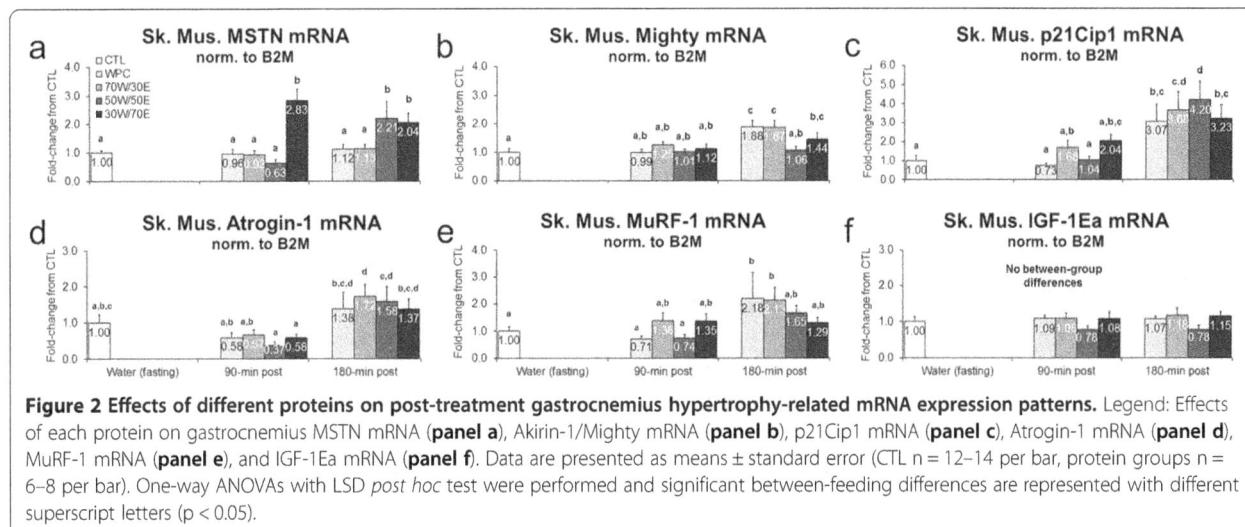

Figure 2 Effects of different proteins on post-treatment gastrocnemius hypertrophy-related mRNA expression patterns. Legend: Effects of each protein on gastrocnemius MSTN mRNA (**panel a**), Akirin-1/Mighty mRNA (**panel b**), p21Cip1 mRNA (**panel c**), Atrogin-1 mRNA (**panel d**), MuRF-1 mRNA (**panel e**), and IGF-1Ea mRNA (**panel f**). Data are presented as means ± standard error (CTL n = 12–14 per bar, protein groups n = 6–8 per bar). One-way ANOVAs with LSD *post hoc* test were performed and significant between-feeding differences are represented with different superscript letters (p < 0.05).

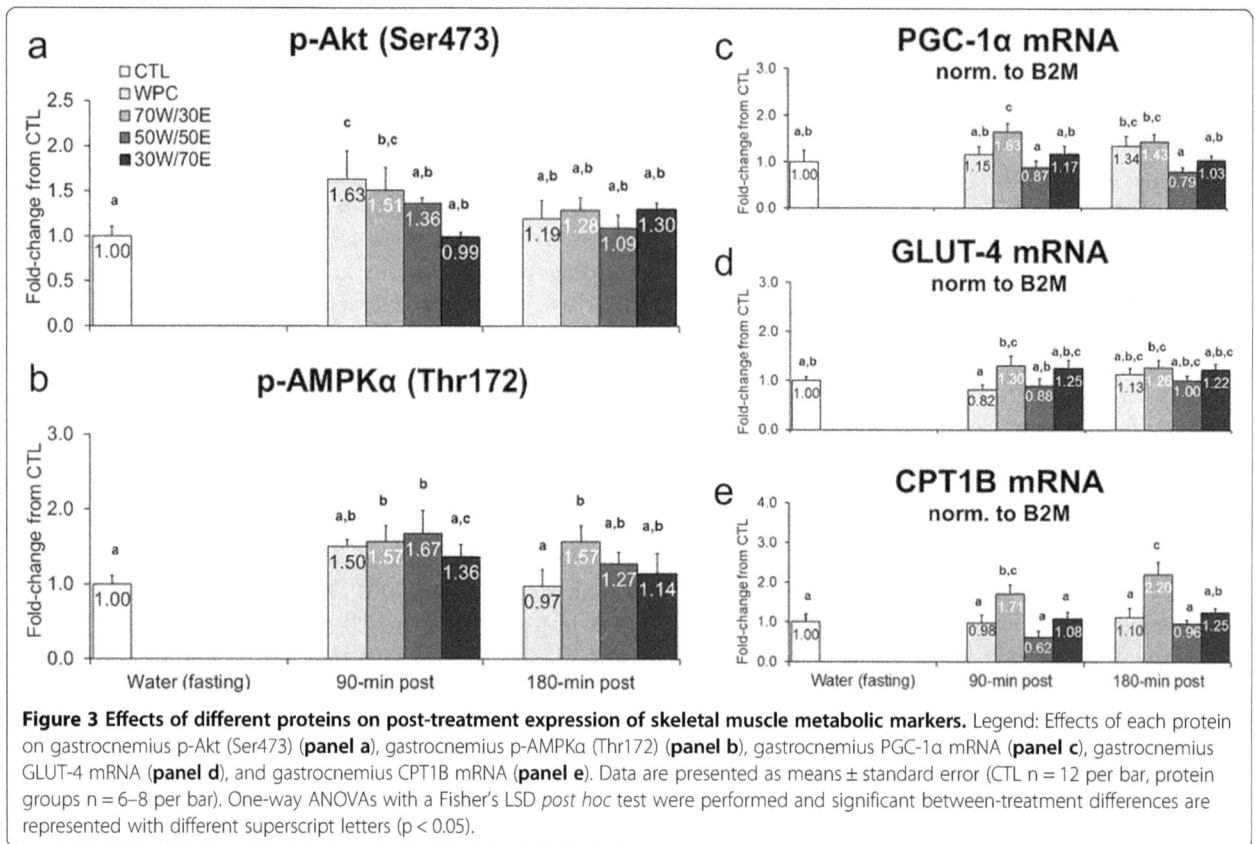

Figure 3 Effects of different proteins on post-treatment expression of skeletal muscle metabolic markers. Legend: Effects of each protein on gastrocnemius p-Akt (Ser473) (**panel a**), gastrocnemius p-AMPKα (Thr172) (**panel b**), gastrocnemius PGC-1α mRNA (**panel c**), gastrocnemius GLUT-4 mRNA (**panel d**), and gastrocnemius CPT1B mRNA (**panel e**). Data are presented as means ± standard error (CTL n = 12 per bar, protein groups n = 6–8 per bar). One-way ANOVAs with a Fisher's LSD post hoc test were performed and significant between-treatment differences are represented with different superscript letters (p < 0.05).

50 W/50E p < 0.001, 70 W/30E vs. 30 W/70E p = 0.005; Figure 3e).

Select lipolysis markers are differentially affected by protein type

Transient alterations in adipose tissue p-HSL and lipolytic/thermogenic gene expression patterns may provide insight into longer-term alterations that occur at the tissue level (i.e., decrements in fat mass size). Protein feeding did not alter OMAT p-HSL (Ser563) 90 min post-treatment, though WPC, 70 W/30E and 50 W/50E significantly increased this marker 3.8 and 6.5-fold, respectively, 180 min post-feeding versus CTL rats (70 W/30E vs. CTL p < 0.001, 50 W/50E vs. CTL p = 0.019; Figure 4a). Likewise, protein feeding did not alter SQ p-HSL (Ser563) 90 min post-treatment, though 70 W/30 W increased SQ p-HSL (Ser563) 3.1-fold versus CTL rats (p = 0.001; Figure 4b) and 1.9-to-4.4-fold versus all other protein groups 180 min post-treatment (70 W/30E vs. WPC p = 0.001, 70 W/30E vs. 50 W/50E p = 0.015, 70 W/30E vs. 30 W/70E p = 0.035; Figure 3e). Interestingly, 70 W/30E increased SQ cAMP 180 min post-treatment versus CTL rats (p = 0.045; Figure 4c) as well as the 30 W/70E group (p = 0.047; Figure 4c) suggesting that a high proportion of WPH in the test protein may facilitate cAMP-mediated p-HSL activation to increase

lipolysis. WPC and 70 W/30E depressed serum free fatty acids 90 min post-treatment versus CTL rats (WPC vs. CTL p = 0.012, 70 W/30E vs CTL p < 0.001; Figure 4e), but this was normalized by 180 min post-treatment. Finally, with regards to thermogenic SQ gene expression markers, 70 W/30E and 50 W/50E tended increase PGC-1α mRNA versus CTL rats 180 min post-treatment (70 W/30E vs. CTL p = 0.083, 50 W/50E vs. CTL p = 0.054; Figure 4f). Furthermore, 50 W/50E increased SQ UCP3 mRNA versus all other protein groups CTL rats 180 min post-treatment (p = 0.004–0.042; Figure 4 g).

Serum lipolysis and thermogenic hormones are minimally affected by protein type

Given that various OMAT and SQ markers of lipolysis and thermogenesis were differentially affected by different protein types, we next examined if protein feedings affected select hormone levels related to these physiological processes. There was no consistent protein feeding effect on serum catecholamines. WPC and 30 W/70E exhibited 40% lower EPI levels compared to CTL rats 90 min post-treatment (WPC vs. CTL p = 0.039, 30 W/70E vs. CTL p = 0.037; Figure 5a), and 50 W/50E exhibited 60% lower EPI levels compared to CTL rats 180 min post-treatment (p = 0.001; Figure 5a). 50 W/50E exhibited 60% lower

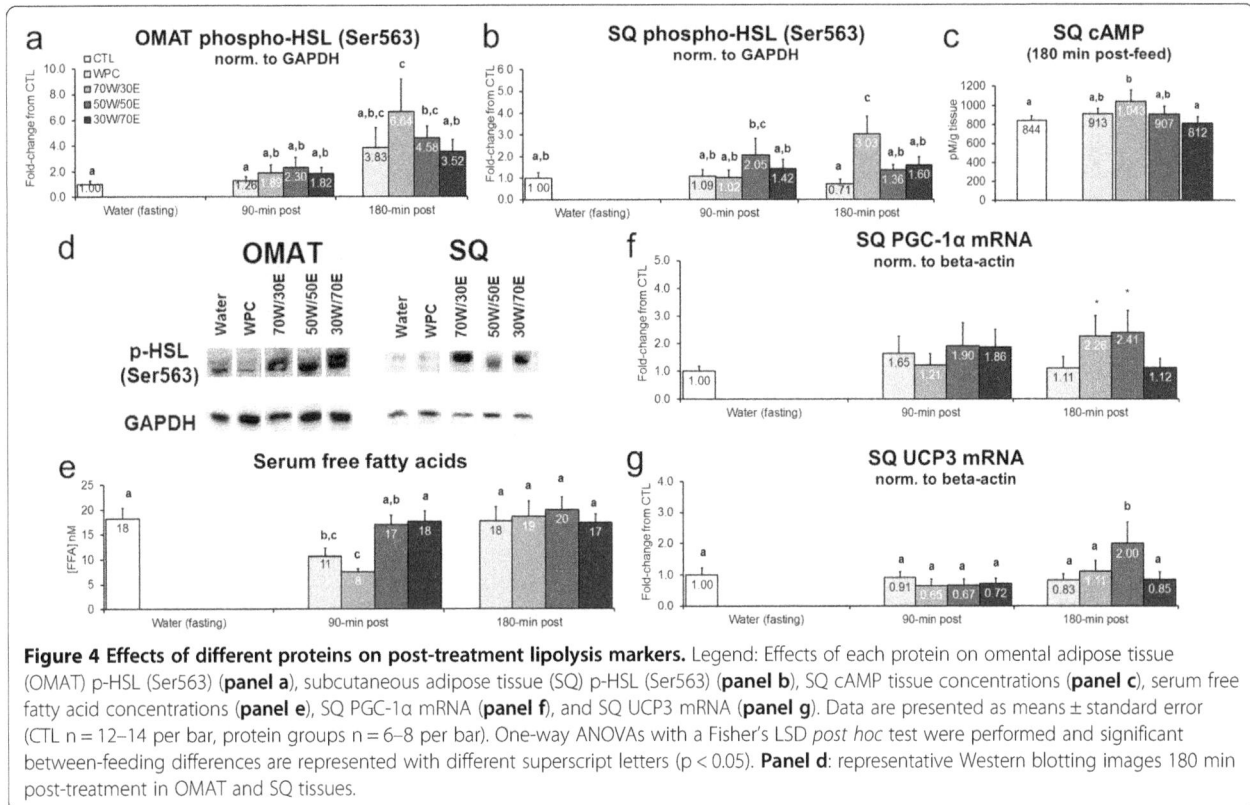

Figure 4 Effects of different proteins on post-treatment lipolysis markers. Legend: Effects of each protein on omental adipose tissue (OMAT) p-HSL (Ser563) (**panel a**), subcutaneous adipose tissue (SQ) p-HSL (Ser563) (**panel b**), SQ cAMP tissue concentrations (**panel c**), serum free fatty acid concentrations (**panel e**), SQ PGC-1α mRNA (**panel f**), and SQ UCP3 mRNA (**panel g**). Data are presented as means ± standard error (CTL n = 12–14 per bar, protein groups n = 6–8 per bar). One-way ANOVAs with a Fisher's LSD *post hoc* test were performed and significant between-feeding differences are represented with different superscript letters (p < 0.05). **Panel d**: representative Western blotting images 180 min post-treatment in OMAT and SQ tissues.

NorEPI values compared to compared to CTL rats 180 min post-treatment (p = 0.006; Figure 5b)

There was also no consistent protein feeding effect on serum T3 levels. WPC generally presented greater serum T3 levels versus other treatments 90 and 180 min post-feeding, though these values were not statistically different from fasting rats (Figure 5c). Moreover, 50 W/50E-fed rats exhibited depressed T3 levels compared to CTL rats 90 min post-feeding (p = 0.020; Figure 5c), though this effect was normalized by 180 min post-feeding. Similarly, 70 W/30E-fed rats presented significantly depressed T3 levels by 180 min post-feeding compared to CTL rats (p = 0.023; Figure 5c).

Effects of different protein feedings on hypothalamic mRNA expression patterns

Transient alterations in anorectic and orexigenic gene expression patterns could suggest that an altered satiety response occurs to different protein types. Interestingly, 70 W/30E and 30 W/70E increased hypothalamic POMC mRNA 90 min post-treatment versus CTL rats suggesting a satiety-related response may have occurred in the former groups (70 W/30E vs. CTL p = 0.008, 30 W/70E vs. CTL p = 0.007; Figure 6a). However, there was a compensatory increase in orexigenic AGRP mRNA in the 70 W/30E group 90 min post-treatment versus CTL rats (p = 0.040; Figure 6b). Likewise, there was a compensatory increase in

orexigenic NPY mRNA in the 30 W/70E group 90 min post-treatment versus CTL rats (p = 0.032; Figure 6c), and a significant increase in this marker in the 50 W/50E group 180 min post-treatment versus CTL rats (p = 0.009; Figure 6c). Though statistical differences existed between groups for hypothalamic LEPR mRNA, fold-changes between protein groups and CTL rats were modest and non-significant (±20–40%, p > 0.05; Figure 6d).

Discussion

Protein type is an important factor in acutely increasing markers of skeletal muscle anabolism

Whey and egg protein consumption has been posited to promote anabolic effects in skeletal muscle via greater post-feeding increases in serum amino acids versus other protein sources [2]. All test proteins in the current study increased the phosphorylation status of mTOR, p70s6k, and rps6 90 min post-feeding compared to CTL rats, though 70 W/30E-fed rats presented sustained elevations in phosphorylated mTOR and rps6 180 min post-feeding. These phosphorylated targets are positive effectors of MPS, and our findings are in agreement with past literature suggesting that whey and egg protein increase the phosphorylation of one or more of these intramuscular signaling markers following feeding with [19,34,20,35] or without [2,1] resistance exercise in rats and humans. However, it is intriguing that higher proportions of EPH (i.e.,

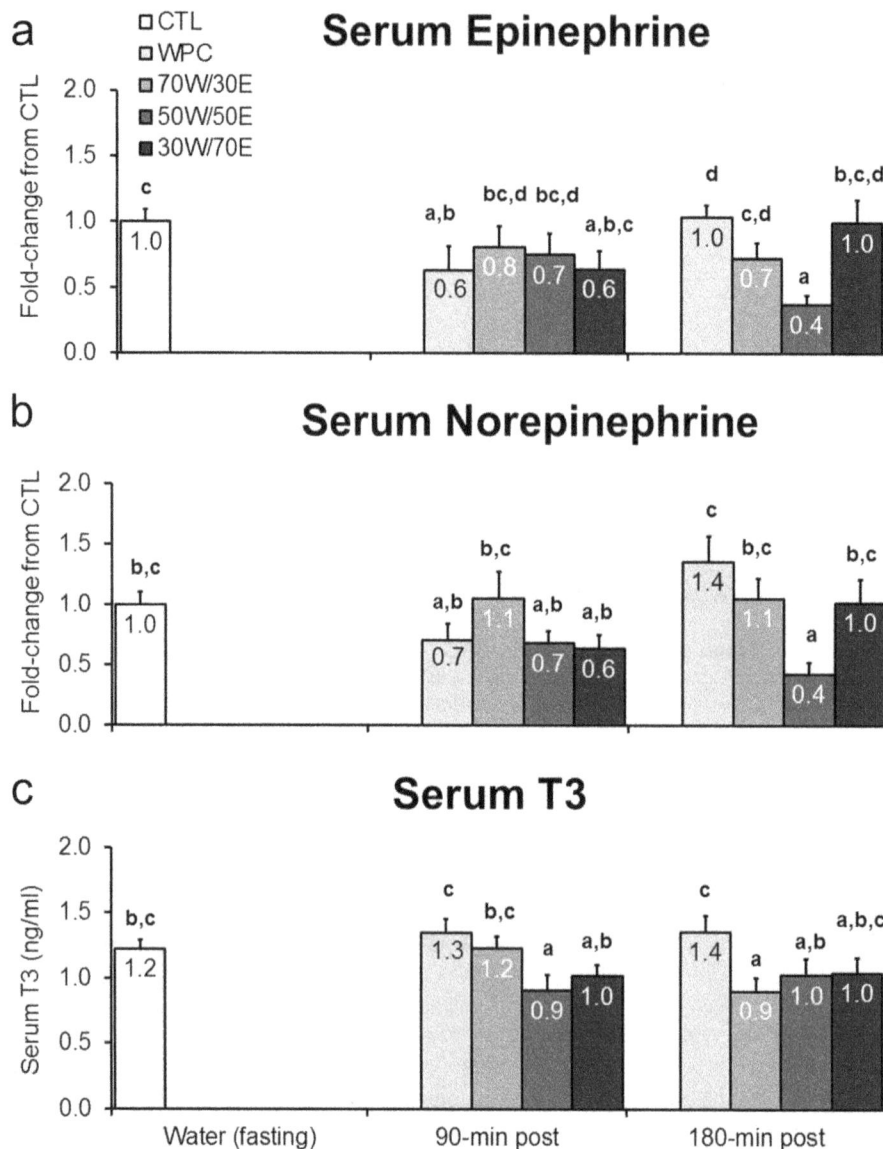

Figure 5 Effects of different proteins on post-treatment lipolytic/thermogenic hormone markers. Legend: Effects of each protein on serum epinephrine (**panel a**), norepinephrine (**panel b**), and triiodothyronine (T3) concentrations (**panel c**). Data are presented as means ± standard error (CTL n = 12–14 per bar, protein groups n = 6–8 per bar). One-way ANOVAs with a Fisher's LSD *post hoc* test were performed and significant between-treatment differences are represented with different superscript letters (p < 0.05).

50–70%) did not statistically increase MPS levels versus CTL rats. Norton et al. [1] demonstrated that a test meal containing 0.64 g of whey or egg protein similarly increases MPS 90 min post-feeding. Our study differs from the findings of Norton et al. given that: a) MPS was measured using two different methodologies; specifically we used the SUnSET method and Norton et al. used an L-^{2}H$_5$-phenylalanine tracer; b) Norton et al. measured post-feeding MPS at 90 min while we measured MPS 180 min post-feeding; and c) Norton et al. fed rats 0.64 g protein in a solid mixed-meal form while we fed rats 0.19 g of unadulterated test protein

solutions. In spite of these methodological differences, we suggest that, relative to CTL rats, a low protein dose comprised mainly of whey protein (i.e., WPC or 70 W/30E) promotes a greater post-feeding increase in MPS relative to a low dose protein solution comprised primarily of egg protein. Alternatively stated, while egg protein is a source of leucine and EAAs, it appears that whey protein is superior at stimulating MPS at lower doses in the current rodent model. While this seems contrary to the conclusions posited by Norton et al. suggesting that the high leucine content in whey and egg equally stimulate MPS, two independent human studies

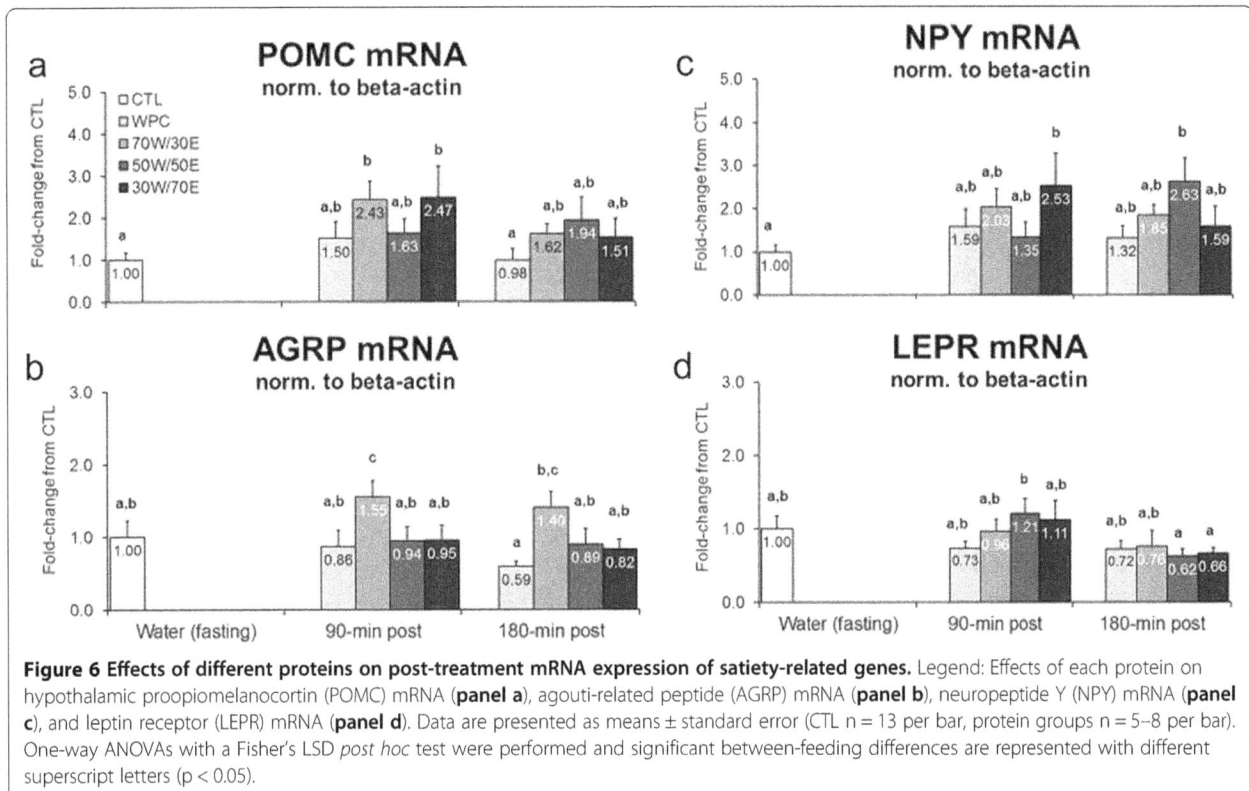

Figure 6 Effects of different proteins on post-treatment mRNA expression of satiety-related genes. Legend: Effects of each protein on hypothalamic proopiomelanocortin (POMC) mRNA (**panel a**), agouti-related peptide (AGRP) mRNA (**panel b**), neuropeptide Y (NPY) mRNA (**panel c**), and leptin receptor (LEPR) mRNA (**panel d**). Data are presented as means ± standard error (CTL n = 13 per bar, protein groups n = 5–8 per bar). One-way ANOVAs with a Fisher's LSD *post hoc* test were performed and significant between-feeding differences are represented with different superscript letters (p < 0.05).

have demonstrated that younger [36] and older subjects [37] consuming supplemental egg protein while resistance training do not experience increases in muscle mass after 8–12-week interventions. Specifically, Hida et al. [36] demonstrated that 15 g/d of egg protein supplementation in female athletes, who were engaged in a resistance training protocol, increased lean body mass by 1.5 kg, whereas a carbohydrate placebo increased lean body mass by 1.6 kg. Likewise, Iglay et al. [37] demonstrated that supplementing the diet with an additional 20 g/d of egg protein did not further increase the lean mass or skeletal muscle cross-sectional area compared to a lower protein group when both groups resistance trained for 12 weeks; of note, both groups gained roughly 1.0 kg of lean body mass.

In contrast, a recent meta-analysis examining several studies [5] clearly demonstrates that whey protein supplementation with resistance exercise is effective at increasing muscle mass in younger and older populations, and Phillips et al. [6] noted that participants engaged in 8–16 weeks of resistance exercise gain, on average, 3.0 kg of lean mass compared to 1.0 kg of lean mass gains in the placebo groups of these studies. One hypothesis deserving of future investigation is whether mammary-derived proteins, due to the inherent purpose of such proteins promoting rapid growth and development of offspring, may offer unique physiological advantages versus what can otherwise be labeled as 'nutritional protein sources' such as egg or other animal proteins. In this regard, future studies

examining why a low dose of whey protein is unique in stimulating muscle anabolism relative to other protein sources that possess a 'leucine-, BCAA-, and EAA-rich profile' are warranted.

Putative anabolic and atrogene gastrocnemius mRNA responses following different protein feedings

Akirin-1/Mighty increased approximately 90% 180 min post-feeding in the WPC and 70 W/30E groups versus CTL rats and other protein groups. Akirin-1/Mighty is a transcriptional target of MSTN that is related to controlling myotube size *in vitro* [32], and resistance exercise has been shown to transiently up-regulate Akirin-1/Mighty mRNA in rodent skeletal muscle [31]. To our knowledge, only one other recent study to date has determined that certain akirin genes are transcriptionally up-regulated in fish that were fasted 21 days and then re-fed [38]. Hence, the aforementioned study along with our current data suggests that Akirin-1/Mighty mRNA is sensitive to protein feeding, and this finding should be further examined at the mechanistic level in order to determine if whey protein affects skeletal muscle hypertrophy through increases in Akirin-1/Mighty mRNA expression.

The expression of select anabolic and catabolic-related gastrocnemius mRNAs responded differently between different treatment groups. Interestingly, higher proportions of EPH caused 90–180 min increases in MSTN mRNA versus CTL rats and/or higher proportions of whey protein.

Preliminary data in humans suggest that the consumption of fertile egg yolk powder reduces circulating MSTN levels [25]. Hence, if one or multiple putative bioactive components in egg protein extract reduce serum MSTN levels then it is possible that skeletal muscle may undergo a compensatory increase in skeletal MSTN mRNA expression to counter systemic down-regulation. Thus, while our data and other limited evidence suggests that MSTN expression is responsive to dietary egg proteins, more research is needed in order to elucidate if egg protein-induced increases in MSTN gene expression and/or signaling in skeletal muscle results in a physiological meaningful response.

All protein sources generally increased the p21Cip1 mRNA expression 180 min post-feeding compared to CTL rats suggesting that protein feeding in general regulates the expression of this gene. p21Cip1 gene expression has been theorized to promote satellite cell differentiation [39,40], though limited information suggests that p21Cip1 gene expression up-regulates protein synthesis and pathological hypertrophy in kidney epithelial cells [41]. Thus, it will be of further interest to examine if protein feeding-induced increases in skeletal muscle p21Cip1 gene expression are related to post-mitotic skeletal muscle protein synthesis mechanisms.

Atrogin-1 was up-regulated in 70 W/30E-fed rats 180 min post-feeding versus CTL rats. Similarly, MuRF-1 was up-regulated in WPC-fed and 70 W/30E-fed rats 180 min post-feeding versus CTL rats. Our finding that test solutions containing predominantly whey protein increase postprandial atrogene (atrogin-1 and MuRF-1) mRNA expression is intriguing given that amino acids are thought to be anti-catabolic [42]. However, ingesting smaller protein ingestion boluses (10–20 g) have been reported to increase MuRF-1 mRNA in human skeletal muscle after resistance exercise versus a larger bolus (40 g) [43]. Thus, our finding that protein ingestion increases the mRNA expression of select atrogenes may represent a stimulation of greater muscle protein turnover rather than an increase in atrophic mechanisms.

Protein source and type as important factors in acutely affecting markers of skeletal muscle metabolism and reduced muscle catabolism

Higher proportions of whey protein in the test solutions (i.e., WPC and 70 W/30E) increased Akt phosphorylation (Ser473) 90 min post-feeding versus CTL rats. Tissue Akt phosphorylation at the Ser473 residues is a common readout for insulin signaling and sensitivity [44], and whey protein feeding following resistance exercise in humans has been shown to increase Akt phosphorylation at the Ser473 residue [19,20]. Our findings are also in partial agreement with West et al. [45] who demonstrated in humans that an EAA bolus increases skeletal muscle Akt phosphorylation (Ser473) 60 min

after feeding. As noted above, however, WPC and EPH are also a rich source of EAAs. Thus, we speculate that the increase in Akt phosphorylation in the WPC and 70 W/30E groups may have been due to the superior ability of whey protein in stimulating insulin secretion and, thus, downstream insulin signaling in skeletal muscle. While we did not measure serum insulin responses in the current study, we have previously shown that WPH feeding to rats causes a robust (>2-fold) rise in insulin 60 min post-feeding [23]. Hence, foods containing a higher proportion of whey protein may stimulate greater intramuscular insulin signaling, and future research should continue to examine if WPC or WPH feeding in acute and long-term settings can enhance insulin sensitivity in insulin-resistant subjects.

Interestingly, 70 W/30E feeding caused a 63% increase in skeletal muscle PGC-1α mRNA expression versus CTL rats, as well as a significant increase in this gene relative to all other groups 90 min post-treatment. Furthermore, rats fed 70 W/30E exhibited a significant increase in skeletal muscle CPT1B mRNA 90- and 180 min post-feeding; this being a gene which is involved with fatty acid transport to the mitochondria for fuel oxidation. Whey protein isolate has been shown to stimulate a further increase in PGC-1α mRNA expression in human skeletal muscle 6 h following cycling [46]. However, to our knowledge, this is the first study to demonstrate that a test protein containing chiefly WPH can increase post-feeding skeletal muscle PGC-1α mRNA expression independent of exercise. We posit that one potential mechanism whereby WPH stimulates the mRNA expression of PGC-1α and CPT1B is through the stimulation of AMPK activity (Figure 3a). To this end, Canto et al. [47] have demonstrated that AMPK activation increases the expression of these two genes, and this would support the hypothesis that whey protein, in particular WPH, can stimulate oxidative metabolism and mitochondrial biogenesis with long-term supplementation. This hypothesis is not unfounded given recent evidence that prolonged whey protein feeding has been shown to increase mitochondrial content and respiration in the brain [48] and liver [49]. Therefore, more mechanistic studies should examine if WPH administration increases the post-feeding expression of mitochondrial-related genes via AMPK activation and/or other mechanisms.

Effects of different proteins on post-feeding markers of lipolysis

As mentioned prior, whey protein ingestion exerts positive effects on body composition and fat mass [14,5]. Furthermore, and as mentioned previously, WPH supplementation during exercise may provide added benefit to reducing body fat versus intact/native protein sources. Despite a transient 90 min post-feeding depression in serum FFAs with 70 W/30E feeding versus CTL rats and other protein groups, 50–70% WPH protein feedings increased select markers of adipose tissue lipolysis and thermogenesis 180 min post-feeding. For instance, rats fed 70 W/30E presented increases in SQ cAMP levels as well as OMAT and SQ p-HSL (Ser563). Likewise, rats that were fed higher proportions of WPH (e.g., 70 W/30E or 50 W/50E) exhibited increases in SQ PGC-1α and UCP3 mRNA expression levels which are putative markers of adipose tissue thermogenesis [50]. Finally, 70 W/30E increased gastrocnemius CPT1B mRNA which could be suggestive of a potential long-term enhancement in fatty acid transport to the mitochondria for oxidation. Conversely, circulating catecholamine levels in response to feeding higher proportions of WPH exhibited no discernable effects. These findings are difficult to reconcile as we have previously reported that WPH increases serum EPI 30 min post-feeding versus WPC-fed and CTL rats [18]. Therefore, the 180-min post-feeding increase in lipolysis markers in the current study may be due to an earlier increase in catecholamines (i.e., within 60 min of feeding) which was not captured due to sampling time points and/or due to WPH-borne bioactives that selectively act upon adipose tissue to stimulate lipolytic mechanisms.

Of note, we measured serum T3 given that it is a well-known stimulator of thermogenesis and cellular respiration. With regards to adipose tissue lipolysis, T3 has been shown to increase adipocyte beta-adrenergic receptor which, in turn, increases lipolytic capabilities over longer-term periods [51]. Notwithstanding, there was no clear protein feeding effect on serum T3 depression, and T3 values did not seem to parallel the increased lipolysis and thermogenesis markers in rats fed 70 W/30E or 50 W/50E which refutes the potential role of thyroid hormones in facilitating this effect.

One final mechanistic explanation as to how higher proportions of WPH increased lipolysis markers is through potential tricarboxylic acid (TCA) cycle modulation. To this end, a recent study by Lillefosse et al. [52] demonstrated that chronic whey protein feeding to obese-prone rodents significantly reduced fat mass gain in response to concomitant high fat feeding. The authors suggested that whey protein feeding increases the urinary excretion of TCA substrates which are stimulators of fatty acid synthesis [53]. Alternatively stated, the ability of WPH to 'extract' TCA cycle intermediates from adipose tissue during the post-feeding period may place adipose tissue in a catabolic state thereby initiating lipolysis-related mechanisms. This is not unfounded, as we have previously noted that WPH significantly increases circulating TCA intermediates (i.e., citrate, succinate, fumarate and malate) 60 min post-feeding versus WPC-fed rats (*supplementary data* in [18]). Hence, more research is needed regarding if the depletion of TCA cycle intermediates within adipose tissue is linked to the WPH-induced lipolysis response.

Effects of different proteins on post-feeding markers of satiety

Sousa et al. [54] recently posited that, regardless of protein source, amino acids may reduce appetite via an increase in gut hormone secretion, an increase in anorexigenic POMC gene expression in the hypothalamus, and/or a reduction in orexigenic NPY gene expression in the hypothalamus. 70 W/30E and 30 W/70E increased hypothalamic POMC mRNA expression patterns 90 min post-feeding; this being a marker that favors satiety signaling in the hypothalamus [55]. However, there was a compensatory increase in the orexigenic AGRP transcript in rats fed a high proportion of WPH. Furthermore, some protein feedings induced an increased expression of hypothalamic NPY mRNA versus CTL rats which, again, suggests a potential orexigenic versus satiety response. Therefore, our mixed findings suggest that two possibilities may exist including: a) the amount of total protein fed to rats, while beneficial in stimulating skeletal muscle anabolism and adipose tissue lipolysis, was not entirely effective at initiating a satiety response; and/or b) hypothalamic signaling is so tightly regulated that a post-feeding increase in anorectic genes is countered with a compensatory increase in orexigenic genes.

Finally, it should be noted that the post-feeding effects of each protein on hypothalamic LEPR mRNA expression patterns was of considerable interest due to the central role of leptin receptor signaling in satiety. Thus, we initially hypothesized that protein-feeding induced alterations in LEPR mRNA expression may be a potential culprit in initiating longer-term body composition alterations through enhanced satiety mechanisms that have been reported to previously occur with chronic protein supplementation. To this end, McAllan et al. [11] recently performed a long-term rodent feeding study whereby C57BL/6 J mice were fed a high fat diet (HFD, 45% energy as fat) enriched with either 20% energy as casein or whey protein isolate. HFD feeding increased the hypothalamic mRNA expression of LEPR; an effect which the authors suggest may be a hallmark feature of hyperphagia and obesity development. However, mice that were co-fed whey protein isolate with the HFD presented a significant reduction in hypothalamic LEPR mRNA expression. Notwithstanding, we demonstrated no noticeable between-group differences in LEPR mRNA expression patterns which suggests that the hypothalamic expression gene is not appreciably altered after one feeding and/or LEPR gene expression may be indiscriminately regulated more so by amino acid concentration alone as opposed to specific bioactive peptides.

Conclusions

We have demonstrated that protein type provide uniquely different physiological responses over a transient postprandial time course. Specifically, and seemingly irrespective of protein type, administering higher concentrations of whey versus egg protein to healthy rodents causes: a) a greater anabolic response in rodents with regards to post-feeding MPS compared to a fasting condition; and b) an increase in intramuscular insulin sensitivity markers (i.e., Akt signaling markers and transient increases in PGC-1α mRNA expression patterns). Alternatively, the administration of higher concentrations of WPH versus EPH increases select markers of post-feeding lipolysis 3 h post-feeding. Of note, while we make assertions that whey protein forms may be more beneficial in facilitating increases in muscle mass and fat loss compared to egg protein per the current findings, the acute nature of this study is a pervading limitation of these hypotheses. Likewise, while several of tissue markers were statistically altered in response to different protein feedings, more research is needed comparing whey versus egg protein supplementation on longer-term physiologically-relevant outcomes (i.e., increases in muscle mass, decreases in fat mass, and/or alterations in satiety as suggested by our transient findings reported herein). Therefore, further research is this nutraceutical arena is warranted with regards to how protein source and type (i.e., native versus hydrolyzed), and varying combinations thereof may affect these physiological parameters in over more chronic periods and in more clinical-based populations.

Additional file

> **Additional file 1: Figure S1** Preliminary testing different WPC doses on post-feeding gastrocnemius phosphorylated mTOR markers and muscle protein synthesis 90 min post-treatment. Legend: data are presented as means ± standard error [CTL n = 8 per bar except for MPS where n = 3 per bar, WPC groups n = 2–3 per bar]. One-way ANOVAs with a Fisher's LSD *post hoc* test was performed; * indicates significance versus water (fasting) rats (p < 0.05). These data show that a low dose of WPC (0.19 g which is 10 human eq. g) is just as effective at stimulating most mTOR substrates and MPS levels versus moderate (0.37 g which is 19 human eq. g) and high (0.93 g which is 19 human eq. g) WPC doses. The relatively low dose (0.19 g which is 10 human eq. g) was subsequently employed for WPC, 70 W/30E, 50 W/50E and 30 W/70E comparisons.

Competing interests

Besides C.M.L., none of the authors have non-finacial and/or financial competing interests. C.M.L. is employed by 4Life, but he intellectually contributed to study design and data write-up. Therefore, all co-authors agreed that his intellectual input into this project warranted co-authorship.

Authors' contributions

CBM, CDF, BSF, CAP, JCH, JSM, CML and MDR: This person has made substantial contributions to conception and design, or acquisition of data, or analysis and interpretation of data. CBM, CML and MDR: This person primarily was involved in drafting the manuscript or revising it critically for important intellectual content. CBM, CDF, BSF, CAP, JCH, JSM, CML and MDR: This person gave final approval of the version to be published. CBM, CDF, BSF, CAP, JCH, JSM, CML and MDR: This person agrees to be accountable for all aspects of the work in ensuring that questions related to the accuracy or integrity of any part of the work are appropriately investigated and resolved. All authors read and approved the final manuscript.

Acknowledgements

The authors thank Dr. David Pascoe and Dr. Andreas Kavazis for intellectual input.

Financial Support

Funding from 4Life Research USA, LLC was used to fund the direct costs of this study, C.A.P.'s graduate assistant stipend, undergraduate technical help, and publication costs of these data.

Author details

[1]School of Kinesiology, Molecular and Applied Sciences Laboratory, Auburn University, 301 Wire Road, Office 286, Auburn, AL 36849, USA. [2]4Life Research USA, LLC, Sandy, UT, USA.

References

1. Norton LE, Wilson GJ, Layman DK, Moulton CJ, Garlick PJ. Leucine content of dietary proteins is a determinant of postprandial skeletal muscle protein synthesis in adult rats. Nutr Metab. 2012;9(1):67. doi:10.1186/1743-7075-9-67.
2. Norton LE, Layman DK, Bunpo P, Anthony TG, Brana DV, Garlick PJ. The leucine content of a complete meal directs peak activation but not duration of skeletal muscle protein synthesis and mammalian target of rapamycin signaling in rats. J Nutr. 2009;139(6):1103–9. doi:10.3945/jn.108.103853.
3. Moore DR, Tang JE, Burd NA, Rerecich T, Tarnopolsky MA, Phillips SM. Differential stimulation of myofibrillar and sarcoplasmic protein synthesis with protein ingestion at rest and after resistance exercise. J Physiol. 2009;587(Pt 4):897–904. doi:10.1113/jphysiol.2008.164087.
4. Witard OC, Jackman SR, Breen L, Smith K, Selby A, Tipton KD. Myofibrillar muscle protein synthesis rates subsequent to a meal in response to increasing doses of whey protein at rest and after resistance exercise. Am J Clin Nutr. 2014;99(1):86–95. doi:10.3945/ajcn.112.055517.
5. Miller PE, Alexander DD, Perez V. Effects of whey protein and resistance exercise on body composition: a meta-analysis of randomized controlled trials. J Am Coll Nutr. 2014;33(2):163–75. doi:10.1080/07315724.2013.875365.
6. Phillips SM, Tang JE, Moore DR. The role of milk- and soy-based protein in support of muscle protein synthesis and muscle protein accretion in young and elderly persons. J Am Coll Nutr. 2009;28(4):343–54.
7. Hulmi JJ, Lockwood CM, Stout JR. Effect of protein/essential amino acids and resistance training on skeletal muscle hypertrophy: A case for whey protein. Nutr Metab. 2010;7:51. doi:10.1186/1743-7075-7-51.
8. Sukkar SG, Vaccaro A, Ravera GB, Borrini C, Gradaschi R, Massa Sacchi-Nemours A, et al. Appetite control and gastrointestinal hormonal behavior (CCK, GLP-1, PYY 1-36) following low doses of a whey protein-rich nutraceutic. Mediterr J Nutr Metab. 2013;6:259–66. doi:10.1007/s12349-013-0121-7.
9. Diepvens K, Haberer D, Westerterp-Plantenga M. Different proteins and biopeptides differently affect satiety and anorexigenic/orexigenic hormones in healthy humans. Int J Obes (Lond). 2008;32(3):510–8. doi:10.1038/sj.ijo.0803758.
10. Luhovyy BL, Akhavan T, Anderson GH. Whey proteins in the regulation of food intake and satiety. J Am Coll Nutr. 2007;26(6):704S–12S.
11. McAllan L, Keane D, Schellekens H, Roche HM, Korpela R, Cryan JF, et al. Whey protein isolate counteracts the effects of a high-fat diet on energy intake and hypothalamic and adipose tissue expression of energy balance-related genes. Br J Nutr. 2013;110(11):2114–26. doi:10.1017/S0007114513001396.
12. Pilvi TK, Storvik M, Louhelainen M, Merasto S, Korpela R, Mervaala EM. Effect of dietary calcium and dairy proteins on the adipose tissue gene expression profile in diet-induced obesity. J Nutrigenet Nutrigenomics. 2008;1(5):240–51. doi:10.1159/000151238.
13. Pilvi TK, Korpela R, Huttunen M, Vapaatalo H, Mervaala EM. High-calcium diet with whey protein attenuates body-weight gain in high-fat-fed C57Bl/6 J mice. Br J Nutr. 2007;98(5):900–7. doi:10.1017/S0007114507764760.
14. Frestedt JL, Zenk JL, Kuskowski MA, Ward LS, Bastian ED. A whey-protein supplement increases fat loss and spares lean muscle in obese subjects: a randomized human clinical study. Nutr Metab. 2008;5:8. doi:10.1186/1743-7075-5-8.
15. Halton TL, Hu FB. The effects of high protein diets on thermogenesis, satiety and weight loss: a critical review. J Am Coll Nutr. 2004;23(5):373–85.
16. Calbet JA, MacLean DA. Plasma glucagon and insulin responses depend on the rate of appearance of amino acids after ingestion of different protein solutions in humans. J Nutr. 2002;132(8):2174–82.
17. Madureira AR, Tavares T, Gomes AM, Pintado ME, Malcata FX. Invited review: physiological properties of bioactive peptides obtained from whey proteins. J Dairy Sci. 2010;93(2):437–55. doi:10.3168/jds. 2009-2566.

18. Roberts MD, Cruthirds CL, Lockwood CM, Pappan K, Childs TE, Company JM, et al. Comparing serum responses to acute feedings of an extensively hydrolyzed whey protein concentrate versus a native whey protein concentrate in rats: a metabolomics approach. Appl Physiol, Nutr Metab =Physiologie appliquee, nutrition et metabolisme. 2014;39(2):158–67. doi:10.1139/apnm–2013–0148.

19. Kakigi R, Yoshihara T, Ozaki H, Ogura Y, Ichinoseki-Sekine N, Kobayashi H, et al. Whey protein intake after resistance exercise activates mTOR signaling in a dose-dependent manner in human skeletal muscle. Eur J Appl Physiol. 2014;114(4):735–42. doi:10.1007/s00421–013–2812–7.

20. Reitelseder S, Agergaard J, Doessing S, Helmark IC, Lund P, Kristensen NB, et al. Whey and casein labeled with L-[1–13C] leucine and muscle protein synthesis: effect of resistance exercise and protein ingestion. Am J Physiol Endocrinol Metab. 2011;300(1):E231–42. doi:10.1152/ajpendo.00513.2010.

21. Morifuji M, Koga J, Kawanaka K, Higuchi M. Branched-chain amino acid-containing dipeptides, identified from whey protein hydrolysates, stimulate glucose uptake rate in L6 myotubes and isolated skeletal muscles. J Nutr Sci Vitaminol. 2009;55(1):81–6.

22. Gaudel C, Nongonierma AB, Maher S, Flynn S, Krause M, Murray BA, et al. A whey protein hydrolysate promotes insulinotropic activity in a clonal pancreatic beta-cell line and enhances glycemic function in ob/ob mice. J Nutr. 2013;143(7):1109–14. doi:10.3945/jn.113.174912.

23. Toedebusch RG, Childs TE, Hamilton SR, Crowley JR, Booth FW, Roberts MD. Postprandial leucine and insulin responses and toxicological effects of a novel whey protein hydrolysate-based supplement in rats. J Int Soc Sports Nutr. 2012;9(1):24. doi:10.1186/1550–2783–9–24.

24. Campbell B, Kreider RB, Ziegenfuss T, La Bounty P, Roberts M, Burke D, et al. International society of sports nutrition position stand: protein and exercise. International Society. 2007;4:8. doi:10.1186/1550–2783–4–8.

25. Colker C. Effect on serum myostatin levels of high-grade handled fertile egg yolk powder (Conference abstract). J Am Coll Nutr. 2009;28 (3).

26. Vander Wal JS, Marth JM, Khosla P, Jen KL, Dhurandhar NV. Short-term effect of eggs on satiety in overweight and obese subjects. J Am Coll Nutr. 2005;24(6):510–5.

27. Vander Wal JS, Gupta A, Khosla P, Dhurandhar NV. Egg breakfast enhances weight loss. Int J Obes (Lond). 2008;32(10):1545–51. doi:10.1038/ijo.2008.130.

28. Reagan-Shaw S, Nihal M, Ahmad N. Dose translation from animal to human studies revisited. FASEB J. 2008;22(3):659–61. doi:10.1096/fj.07–9574LSF.

29. Goodman CA, Hornberger TA. Measuring protein synthesis with sunset: a valid alternative to traditional techniques? Exerc Sport Sci Rev. 2013;41 (2):107–15. doi:10.1097/JES.0b013e3182798a95.

30. Roberts MD, Gilpin L, Parker KE, Childs TE, Will MJ, Booth FW. Dopamine D1 receptor modulation in nucleus accumbens lowers voluntary wheel running in rats bred to run high distances. Physiol Behav. 2012;105(3):661–8. doi:10.1016/j.physbeh.2011.09.024.

31. MacKenzie MG, Hamilton DL, Pepin M, Patton A, Baar K. Inhibition of myostatin signaling through Notch activation following acute resistance exercise. PLoS One. 2013;8(7):e68743. doi:10.1371/journal.pone.0068743.

32. Mobley CB, Fox CD, Ferguson BS, Amin RH, Dalbo VJ, Baier S, et al. L-leucine, beta-hydroxy-beta-methylbutyric acid (HMB) and creatine monohydrate prevent myostatin-induced Akirin-1/Mighty mRNA down-regulation and myotube atrophy. J Int Soc Sports Nutr. 2014;11:38. doi:10.1186/1550–2783–11–38.

33. Roberts MD, Dalbo VJ, Kerksick CM. Postexercise myogenic gene expression: are human findings lost during translation? Exerc Sport Sci Rev. 2011;39(4):206–11. doi:10.1097/JES.0b013e31822dad1f.

34. Farnfield MM, Carey KA, Gran P, Trenerry MK, Cameron-Smith D. Whey protein ingestion activates mTOR-dependent signalling after resistance exercise in young men: a double-blinded randomized controlled trial. Nutrients. 2009;1(2):263–75. doi:10.3390/nu1020263.

35. Farnfield MM, Breen L, Carey KA, Garnham A, Cameron-Smith D. Activation of mTOR signalling in young and old human skeletal muscle in response to combined resistance exercise and whey protein ingestion. Applied physiology, nutrition, and metabolism =. Physiol Appl Nutr Metab. 2012;37(1):21–30. doi:10.1139/h11–132.

36. Hida A, Hasegawa Y, Mekata Y, Usuda M, Masuda Y, Kawano H, et al. Effects of egg white protein supplementation on muscle strength and serum free amino acid concentrations. Nutrients. 2012;4(10):1504–17. doi:10.3390/nu4101504.

37. Iglay HB, Apolzan JW, Gerrard DE, Eash JK, Anderson JC, Campbell WW. Moderately increased protein intake predominantly from egg sources does not influence whole body, regional, or muscle composition responses to resistance training in older people. J Nutr Health Aging. 2009;13(2):108–14.

38. Macqueen DJ, Kristjansson BK, Johnston IA. Salmonid genomes have a remarkably expanded akirin family, coexpressed with genes from conserved pathways governing skeletal muscle growth and catabolism. Physiol Genomics. 2010;42(1):134–48. doi:10.1152/physiolgenomics.00045.2010.

39. Hawke TJ, Jiang N, Garry DJ. Absence of p21CIP rescues myogenic progenitor cell proliferative and regenerative capacity in Foxk1 null mice. J Biol Chem. 2003;278(6):4015–20. doi:10.1074/jbc.M209200200.

40. Hawke TJ, Meeson AP, Jiang N, Graham S, Hutcheson K, DiMaio JM, et al. p21 is essential for normal myogenic progenitor cell function in regenerating skeletal muscle. Am J Physiol Cell Physiol. 2003;285(5):C1019–27. doi:10.1152/ajpcell.00055.2003.

41. Fan YP, Weiss RH. Exogenous attenuation of p21 (Waf1/Cip1) decreases mesangial cell hypertrophy as a result of hyperglycemia and IGF-1. J Am Soc Nephrol: JASN. 2004;15(3):575–84.

42. Herningtyas EH, Okimura Y, Handayaningsih AE, Yamamoto D, Maki T, Iida K, et al. Branched-chain amino acids and arginine suppress MaFbx/atrogin-1 mRNA expression via mTOR pathway in C2C12 cell line. Biochim Biophys Acta. 2008;1780(10):1115–20. doi:10.1016/j.bbagen.2008.06.004.

43. Areta JL, Burke LM, Ross ML, Camera DM, West DW, Broad EM, et al. Timing and distribution of protein ingestion during prolonged recovery from resistance exercise alters myofibrillar protein synthesis. J Physiol. 2013;591(Pt 9):2319–31. doi:10.1113/jphysiol.2012.244897.

44. Hojlund K, Glintborg D, Andersen NR, Birk JB, Treebak JT, Frosig C, et al. Impaired insulin-stimulated phosphorylation of Akt and AS160 in skeletal muscle of women with polycystic ovary syndrome is reversed by pioglitazone treatment. Diabetes. 2008;57(2):357–66. doi:10.2337/db07–0706.

45. West DW, Burd NA, Coffey VG, Baker SK, Burke LM, Hawley JA, et al. Rapid aminoacidemia enhances myofibrillar protein synthesis and anabolic intramuscular signaling responses after resistance exercise. Am J Clin Nutr. 2011;94(3):795–803. doi:10.3945/ajcn.111.013722.

46. Hill KM, Stathis CG, Grinfeld E, Hayes A, McAinch AJ. Co-ingestion of carbohydrate and whey protein isolates enhance PGC-1alpha mRNA expression: a randomised, single blind, cross over study. J Int Soc Sports Nutr. 2013;10(1):8. doi:10.1186/1550–2783–10–8.

47. Canto C, Gerhart-Hines Z, Feige JN, Lagouge M, Noriega L, Milne JC, et al. AMPK regulates energy expenditure by modulating NAD+ metabolism and SIRT1 activity. Nat. 2009;458(7241):1056–60. doi:10.1038/nature07813.

48. Shertzer HG, Krishan M, Genter MB. Dietary whey protein stimulates mitochondrial activity and decreases oxidative stress in mouse female brain. Neurosci Lett. 2013;548:159–64. doi:10.1016/j.neulet.2013.05.061.

49. Shertzer HG, Woods SE, Krishan M, Genter MB, Pearson KJ. Dietary whey protein lowers the risk for metabolic disease in mice fed a high-fat diet. J Nutr. 2011;141(4):582–7. doi:10.3945/jn.110.133736.

50. Bostrom P, Wu J, Jedrychowski MP, Korde A, Ye L, Lo JC, et al. A PGC1-alpha-dependent myokine that drives brown-fat-like development of white fat and thermogenesis. Nat. 2012;481(7382):463–8. doi:10.1038/nature10777.

51. Fain JN, Coronel EC, Beauchamp MJ, Bahouth SW. Expression of leptin and beta 3-adrenergic receptors in rat adipose tissue in altered thyroid states. Biochem J. 1997;322(Pt 1):145–50.

52. Lillefosse HH, Clausen MR, Yde CC, Ditlev DB, Zhang X, Du ZY, et al. Urinary loss of tricarboxylic Acid cycle intermediates as revealed by metabolomics studies: an underlying mechanism to reduce lipid accretion by whey protein ingestion? J Proteome Res. 2014;13(5):2560–70. doi:10.1021/pr500039t.

53. Martin DB, Vagelos PR. The mechanism of tricarboxylic acid cycle regulation of fatty acid synthesis. J Biol Chem. 1962;237:1787–92.

54. Sousa GT, Lira FS, Rosa JC, de Oliveira EP, Oyama LM, Santos RV, et al. Dietary whey protein lessens several risk factors for metabolic diseases: a review. Lipids Health Dis. 2012;11:67. doi:10.1186/1476–511X–11–67.

55. Mizuno TM, Kleopoulos SP, Bergen HT, Roberts JL, Priest CA, Mobbs CV. Hypothalamic pro-opiomelanocortin mRNA is reduced by fasting and [corrected] in ob/ob and db/db mice, but is stimulated by leptin. Diabetes. 1998;47(2):294–7.

21

Influence of a montmorency cherry juice blend on indices of exercise-induced stress and upper respiratory tract symptoms following marathon running—a pilot investigation

Lygeri Dimitriou[1*], Jessica A Hill[2], Ahmed Jehnali[3], Joe Dunbar[3], James Brouner[4], Malachy P. McHugh[5] and Glyn Howatson[6,7]

Abstract

Background: Prolonged exercise, such as marathon running, has been associated with an increase in respiratory mucosal inflammation. The aim of this pilot study was to examine the effects of Montmorency cherry juice on markers of stress, immunity and inflammation following a Marathon.

Methods: Twenty recreational Marathon runners consumed either cherry juice (CJ) or placebo (PL) before and after a Marathon race. Markers of mucosal immunity secretory immunoglobulin A (sIgA), immunoglobulin G (IgG), salivary cortisol, inflammation (CRP) and self-reported incidence and severity of upper respiratory tract symptoms (URTS) were measured before and following the race.

Results: All variables except secretory IgA and IgG concentrations in saliva showed a significant time effect ($P < 0.01$). Serum CRP showed a significant interaction and treatment effect ($P < 0.01$). The CRP increase at 24 and 48 h post-Marathon was lower ($P < 0.01$) in the CJ group compared to PL group. Mucosal immunity and salivary cortisol showed no interaction effect or treatment effect. The incidence and severity of URTS was significantly greater than baseline at 24 h and 48 h following the race in the PL group and was also greater than the CJ group ($P < 0.05$). No URTS were reported in the CJ group whereas 50 % of runners in the PL group reported URTS at 24 h and 48 h post-Marathon.

Conclusions: This is the first study that provides encouraging evidence of the potential role of Montmorency cherries in reducing the development of URTS post-Marathon possibly caused by exercise-induced hyperventilation trauma, and/or other infectious and non-infectious factors.

Keywords: Recovery, URTS, Exercise-induced inflammation, Muscle damage

Background

Prolonged and exhaustive exercise is often associated with symptoms and signs of respiratory mucosal inflammation [1, 2]. The upper respiratory tract symptoms (URTS) usually seen following prolonged and exhaustive exercise [3, 4] have conventionally been attributed to a transient depression of the innate and adaptive immunity that eventually progresses into infection [5]. However, recent studies that

examined the aetiology of URTS following Marathon running reported that half or more than two-thirds of symptomatic cases were attributable to inflammation [6] and/or allergy [7]. This non-infectious hypothesis can be further supported due to the fact, episodes of URTS in athletes are not characterised by usual seasonal patterns and show an unusual short-term duration [8]. Exercise-induced airway inflammation, common in endurance athletes [1, 9-11] can be mediated by a number of factors including the synergistic effect of hyperventilation trauma [2, 12], oxidative stress [13] and inhaled allergens and pollutants [7, 10, 14].

Exercise has shown to up-regulate the chemotactic cytokine expression in the airways [15] causing inflammation,

* Correspondence: l.dimitriou@mdx.ac.uk
[1]London Sport Institute, Middlesex University, Allianz Park, Greenland Way, NW4 1RLE, London, UK
Full list of author information is available at the end of the article

allergic reactions in bronchi, increasing the likelihood of bronchoconstriction and possibly imitating symptoms that resemble respiratory infections [8]. For example, interleukin-8 (IL-8) has been implicated in pulmonary inflammation and hyper-responsiveness under acute oxidative stress [16, 17]. Previous studies have shown a unanimous increase in IL-8 following prolonged and exhaustive exercise [18, 19]. IL-8 is known to be a potent mediator of chemotaxis, and activates neutrophils resulting in the generation of reactive oxygen species (ROS) [20], which might lead to pulmonary inflammation and trauma [13]. Neutrophils increase markedly post-Marathon [19, 21], and pulmonary inflammation is characterised by the migration and activation of neutrophils into the airways [22]. Increased neutrophils in induced sputum post-Marathon have been reported in healthy athletes [1].

Tart Montmorency cherries are purported to be high in numerous phytochemicals, such as anthocyanins, and other polyphenolic compounds such as quercetin that possess anti-inflammatory and anti-oxidative properties [23, 24]. Growing interest in these functional foods has gained momentum in recent years and there is a mounting body of evidence to suggest Montmorency cherries can facilitate exercise recovery [24-28]; this is likely attributable to the increased bioavailability of these anti-inflammatory and anti-oxidative phytochemicals following ingestion [29, 30]. In a recent addition to the literature, Bell *et al.* [24] showed that in trained cyclists, consumption of a Montmorency cherry concentrate (in comparison to a calorific matched placebo) resulted in a reduction in lipid hyperoxides and a concomitant reduction in inflammation (IL-6 and C-reactive protein) following repeated days strenuous cycling. Additionally, polyphenols such as quercetin (also found in Montmorency cherries), modulate the expression of transcription nuclear factor-kappa B (NF-kappaB), [31, 32], which may in turn decreased the exercised-induced IL-6 production by an attenuation of cytokine transcription for IL-6. Previous studies have also shown these polyphenols to reduce other inflammatory biomarkers such as tumor necrosis factor alpha [32, 33], and macrophage inflammatory protein [33]. Consequently, it is conceivable that the anti-inflammatory and anti-oxidative potential of Montmorency cherries could attenuate the exercise-induced 'stress' response, immunity and URTS. Therefore, the aim of the current pilot study was to explore the possibility that Montmorency CJ supplementation before and following Marathon running could modulate markers of stress, immunity and self-reported upper respiratory tract symptoms.

Methods

Participants

Twenty Marathon runners (characteristics presented in Table 1) volunteered to participate. The subjects were the same cohort as those from previously published work [30] that examined the impact of Montmorency cherry juice blend on recovery following Marathon running. Eighteen completed the 2008 London Marathon (temp: 7 °C, humidity: 56 %, wind speed: 4 km/h) and remaining two completed the same distance in West London two weeks later in similar conditions (temperature: 7 °C, humidity: 50 %, wind speed: 12 km/h). Following completion of written informed consent, all participants were asked to refrain from taking nutritional supplements, pharmacological interventions and strenuous exercise (other than completing training runs prior to the Marathon) for the duration of the study. All procedures were granted ethical approval from the Institutional Research Ethics Committee, in accordance with the Helsinki Declaration.

Experimental overview

Participants were randomly assigned to either a placebo (PL) or cherry juice blend (CJ) group based upon predicted Marathon finish time. Possible sex differences in response to Marathon running were controlled by balancing the number of male and female participants in each group (3 CJ, 4 PL). Markers of stress, inflammation, mucosal immunity and upper respiratory tract symptoms were measured on four occasions; the day before the Marathon, immediately after, and at 24 h and 48 h after the Marathon. Following an initial visit to the laboratory, six days prior to the Marathon, participants were allocated to treatment groups and were instructed to take the supplement for five days prior to, the day of the Marathon and for the 48 h following the Marathon (total eight days).

Treatment groups

The CJ group consumed 2 servings x 236 ml (taken morning and afternoon) of a fresh pressed blend (Cherrypharm Inc., Geneva, New York, USA) of tart Montmorency CJ combined with proprietary apple juice (which the manufacturers add to increase palatability). According to previous work [26, 28] each serving equated to 50-60 whole cherries and contained ~600 mg of phenolic compounds of which at least 40 mg were anthocyanins. The remaining compounds consisted of flavonoids such as quercetin, kaempferol and isoramnetin; flavanols such as catechin and epicatechin procyanidins and phenolic acids such as neochlorogenic acid, chlorogenic acid and ellagic acid. The estimated oxygen radical absorbance capacity (ORAC) value per serving was estimated as 55 mMol/L Trolox equivalents [26]. The PL group consumed 2 x 236 ml per day of a pre-made, sugar-free fruit flavored drink (Summer Fruits Squash, Tesco, UK) of similar appearance, but lacking the phytonutrient content and contained only a trace of anthocyanin.

Table 1 Study's participant's characteristics. No statistical differences found between groups for any variable; Values are mean ± SD

Group	Gender (M/F)	Age (years)	Stature (m)	Mass (kg)	Predicted time (h:min:ss)	Actual time (h:min:ss)	Highest weekly mileage	Longest training run (miles)	Past Marathons
CJ	7/3	37 ± 13	1.77 ± 0.06	72.9 ± 9.8	3:41:00 ± 0:26:01	3:48:04 ± 0:48:58	33.0 ± 11.6	20.9 ± 2.6	7 ± 9
PL	6/4	38 ± 5	1.75 ± 0.09	73.8 ± 9.5	3:56:40 ± 0:40:37	4:15:48 ± 1:01:22	31.7 ± 8.2	19.3 ± 3.1	2 ± 7

Incidence and severity of upper respiratory tract symptoms (URTS)

Runners were asked to report (adapted from Reid et al., [34]) any incidence of cough; colored discharge; sore throat; watery eyes; nasal symptoms (congestion and/or discharge); sneezing and rate their severity on a 5-point Likert scale anchored by 1 (very mild) to 5 (very strong) as described by Nieman et al. [35]. Participants with two or more of the above symptoms present for a minimum of two consecutive days in the study period were identified as symptomatic [36].

Saliva sampling procedures

Ten minutes before saliva collection, participants rinsed their mouths thoroughly for 30 s with water [37], and swallowed any saliva present in the mouth. Participants then actively swabbed their mouths, around their gums, tongue and inside their cheek, with an oral fluid collector (OFC; IPRO Interactive, Oxfordshire, UK) consisting of a synthetic polymer based material on a polypropylene tube, to collect saliva. The OFC has a volume adequacy indicator, giving a clear colour change when 1.0 mL (±20 %) is collected. Analyte recovery from the OFC is in excess of 85 % within 1 min of gentle shaking [38]. Saliva sample collection time was recorded (s), to facilitate the calculation of saliva flow rate (Sal_{fr}), as described elsewhere [37], and was dependent on the time required by each individual to collect ~0.5 ml of saliva. The OFC was then inserted immediately in to an extraction buffer containing sodium phosphate, salts, detergents and preservatives designed to prevent growth of microorganisms and facilitate extraction of proteins and small mass molecular analytes from the swab. Samples were frozen immediately and stored at—20C until analysis [37].

Salivary analyses

Secretory immunoglobulin A (sIgA), salivary immunoglobulin G (IgG) and salivary cortisol were determined in duplicate from the same sample, using enzyme immunoassay (EIA) test kits (IPRO Interactive Ltd., Oxfordshire, England), in an automated analyser (Tecan Nanoquant). The assay ranges were: sIgA 18.75–600 μg/mL; IgG 2.0–120 μg/mL; and cortisol 0.25–32.0 ng/mL. The intra-assay CV was: sIgA < 5.77 %; IgG < 3.37 %; cortisol < 7.85 %. The inter-assay CV was: sIgA < 12.52 %; IgG <10.77 %; and cortisol < 13.10 %. sIgA data is expressed as concentration (μg/mL) and as output/secretory rate (μg/min).

Serum analyses

Serum C-reactive protein was determined using an automated analyser (c800, Abbott Architect). These data are published elsewhere [28], but are presented here as a global index of the exercise-induced inflammatory response. Normal ranges for this assay are <0.8 mg.L^{-1}with minimum detection concentration (mdc) 0.3 mg.L^{-1}. The CV of the intra-sample variability was 3.7 %. Samples with values below the mdc for any of the above markers were reported as equal to 0.5 mdc [39].

Statistical analyses

Statistical analyses were performed using SPSS version 19.0. Values are reported as means and ± SD. An alpha level of 0.05 was chosen a priori. Independent T-tests were used to assess for demographic characteristics, predicted and actual Marathon time, Marathon history and training mileage leading up to the race between treatment groups. Differences between treatments were analysed using a 2 x 4 mixed model analyses of variance ANOVA with Treatment: CJ versus PL and Time as the within subject factor (pre, post, 24 h and 48 h). Mauchly's sphericity test was used to assess if the variances of the differences between conditions were homogeneous. Simple main effects analyses were calculated for significant interaction effects between treatment and time. Violations of the sphericity assumption were corrected using the Greenhouse-Geisser estimate.

Results

There were no differences between groups for age, stature, mass, previous Marathon history, weekly mileage, longest single training run, predicted and actual Marathon time (Table 1). Post-race body mass was lower than body mass the day before the race (P < 0.001) with similar declines in the CJ group and PL group (1.2 ± 1.3 kg vs. 1.7 ± 1.5 kg, respectively).

Secretory IgA concentration showed no time or interaction effects (Fig. 1A). Conversely, there was a time effect for output ($F_{(3,54)}$ = 7.560, P < 0.001, η_p^2 = 0.296) and decreased immediately post-race in both groups when compared to pre-race levels, and returned to baseline by 24 h post-race. No treatment or interaction effects

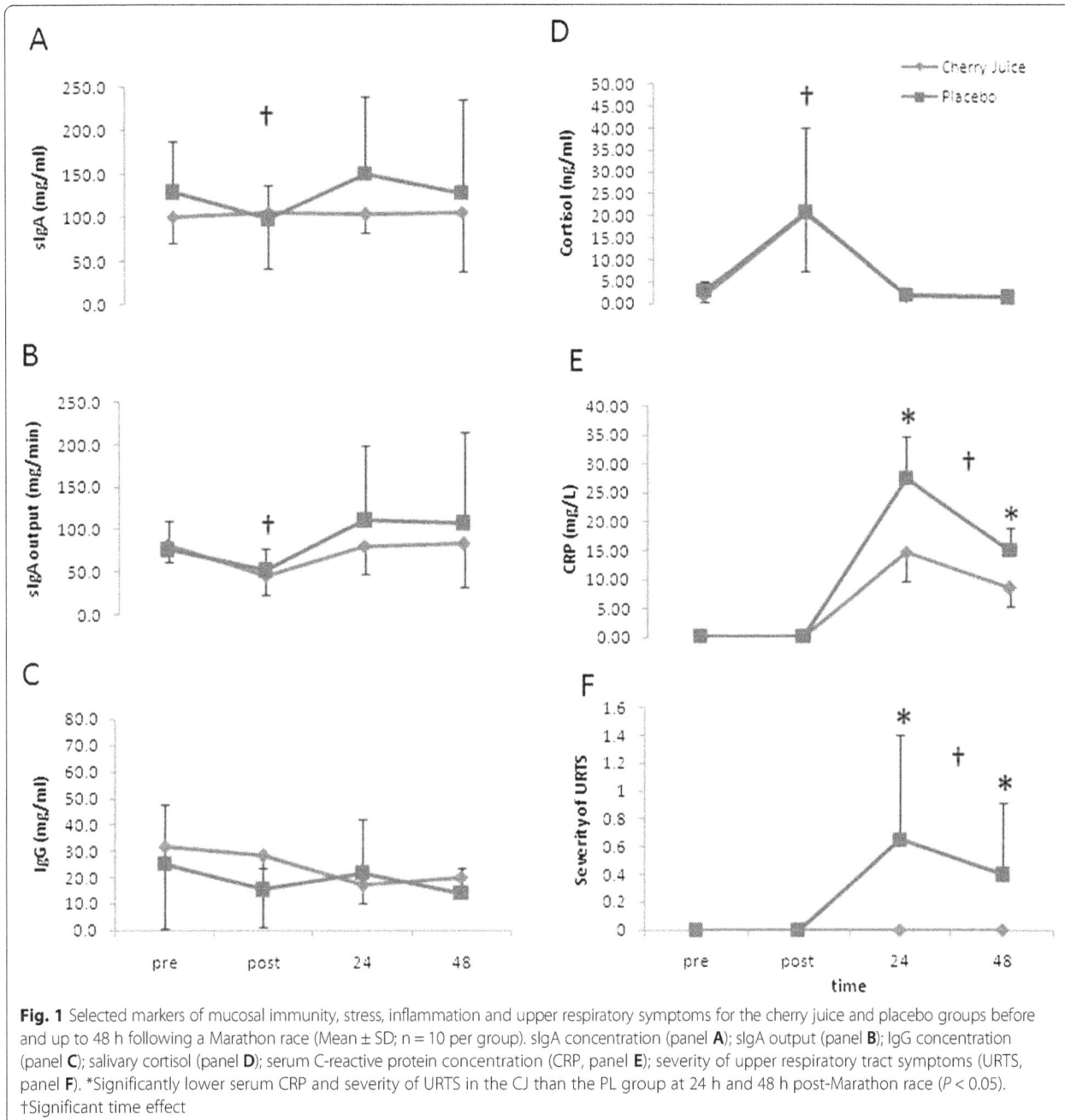

Fig. 1 Selected markers of mucosal immunity, stress, inflammation and upper respiratory symptoms for the cherry juice and placebo groups before and up to 48 h following a Marathon race (Mean ± SD; n = 10 per group). sIgA concentration (panel **A**); sIgA output (panel **B**); IgG concentration (panel **C**); salivary cortisol (panel **D**); serum C-reactive protein concentration (CRP, panel **E**); severity of upper respiratory tract symptoms (URTS, panel **F**). *Significantly lower serum CRP and severity of URTS in the CJ than the PL group at 24 h and 48 h post-Marathon race (P < 0.05). †Significant time effect

($P > 0.05$) for sIgA were shown (Fig. 1B). Salivary IgG concentration showed no time, treatment or interaction effects (Fig. 1C).

Salivary Cortisol showed a significant time effect and was elevated immediately post-race in both groups, ($F_{(1,18)} = 26.291$, P < 0.001, $\eta_p^2 = 0.594$) when compared to pre-race levels, and returned to baseline by 24 h post-race. No significant treatment or treatment by time interaction effects were observed (see Fig. 1D).

Serum CRP showed a significant time effect ($F_{(3,54)} = 247.138$, P < 0.001, $\eta_p^2 = 0.932$), a treatment by time interaction effect ($F_{(3,54)} = 10.667$, P < 0.01, $\eta_p^2 = 0.372$), and a

treatment effect $F_{(1,18)} = 12.920$, P < 0.01, $\eta_p^2 = 0.418$). The increase in CRP at 24 and 48 h post-Marathon was significantly lower ($F_{(1,18)} = 12.14$, P < 0.01 and $F_{(1,18)} = 9.88$, P < 0.01, respectively) in the CJ group compared to PL group (see Fig. 1E).

The incidence and severity of URTS showed a time effect ($F_{(3,54)} = 6.359$, P < 0.01, $\eta_p^2 = 0.261$). URTS were increased at 24 h and 48 h following the race when compared to pre-race levels in the PL group only. A treatment ($F(1,18) = 7.826$, P < 0.05, $\eta_p^2 = 0.303$) and interaction effect ($F_{(3,54)} = 6.359$, P < 0.01, $\eta_p^2 = 0.261$) was observed, whereby URTS were significantly higher in the PL group at 24 h ($F_{(1,18)}$ = 7.57, $P < 0.05$) and 48 h post-race ($F_{(1,18)}$ = 5.44, $P < 0.05$) compared to CJ group (Fig. 1F). No URTS were reported in the CJ group at 24 h and 48 h post-Marathon as opposed to the PL group whom 50 % (5/10) of the runners developed URTS.

Discussion

In this pilot study, we investigated the effects of a Montmorency tart cherry juice on markers of stress, immunity, and self-reported incidence and severity of upper respiratory tract symptoms following a Marathon. It was hypothesised that CJ supplementation would attenuate the cortisol and inflammatory response, reduce transient suppression of mucosal immunity and lower the development of URTS by protecting the respiratory tract from symptoms associated with infectious and non-infectious inflammatory agents following a Marathon. Despite no apparent change in cortisol or mucosal immunity between groups, runners that consumed Montmorency CJ had a lower CRP response at 24 and 48 h post–Marathon and had zero incidence of reported URTS up to 48 h after the Marathon, suggesting that CJ attenuated the exercise-induced inflammatory response and the subsequent development of URTS compared to the PL group following the race.

The development of URTS observed at 24 and 48 h post-Marathon in the PL group only, might be of a non-infectious nature reflecting a synergistic effect of pulmonary inflammation mediated by exercise-induced hyperventilation trauma [2, 12], oxidative stress [13], allergies [7] and air pollution [14]. A limitation with the current study is that we did not examine the prevalence of URTS beyond 48 h and this could be explored in future work given that URTS might become evident well beyond 48 h. Enhanced airway exposure to inhaled pollutants and/or allergens has been associated with airway hyper-responsiveness in many athletes of different sports [10]. Hyperventilation can cause bronchial dehydration injuries, excessive mucus production and/or airway oedema [40]; symptoms that could resemble an URTI. Airway inflammation is commonly reported in endurance athletes [1, 9-11], and heavy exercise is associated with pulmonary mucosal inflammation [2] induced by repetitive hyperventilation, bronchial dehydration [40], and increased airway osmolarity. Speculatively, these in turn might stimulate the release of chemotactic factors from bronchial epithelial cells [15], further supporting an exercise-induced URTS development attributable to non-infective inflammatory factors [41] in this study. The URTS usually seen following prolonged and exhaustive exercise [3] have conventionally been attributed to a transient immune depression that eventually progresses into infection [5]. However, recent studies that examined the aetiology of URTS following Marathon

running reported that equal or more than two-thirds of symptomatic cases were attributable to inflammation [6] and/or allergy [7]. In the present study, CRP was significantly elevated in both groups but its response at 24 and 48 h following the Marathon was blunted in the CJ group compared to the PL. This is consistent with previous studies that used cherry supplementation [24, 28, 42, 43]. Furthermore, the CJ group did not report any URTS at 24 and 48 h post-Marathon as opposed to the PL group that reported a 50 % development of URTS. Further studies are needed to explore this in larger samples using techniques such as endobronchial biopsies and induced bronchoalveolar lavage fluid (BALF) to elucidate this possibility.

Findings from a previously published study that used the same cohort [28] showed a blunted IL-6 response immediately post-Marathon, and lower uric acid immediately and 24 h post-Marathon in the CJ group compared to the PL group. The bioactive food components (BAFC) contained in cherries have shown, in vitro, to inhibit cyclooxygenase (COX)-1 and COX-2 enzyme activity, by an average of 28 % and 47 % respectively, which is responsible for the inflammatory response [44]. A subsequent study further supported this by showing a COX-2 inhibitory effect of anthocyanins [45]. These aforementioned studies and the results from the cohort of this study suggest that the anti-inflammatory activities in tart cherries could attenuate the exercise-induced inflammatory response, its exacerbation and therefore the development of URTS. This observation adds to the growing body of evidence that shows the potential of tart Montmorency cherries in aiding exercise recovery and improving health indices [23, 24, 30, 32, 46, 47].

The prevalence of allergy and atopy (sensitization to common inhalant allergens) in long-distance runners has been reported to be 40 % and 49 %, respectively [7, 10]. In allergic diseases associated with the respiratory tract (i.e., asthma and rhinitis) the migration of eosinophils to the mucosal surfaces is enhanced [48]. The respiratory tract is rich in cytokines and chemokines (e.g., IL-8), which in turn could activate the eosinophils and possibly participate in the modulation of the local immune response via degranulation [49]. Eosinophil activation has been reported to be a crucial element in upper and lower respiratory inflammation [50]. Exercise-induced recruitment and degranulation of eosinophils and basophils to the respiratory tract due to airway inflammation may possibly explain the exercise-induced URTS development seen in the PL group in this study and the increased incidence of URTI reported previously [3]. Furthermore, a more recent in vitro study showed that the polyphenol quercetin suppresses eosinophil activation [51], suggesting that various BAFC of cherries might modulate eosinophil-mediated diseases, such as allergic rhinitis and asthma, which are very common pathologies in athletes. This idea is further supported by a study that showed that 58 % of runners with reported URTS following the 2010 London Marathon had allergy, as defined by a positive Allergy Questionnaire for Athletes (AQUA) and specific immunoglobulin E (IgE) response to various inhalant allergens [7]. The prevalence of the reported URTS following the 2008 London Marathon in this study were considerably lower (25 %) than previously reported (47 %) by Robson-Ansley *et al.* [7]. This difference could be partly explained by the daily average tree pollen counts on the day of the 2008 London Marathon that were approximately 9-fold less (Robson-Ansley *et al.* [7]) than those reported in the 2010 Marathon. Although this suggests a dose-dependent response between pollen counts and URTS, the antioxidant and anti-inflammatory properties of CJ offers a plausible explanation for the complete absence of reported URTS in the CJ group.

Pulmonary inflammation can be exacerbated by concurrent exposure to tropospheric ozone and other pollutants present in Metropolitan cities [14]. Exposure to air pollutants is greater in endurance athletes as they train mostly outdoors, and compete in Marathons that commonly take place in big cities. Furthermore, the shifting from nasal to oronasal or oral breathing leads to a greater inhalation of airborne allergens, pollutants, antigens and untreated air [7]. Pollutants increase the susceptibility to bacterial respiratory infections [14]. However, CJ ingestion could reduce exercise-induced URTI susceptibility since there are several cell culture studies that show the polyphenol quercetin to exert antipathogenic activities against a wide variety of viruses and bacteria, and to reduce infectivity of target cells and virus replication [52]. The results of the present study showed an absence of reported URTS development in the CJ group and might signify a down-regulation of the inflammatory pathways involved in pollutant inhalation. Furthermore, we cannot rule out that the absence of reported URTS in the CJ group might indicate an enhanced anti-pathogenic activity compared to PL. Future studies could investigate the interaction effect between air pollution and prolonged exhaustive exercise on the incidence of respiratory symptoms and bronchoconstriction, and identify possible prophylactic measures against them.

Conclusions

The results of this pilot study showed that a Montmorency cherry juice blend appears to protect the URT from inflammatory symptoms caused by infectious and non-infectious agents, by possibly reducing the exercise-induced pulmonary inflammation. Modulation of the exercise-induced pulmonary inflammation by natural plant products might represent an attractive strategy to protect or alleviate the URT from inflammatory symptoms. This pilot investigation is the first to demonstrate preliminary evidence of the potential role of Montmorency cherry juice in reducing the development of URTS following long duration endurance exercise. Considering the limited sample size and healthy state of this study's cohort, further studies with a larger sample size and participants with asthma, atopy, allergic rhinitis, exercise induced bronchoconstriction, airway hyper-responsiveness, and other pulmonary pathologies could be performed to explore the potential of cherries and other functional foods that might exert a similar effect.

Abbreviations

AQUA: Allergy questionnaire for athletes; BAFC: Bioactive food components; CJ: Cherry juice; COX: Cyclooxygenase; EIA: Enzyme immunoassay; IgE: Immunoglobulin E; IgG: Immunoglobulin G; IL-6: Interleukin-6; IL-8: Interleukin-8; OFC: Oral fluid collector; PL: Placebo; ROS: Reactive oxygen species; Sal$_{fr}$: Saliva flow rate; sIgA: Secretory immunoglobulin A; URTS: Upper respiratory tract symptoms.

Competing interests

The authors declare that they have no competing interests.

Authors' contributions

LD, JH, MPM and GH contributed to the study design. Data collection was conducted by LD, JH, JD, JB and GH. Data analysis was conducted by LD, JH, JD, JA, MPM, and GH. LD and GH drafted the initial manuscript. All authors contributed to data interpretation, editing and approval of the final article.

Acknowledgments

The authors would like to thank the participants for their commitment in completing this investigation. We would also like to extend our gratitude to Julia Atkin, John Eagle, Sarah Brouner, Sunny Pottay, Louise Ross and Natalie Ross for their valuable contributions on day of the Marathon. This work was supported by Northumbria University, Middlesex University and St Mary's University College.

Author details

[1]London Sport Institute, Middlesex University, Allianz Park, Greenland Way, NW4 1RLE, London, UK. [2]School of Sport, Health and Applied Science, St Mary's University College, Twickenham, UK. [3]Ipro Interactive Ltd, Oxfordshire, UK. [4]School of Life Sciences, Kingston University, London, UK. [5]Nicholas Institute of Sports Medicine and Athletic Trauma, Lenox Hill Hospital, New York, NY, UK. [6]Faculty of Health and Life Sciences, Northumbria University, Newcastle-upon-Tyne, UK. [7]Water Research Group, School of Biological Sciences, North West University, Potchefstroom, South Africa.

References

1. Bonsignore MR, Morici G, Riccobono L, Insalaco G, Bonanno A, Profita M, et al. Airway inflammation in nonasthmatic amateur runners. American J Physiol. 2001;281(3):L668–76.
2. Helenius I, Lumme A, Haahtela T. Asthma, airway inflammation and treatment in elite athletes. Sports Med. 2005;35(7):565–74.
3. Peters EM, Bateman E. Ultramarathon running and upper respiratory tract infections. S Afr Med J. 1983;64(15):582–4.
4. Nieman D, Johanssen L, Lee J, Arabatzis K. Infectious episodes in runners before and after the Los Angeles Marathon. J Sports Med Phys Fitness. 1990;30(3):316–28.
5. Nieman DC. Exercise, upper respiratory tract infection, and the immune system. Med Sci Sports Exerc. 1994;26(2):128–39.
6. Spence L, Brown WJ, Pyne DB, Nissen MD, Sloots TP, McCormack JG, et al. Incidence, etiology, and symptomatology of upper respiratory illness in elite athletes. Med Sci Sports Exerc. 2007;39(4):577.
7. Robson-Ansley P, Howatson G, Tallent J, Mitcheson K, Walshe I, Toms C, et al. Prevalence of allergy and upper respiratory tract symptoms in runners of the London marathon. Med Sci Sports Exerc. 2012;44(6):999–1004.

8. Kuchar E, Miskiewicz K, Nitsch-Osuch A, Kurpas D, Han S, Szenborn L. Immunopathology of exercise-induced bronchoconstriction in athletes—A new modified inflammatory hypothesis. Respir Physiol Neurobiol. 2013;187(1):82–7.

9. Verges S, Devouassoux G, Flore P, Rossini E, Fior-Gozlan M, Levy P, et al. Bronchial hyperresponsiveness, airway inflammation, and airflow limitation in endurance athletes. CHEST J. 2005;127(6):1935–41.

10. Helenius I, Rytilä P, Metso T, Haahtela T, Venge P, Tikkanen H. Respiratory symptoms, bronchial responsiveness, and cellular characteristics of induced sputum in elite swimmers. Allergy. 1998;53(4):346–52.

11. Karjalainen E-M, Laitinen A, Sue-Chu M, Altraja A, Bjermer L, Laitinen LA. Evidence of airway inflammation and remodeling in ski athletes with and without bronchial hyperresponsiveness to methacholine. Am J Respir Crit Care Med. 2000;161(6):2086–91.

12. Bermon S. Airway inflammation and upper respiratory tract infection in athletes: is there a link. Exerc Immunol Rev. 2007;13:6–14.

13. Guo R-F, Ward PA. Mediators and regulation of neutrophil accumulation in inflammatory responses in lung: insights from the IgG immune complex model < sup > 1, 2</sup> Free Radical Biol Med. 2002;33(3):303–10.

14. Spannhake EW, Reddy SP, Jacoby DB, Yu X-Y, Saatian B, Tian J. Synergism between rhinovirus infection and oxidant pollutant exposure enhances airway epithelial cell cytokine production. Environ Health Perspect. 2002;110(7):665.

15. Bonsignore M, Morici G, Vignola A, Riccobono L, Bonanno A, Profita M, et al. Increased airway inflammatory cells in endurance athletes: what do they mean? Clin Experimental Allergy. 2003;33(1):14–21.

16. Ayyagari VN, Januszkiewicz A, Nath J. Pro-inflammatory responses of human bronchial epithelial cells to acute nitrogen dioxide exposure. Toxicology. 2004;197(2):148–63. doi:http://dx.doi.org/10.1016/j.tox.2003.12.017.

17. Epstein FH, Luster AD. Chemokines—chemotactic cytokines that mediate inflammation. New England J Med. 1998;338(7):436–45.

18. Ostrowski K, Rohde T, Asp S, Schjerling P, Klarlund Pedersen B. Chemokines are elevated in plasma after strenuous exercise in humans. Eur J Appl Physiol. 2001;84(3):244–5. 10.1007/s004210170012.

19. Suzuki K, Nakaji S, Yamada M, Liu Q, Kurakake S, Okamura N, et al. Impact of a competitive marathon race on systemic cytokine and neutrophil responses. Med Sci Sports Exerc. 2003;35(2):348–55.

20. Gregory H, Young J, Schröder J-M, Mrowietz U, Christophers E. Structure determination of a human lymphocyte derived neutrophil activating peptide (LYNAP). Biochem Biophys Res Commun. 1988;151(2):883–90.

21. Niess AM, Sommer M, Schlotz E, Northoff H, Dickhuth H-H, Fehrenbach E. Expression of the inducible nitric oxide synthase (iNOS) in human leukocytes: responses to running exercise. Med Sci Sports Exerc. 2000;32(7):1220–5.

22. Knaapen AM, Güngör N, Schins RP, Borm PJ, Van Schooten FJ. Neutrophils and respiratory tract DNA damage and mutagenesis: a review. Mutagenesis. 2006;21(4):225–36.

23. McCune LM, Kubota C, Stendell-Hollis NR, Thomson CA. Cherries and health: a review. Crit Rev Food Sci Nutr. 2010;51(1):1–12.

24. Bell PG, Walshe IH, Davison GW, Stevenson E, Howatson G. Montmorency Cherries reduce the oxidative stress and inflammatory responses to repeated days high-intensity stochastic cycling. Nutrients. 2014;6(2):829–43.

25. Kuehl KS, Perrier ET, Elliot DL, Chesnutt JC. Research article Efficacy of tart cherry juice in reducing muscle pain during running: a randomized controlled trial. 2010.

26. Connolly D, McHugh M, Padilla-Zakour O. Efficacy of a tart cherry juice blend in preventing the symptoms of muscle damage. Br J Sports Med. 2006;40(8):679–83.

27. Sumners D, Dyer A, Fox P, Mileva K, Bowtell J. Montmorency cherry juice reduces muscle damage caused by intensive strength exercise. Med Sci Sports Exerc. 2011;43(8):1544–51.

28. Howatson G, McHugh M, Hill J, Brouner J, Jewell A, Van Someren KA, et al. Influence of tart cherry juice on indices of recovery following marathon running. Scand J Med Sci Sports. 2010;20(6):843–52.

29. Bell PG, Gaze DC, Davison GW, George TW, Scotter MJ, Howatson G. Montmorency tart cherry (< i > Prunus cerasus L.</i>) concentrate lowers uric acid, independent of plasma cyanidin-3-O-glucosiderutinoside. J Functional Foods. 2014;11:82–90.

30. Bell P, McHugh M, Stevenson E, Howatson G. The role of cherries in exercise and health. Scand J Med Sci Sports. 2014;24(3):477–90.

31. Chen J-C, Ho F-M, Pei-Dawn Lee C, Chen C-P, Jeng K-CG, Hsu H-B, et al. Inhibition of iNOS gene expression by quercetin is mediated by the inhibition of IκB kinase, nuclear factor-kappa B and STAT1, and depends on heme oxygenase-1 induction in mouse BV-2 microglia. Eur J Pharmacol. 2005;521(1–3):9–20. doi:http://dx.doi.org/10.1016/j.ejphar.2005.08.005.

32. Nair MP, Mahajan S, Reynolds JL, Aalinkeel R, Nair H, Schwartz SA, et al. The flavonoid quercetin inhibits proinflammatory cytokine (tumor necrosis factor alpha) gene expression in normal peripheral blood mononuclear cells via modulation of the NF-κβ system. Clin Vaccine Immunol. 2006;13(3):319–28.

33. Comalada M, Ballester I, Bailón E, Sierra S, Xaus J, Gálvez J, et al. Inhibition of pro-inflammatory markers in primary bone marrow-derived mouse macrophages by naturally occurring flavonoids: analysis of the structure–activity relationship. Biochem Pharmacol. 2006;72(8):1010–21.

34. Reid V, Gleeson M, Williams N, Clancy R. Clinical investigation of athletes with persistent fatigue and/or recurrent infections. Br J Sports Med. 2004;38(1):42–5.

35. Nieman DC, Nehlsen-Cannarella SL, Fagoaga OR, Henson DA, Shannon M, Hjertman JM, et al. Immune function in female elite rowers and non-athletes. Br J Sports Med. 2000;34(3):181–7.

36. Nieman DC, Henson DA, Gross SJ, Jenkins DP, Davis JM, Murphy EA, et al. Quercetin reduces illness but not immune perturbations after intensive exercise. Med Sci Sports Exerc. 2007;39(9):1561.

37. Dimitriou L, Sharp N, Doherty M. Circadian effects on the acute responses of salivary cortisol and IgA in well trained swimmers. Br J Sports Med. 2002;36(4):260–4.

38. Jehanli A, Dunbar J. Skelhorn S, editors. International Society of Exercise Immunology Symposium: Development and validation of an oral fluid collection device and its use in the immunoassay of salivary steroids and immunoglobulins in sports persons; 2011.

39. Minetto M, Rainoldi A, Gazzoni M, Terzolo M, Borrione P, Termine A, et al. Differential responses of serum and salivary interleukin-6 to acute strenuous exercise. Eur J Appl Physiol. 2005;93(5-6):679–86.

40. Anderson SD, Holzer K. Exercise-induced asthma: Is it the right diagnosis in elite athletes? J Allergy Clin Immun. 2000;106(3):419–28. doi:http://dx.doi.org/10.1067/mai.2000.108914.

41. Walsh NP, Gleeson M, Shephard RJ, Gleeson M, Woods JA, Bishop N, et al. Position statement part one: immune function and exercise. 2011.

42. Jacob RA, Spinozzi GM, Simon VA, Kelley DS, Prior RL, Hess-Pierce B, et al. Consumption of cherries lowers plasma urate in healthy women. J Nutr. 2003;133(6):1826–9.

43. Kelley DS, Rasooly R, Jacob RA, Kader AA, Mackey BE. Consumption of Bing sweet cherries lowers circulating concentrations of inflammation markers in healthy men and women. J Nutr. 2006;136(4):981–6.

44. Seeram N, Momin R, Nair M, Bourquin L. Cyclooxygenase inhibitory and antioxidant cyanidin glycosides in cherries and berries. Phytomedicine. 2001;8(5):362–9.

45. Hou D-X, Yanagita T, Uto T, Masuzaki S, Fujii M. Anthocyanidins inhibit cyclooxygenase-2 expression in LPS-evoked macrophages: Structure–activity relationship and molecular mechanisms involved. Biochem Pharmacol. 2005;70(3):417–25. doi:http://dx.doi.org/10.1016/j.bcp.2005.05.003.

46. Seeram NP, Aviram M, Zhang Y, Henning SM, Feng L, Dreher M, et al. Comparison of antioxidant potency of commonly consumed polyphenol-rich beverages in the United States. J Agric Food Chem. 2008;56(4):1415–22.

47. Howatson G, Bell PG, Tallent J, Middleton B, McHugh MP, Ellis J. Effect of tart cherry juice (Prunus cerasus) on melatonin levels and enhanced sleep quality. Eur J Nutr. 2012;51(8):909–16.

48. Djukanović R, Roche W, Wilson J, Beasley C, Twentyman O, Howarth P, et al. Mucosal inflammation in asthma. American Rev Respiratory Dis. 1990;142(2):434–57.

49. MacKenzie JR, Mattes J, Dent LA, Foster PS. Eosinophils promote allergic disease of the lung by regulating CD4+ Th2 lymphocyte function. J Immun. 2001;167(6):3146–55.

50. Choi GS, Kim JH, Shin YS, Ye YM, Kim SH, Park HS. Eosinophil activation and novel mediators in the aspirin-induced nasal response in AERD. Clin Experimental Allergy. 2013;43(7):730–40.

51. Sakai-Kashiwabara M, Asano K. Inhibitory Action of Quercetin on Eosinophil Activation In Vitro. Evidence-Based Complementary Alternative Med. 2013;2013.

52. Cushnie T, Lamb AJ. Antimicrobial activity of flavonoids. Int J Antimicrob Agents. 2005;26(5):343–56.

Permissions

List of Contributors

Selma C Liberato
Menzies School of Health Research, Charles Darwin University, Darwin, NT, Australia

Josefina Bressan
Departamento de Nutrição e Saúde, Universidade Federal de Viçosa, Viçosa, MG, Brazil

Andrew P Hills
Mater Mother's Hospital/Mater Research Institute, Griffith Health Institute/Griffith University, Brisbane, QLD, Australia

Daniela Chlíbková
Centre of Sports Activities, Brno University of Technology, Brno, Czech Republic

Beat Knechtle
Institute of General Practise and for Health Services Research, University of Zurich, Zurich, Switzerland

Thomas Rosemann
Institute of General Practise and for Health Services Research, University of Zurich, Zurich, Switzerland

Alena Žákovská
Institute of Experimental Biology, Faculty of Science, Masaryk University, Brno, Czech Republic

Ivana Tomášková
Faculty of Forestry and Wood Sciences, Czech University of Life Sciences, Prague, Czech Republic

Marcus Shortall
Institute of Technology Tallaght, Dublin, Ireland

Iva Tomášková
SurGal clinic s.r.o., Center for Sports Medicine, Brno, Czech Republic

Michael J Ormsbee
Department of Nutrition, Food and Exercise Sciences, Florida State University, Tallahassee, FL 32306, USA
University of KwaZulu-Natal, Durban, South Africa
Institute of Sports Science & Medicine, Florida State University, Tallahassee, FL, USA

Shweta R Rawal
Department of Nutrition, Food and Exercise Sciences, Florida State University, Tallahassee, FL 32306, USA

Daniel A Baur
Department of Nutrition, Food and Exercise Sciences, Florida State University, Tallahassee, FL 32306, USA

Amber W Kinsey
Department of Nutrition, Food and Exercise Sciences, Florida State University, Tallahassee, FL 32306, USA

Marcus L Elam
Department of Nutrition, Food and Exercise Sciences, Florida State University, Tallahassee, FL 32306, USA

Maria T Spicer
Department of Nutrition, Food and Exercise Sciences, Florida State University, Tallahassee, FL 32306, USA

Nicholas T Fischer
Department of Nutrition, Food and Exercise Sciences, Florida State University, Tallahassee, FL 32306, USA

Takudzwa A Madzima
Department of Nutrition, Food and Exercise Sciences, Florida State University, Tallahassee, FL 32306, USA

D David Thomas
Department of Nutrition, Food and Exercise Sciences, Florida State University, Tallahassee, FL 32306, USA

Juan Mielgo-Ayuso
Department of Nutrition and Dietetics, Haro Volleyball Club, Nutrition Centre of La Rioja, C/ Donantes de sangre, 14.26200 Haro, La Rioja, Spain

Pilar S Collado
Department of Biomedical Sciences, University of Leon, Leon, Spain
Institute of Biomedicine (IBIOMED), University of Leon, Leon, Spain

Aritz Urdampilleta
Public Sports Education Center, Kirolene, Basque Government, Scientific-Technical Planning for Sports, Nutriaktive, Vitoria-Gasteiz, Spain

José Miguel Martínez-Sanz
Department of Nursing, Faculty of Health Sciences, University of Alicante, Alicante, Spain

Jesús Seco
Institute of Biomedicine (IBIOMED), University of Leon, Leon, Spain
Visiting Researcher at the University of the Basque Country, Leioa, Bizkaia, Spain

Julie Y Kresta
Department of Sports Medicine and Nutrition, School of Health and Rehabilitation Sciences, University of Pittsburgh, Pittsburgh, PA 15260, USA

Jonathan M Oliver
Kinesiology Department, Texas Christian University, Fort Worth, TX 76129, USA

Andrew R Jagim
Department of Exercise & Sport Science, University of Wisconsin – La Crosse, La Crosse, WI 54601, USA

James Fluckey
Department of Health and Kinesiology, Muscle Biology Laboratory, Texas A&M University, College Station, TX 77843-4243, USA

Steven Riechman
Department of Health and Kinesiology, Human Countermeasures Laboratory, Texas A&M University, College Station, TX 77843-4243, USA

Katherine Kelly
Department of Medical Physiology, Texas A&M Health Science Center, College Station, TX 77843-1114, USA

Cynthia Meininger
Department of Medical Physiology, Texas A&M Health Science Center, College Station, TX 77843-1114, USA

Susanne U Mertens-Talcott
Department of Nutrition and Food Science, Institute for Obesity Research and Program Evaluation, Texas A&M University, College Station, TX 77843-4243, USA

Christopher Rasmussen
Department of Health and Kinesiology, Exercise and Sport Nutrition Lab, Texas A&M University, College Station, TX 77843-4243, USA

Richard B Kreider
Department of Health and Kinesiology, Exercise and Sport Nutrition Lab, Texas A&M University, College Station, TX 77843-4243, USA

Henrique Bortolotti
Metabolism, Nutrition, and Exercise Research Group, Londrina State University, Londrina, Paraná, Brazil
Neuromuscular System and Exercise Research Group, Londrina State University, Londrina, Paraná, Brazil
School of Physical Education and Sport, University of São Paulo, São Paulo, Brazil

Leandro Ricardo Altimari
Metabolism, Nutrition, and Exercise Research Group, Londrina State University, Londrina, Paraná, Brazil
Neuromuscular System and Exercise Research Group, Londrina State University, Londrina, Paraná, Brazil
Department of Physical Education, Centre for Physical Education and Sport, Londrina State University, Londrina, Paraná, Brazil

Marcelo Vitor-Costa
Metabolism, Nutrition, and Exercise Research Group, Londrina State University, Londrina, Paraná, Brazil
Neuromuscular System and Exercise Research Group, Londrina State University, Londrina, Paraná, Brazil

Edilson Serpeloni Cyrino
Metabolism, Nutrition, and Exercise Research Group, Londrina State University, Londrina, Paraná, Brazil
Neuromuscular System and Exercise Research Group, Londrina State University, Londrina, Paraná, Brazil
Department of Physical Education, Centre for Physical Education and Sport, Londrina State University, Londrina, Paraná, Brazil

Jonathan M Kurka
Exercise and Wellness Program, School of Nutrition and Health Promotion, Arizona State University, 500 N Third Street, Mail Code 3020, Phoenix, AZ 85004, USA

Matthew P Buman
Exercise and Wellness Program, School of Nutrition and Health Promotion, Arizona State University, 500 N Third Street, Mail Code 3020, Phoenix, AZ 85004, USA

Barbara E Ainsworth
Exercise and Wellness Program, School of Nutrition and Health Promotion, Arizona State University, 500 N Third Street, Mail Code 3020, Phoenix, AZ 85004, USA

José Vítor Vieira Salgado
Exercise Physiology Laboratory - FISEX, FEF-UNICAMP Cidade Universitária, Physical Education Faculty, State University of Campinas, Cep:13083-851, Campinas SP 6134, Brazil
Sport's Sciences Department, University of Campinas, Physical Education Faculty, Erico Veríssimo Av., 701., Campinas, Brazil

Pablo Christiano Barboza Lollo
Food's Engineering Faculty, Department of Food and Nutrition, State University of Campinas - UNICAMP, Campinas, SP, Brazil

Jaime Amaya-Farfan
Food's Engineering Faculty, Department of Food and Nutrition, State University of Campinas - UNICAMP, Campinas, SP, Brazil

Mara PatríciaTraina Chacon-Mikahil
Exercise Physiology Laboratory - FISEX, FEF-UNICAMP Cidade Universitária, Physical Education Faculty, State University of Campinas, Cep:13083-851, Campinas SP 6134, Brazil

Adam J Wells, Jay R Hoffman
Institute of Exercise Physiology and Wellness, University of Central Florida, 4000 Central Florida Blvd., Orlando, FL 32816, USA

Adam M Gonzalez
Institute of Exercise Physiology and Wellness, University of Central Florida, 4000 Central Florida Blvd., Orlando, FL 32816, USA

Kyle S Beyer
Institute of Exercise Physiology and Wellness, University of Central Florida, 4000 Central Florida Blvd., Orlando, FL 32816, USA

Adam R Jajtner
Institute of Exercise Physiology and Wellness, University of Central Florida, 4000 Central Florida Blvd., Orlando, FL 32816, USA

Jeremy R Townsend
Institute of Exercise Physiology and Wellness, University of Central Florida, 4000 Central Florida Blvd., Orlando, FL 32816, USA

Leonardo P Oliveira
Institute of Exercise Physiology and Wellness, University of Central Florida, 4000 Central Florida Blvd., Orlando, FL 32816, USA

David H Fukuda
Institute of Exercise Physiology and Wellness, University of Central Florida, 4000 Central Florida Blvd., Orlando, FL 32816, USA

Maren S Fragala
Institute of Exercise Physiology and Wellness, University of Central Florida, 4000 Central Florida Blvd., Orlando, FL 32816, USA

Jeffrey R Stout
Institute of Exercise Physiology and Wellness, University of Central Florida, 4000 Central Florida Blvd., Orlando, FL 32816, USA

Nicole Walker
Department of Human Nutrition, University of Otago, PO Box 56, Dunedin 9054, New Zealand

Thomas D Love
College of Engineering, Swansea University, Swansea, UK

Dane Francis Baker
Chiefs Super Rugby Franchise, Hamilton, New Zealand

Phillip Brian Healey
Chiefs Super Rugby Franchise, Hamilton, New Zealand

Jillian Haszard
Department of Human Nutrition, University of Otago, PO Box 56, Dunedin 9054, New Zealand

Antony S Edwards
High Performance Sport New Zealand, Auckland, New Zealand

Katherine Elizabeth Black
Department of Human Nutrition, University of Otago, PO Box 56, Dunedin 9054, New Zealand

Nicolas Babault
National Institute for health and medical research (INSERM), unit 1093, Cognition, Action and sensorimotor plasticity, Dijon, France
Centre for Performance Expertise, UFR STAPS, Dijon, France
Faculté des Sciences du Sport, Université de Bourgogne, BP 27877, 21078 Dijon, Cedex, France

Gaëlle Dele
National Institute for health and medical research (INSERM), unit 1093, Cognition, Action and sensorimotor plasticity, Dijon, France
Centre for Performance Expertise, UFR STAPS, Dijon, France

Pascale Le Ruyet
Lactalis R&D, Retiers, France

François Morgan
Lactalis R&D, Retiers, France

François André Allaert
Chair of Medical Evaluation ESC, Dijon, France
CEN Nutriment, Dijon, France

Joseph N Sciberras
Sport Nutrition graduate from the University of Stirling, 74, San Anton Court, Pope John XXIII street, Birkirkara BKR1033, Malta

Stuart DR Galloway
Health and Exercise Sciences Research Group, School of Sport, University of Stirling, Stirling, Scotland

Anthony Fenech
Department of Clinical Pharmacology and Therapeutics, University of Malta, Msida, Malta

Godfrey Grech
Department of Pathology, University of Malta, Msida, Malta

Claude Farrugia
Department of Chemistry, University of Malta, Msida, Malta

Deborah Duca
Department of Chemistry, University of Malta, Msida, Malta

Janet Mifsud
Department of Clinical Pharmacology and Therapeutics, University of Malta, Msida, Malta

Vinicius Fernandes Cruzat
CHIRI Biosciences Research Precinct, Faculty of Health Sciences, School of Biomedical Sciences, Curtin University, GPO Box U1987, Perth, Western Australia, Australia

Maurício Krause
Laboratory of Cellular Physiology, Department of Physiology, Institute of Basic Health Sciences, Federal University of Rio Grande do Sul, Porto Alegre, RS, Brazil

Philip Newsholme
CHIRI Biosciences Research Precinct, Faculty of Health Sciences, School of Biomedical Sciences, Curtin University, GPO Box U1987, Perth, Western Australia, Australia

Jordan M Joy
Department of Health Sciences and Human Performance, The University of Tampa, Tampa, FL, USA
MusclePharm Sports Science Institute, MusclePharm Corp., Denver, CO, USA

Ryan P Lowery
Department of Health Sciences and Human Performance, The University of Tampa, Tampa, FL, USA

Paul H Falcone
MusclePharm Sports Science Institute, MusclePharm Corp., Denver, CO, USA

MattM Mosman
MusclePharm Sports Science Institute, MusclePharm Corp., Denver, CO, USA

Roxanne M Vogel
MusclePharm Sports Science Institute, MusclePharm Corp., Denver, CO, USA

Laura R Carson
MusclePharm Sports Science Institute, MusclePharm Corp., Denver, CO, USA

Chih-Yin Tai
MusclePharm Sports Science Institute, MusclePharm Corp., Denver, CO, USA

David Choate
Metropolitan State University, Denver, CO, USA

Dylan Kimber
Metropolitan State University, Denver, CO, USA

Jacob A Ormes
Department of Health Sciences and Human Performance, The University of Tampa, Tampa, FL, USA

Jacob M Wilson
Department of Health Sciences and Human Performance, The University of Tampa, Tampa, FL, USA

Jordan R Moon
MusclePharm Sports Science Institute, MusclePharm Corp., Denver, CO, USA
Department of Sports Exercise Science, United States Sports Academy, Daphne, AL, USA

Justin D Roberts
Department of Life Sciences, Anglia Ruskin University, East Road, Cambridge, UK
School of Life & Medical Sciences, University of Hertfordshire, College Lane, Hatfield, Hertfordshire, UK

Michael G Roberts
School of Life & Medical Sciences, University of Hertfordshire, College Lane, Hatfield, Hertfordshire, UK

Michael D Tarpey
School of Life & Medical Sciences, University of Hertfordshire, College Lane, Hatfield, Hertfordshire, UK

Jack C Weekes
School of Life & Medical Sciences, University of Hertfordshire, College Lane, Hatfield, Hertfordshire, UK

Clare H Thomas
School of Life & Medical Sciences, University of Hertfordshire, College Lane, Hatfield, Hertfordshire, UK

James P Lugo
InterHealth Nutraceuticals, Benicia, CA 94510, USA

Zainulabedin M Saiyed
InterHealth Nutraceuticals, Benicia, CA 94510, USA

Francis C Lau
InterHealth Nutraceuticals, Benicia, CA 94510, USA

Jhanna Pamela L Molina
Medicus Research LLC, 28720 Roadside Drive, Suite 310, Agoura Hills, CA 91301, USA

Michael N Pakdaman
Medicus Research LLC, 28720 Roadside Drive, Suite 310, Agoura Hills, CA 91301, USA

Arya Nick Shamie
UCLA Medical Center, Santa Monica, CA 90401, USA

Jay K Udani
Medicus Research LLC, 28720 Roadside Drive, Suite 310, Agoura Hills, CA 91301, USA

Northridge Hospital Integrative Medicine Program, Northridge, CA 91325, USA

Timothy D Mickleborough
Department of Kinesiology, Human Performance and Exercise Biochemistry Laboratory, School of Public Health-Bloomington, 1025 E. 7th St. SPH 112, Bloomington, Indiana 47401, USA

Jacob A Sinex
Department of Kinesiology, Human Performance and Exercise Biochemistry Laboratory, School of Public Health-Bloomington, 1025 E. 7th St. SPH 112, Bloomington, Indiana 47401, USA

David Platt
Department of Kinesiology, Human Performance and Exercise Biochemistry Laboratory, School of Public Health-Bloomington, 1025 E. 7th St. SPH 112, Bloomington, Indiana 47401, USA

Robert F Chapman
Department of Kinesiology, Human Performance and Exercise Biochemistry Laboratory, School of Public Health-Bloomington, 1025 E. 7th St. SPH 112, Bloomington, Indiana 47401, USA

Molly Hirt
Department of Kinesiology, Human Performance and Exercise Biochemistry Laboratory, School of Public Health-Bloomington, 1025 E. 7th St. SPH 112, Bloomington, Indiana 47401, USA

Lindsy S Kass
University of Hertfordshire, School of Life and Medical Science, College Lane, Hatfield, Hertfordshire AL10 9AB, UK

Filipe Poeira
University of Hertfordshire, School of Life and Medical Science, College Lane, Hatfield, Hertfordshire AL10 9AB, UK

Scott Lloyd Robinson
Guru Performance LTD, 58 South Molton St, London W1K 5SL, UK

Anneliese Lambeth-Mansell
Institute of Sport & Exercise Science, University of Worcester, Henwick Grove, Worcester WR2 6AJ, UK

Gavin Gillibrand
Ultimate City Fitness, 1-3 Cobb Street, London E1 7LB, UK

Abbie Smith-Ryan
Department of Exercise and Sport Science, University of North Carolina Chapel Hill, Office: 303A Woolen, 209 Fetzer Hall, Chapel Hill, NC, USA

Laurent Bannock
Guru Performance LTD, 58 South Molton St, London W1K 5SL, UK

Christopher Brooks Mobley
School of Kinesiology, Molecular and Applied Sciences Laboratory, Auburn University, 301 Wire Road, Office 286, Auburn, AL 36849, USA

Carlton D Fox
School of Kinesiology, Molecular and Applied Sciences Laboratory, Auburn University, 301 Wire Road, Office 286, Auburn, AL 36849, USA

Brian S Ferguson
School of Kinesiology, Molecular and Applied Sciences Laboratory, Auburn University, 301 Wire Road, Office 286, Auburn, AL 36849, USA

Corrie A Pascoe
School of Kinesiology, Molecular and Applied Sciences Laboratory, Auburn University, 301 Wire Road, Office 286, Auburn, AL 36849, USA

James C Healy
School of Kinesiology, Molecular and Applied Sciences Laboratory, Auburn University, 301 Wire Road, Office 286, Auburn, AL 36849, USA

Jeremy S McAdam
School of Kinesiology, Molecular and Applied Sciences Laboratory, Auburn University, 301 Wire Road, Office 286, Auburn, AL 36849, USA

Christopher M Lockwood
4Life Research USA, LLC, Sandy, UT, USA

Michael D Roberts
School of Kinesiology, Molecular and Applied Sciences Laboratory, Auburn University, 301 Wire Road, Office 286, Auburn, AL 36849, USA

Lygeri Dimitriou
London Sport Institute, Middlesex University, Allianz Park, Greenland Way, NW4 1RLE, London, UK

Jessica A Hill
School of Sport, Health and Applied Science, St Mary's University College, Twickenham, UK

Ahmed Jehnali
Ipro Interactive Ltd, Oxfordshire, UK

Joe Dunbar
Ipro Interactive Ltd, Oxfordshire, UK

James Brouner
School of Life Sciences, Kingston University, London, UK

Malachy P. McHugh
Nicholas Institute of Sports Medicine and Athletic Trauma, Lenox Hill Hospital, New York, NY, UK

Glyn Howatson
Faculty of Health and Life Sciences, Northumbria University, Newcastle-upon-Tyne, UK
Water Research Group, School of Biological Sciences, North West University, Potchefstroom, South Africa